THE SOCIAL DETERMINANTS OF HEALTH AND HEALTH DISPARITIES

THE SOCIAL DETERMINANTS OF HEALTH AND HEALTH DISPARITIES

PAULA BRAVEMAN, MD, MPH

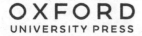

OXFORD
UNIVERSITY PRESS

OXFORD
UNIVERSITY PRESS

Oxford University Press is a department of the University of Oxford. It furthers
the University's objective of excellence in research, scholarship, and education
by publishing worldwide. Oxford is a registered trade mark of Oxford University
Press in the UK and certain other countries.

Published in the United States of America by Oxford University Press
198 Madison Avenue, New York, NY 10016, United States of America.

© Oxford University Press 2023

Library of Congress Cataloging-in-Publication Data
Names: Braveman, Paula, author.
Title: The social determinants of health and health disparities / by Paula Braveman.
Description: New York, NY : Oxford University Press, [2023] |
Includes bibliographical references and index.
Identifiers: LCCN 2022027329 (print) | LCCN 2022027330 (ebook) |
ISBN 9780190624118 (hardback) | ISBN 9780190624132 (epub) | ISBN 9780190624149 (online)
Subjects: MESH: Social Determinants of Health | Health Inequities |
Healthcare Disparities | Socioeconomic Factors
Classification: LCC RA563.M56 (print) | LCC RA563.M56 (ebook) | NLM WA 30 |
DDC 362.1089—dc23/eng/20220914
LC record available at https://lccn.loc.gov/2022027329
LC ebook record available at https://lccn.loc.gov/2022027330

DOI: 10.1093/oso/9780190624118.001.0001

This material is not intended to be, and should not be considered, a substitute for medical or other
professional advice. Treatment for the conditions described in this material is highly dependent on the
individual circumstances. And, while this material is designed to offer accurate information with respect
to the subject matter covered and to be current as of the time it was written, research and knowledge
about medical and health issues is constantly evolving and dose schedules for medications are being
revised continually, with new side effects recognized and accounted for regularly. Readers must therefore
always check the product information and clinical procedures with the most up-to-date published
product information and data sheets provided by the manufacturers and the most recent codes of
conduct and safety regulation. The publisher and the authors make no representations or warranties to
readers, express or implied, as to the accuracy or completeness of this material. Without limiting the
foregoing, the publisher and the authors make no representations or warranties as to the accuracy or
efficacy of the drug dosages mentioned in the material. The authors and the publisher do not accept,
and expressly disclaim, any responsibility for any liability, loss, or risk that may be claimed or incurred
as a consequence of the use and/or application of any of the contents of this material.

Printed by Integrated Books International, United States of America

CONTENTS

ACKNOWLEDGMENTS

I wish to acknowledge the Robert Wood Johnson Foundation, which supported the production of several issue briefs that provided a basis for many chapters in this book. The Foundation has made important contributions to knowledge and action addressing the social determinants of health.

I also acknowledge my longtime colleague and friend Susan Egerter, PhD, who co-authored those issue briefs and other publications on which many of the chapters build; and Miranda Brillante, MPH, who, along with Susan Egerter, provided valuable substantive editing of drafts of some of the chapters. Elaine Arkin also co-authored a number of the issue briefs. Julia Acker and Nicole Holm, provided valuable assistance with the research. Many other individuals made contributions to one or more chapters and are acknowledged in each chapter. My husband John Levin provided moral and intellectual support throughout the years of working on this book.

The order of presentation of the chapters does not reflect differences in importance. All the chapter themes are essential, and they are interrelated, including causally.

There is some deliberate overlap of content across the chapters, in an effort to make each chapter cover essential issues and be able to stand on its own.

An effort was made to provide current references. In some cases, however, older sources were cited because they are classics and/or the best references for a given statement.

CHAPTER 1

Introduction

What Influences Health? And What Influences the Influences?

1.1. WHY DEVOTE A BOOK TO THE SOCIAL DETERMINANTS OF HEALTH?

If you ask most people what influences health, almost invariably the first reply will be health (or medical) *care*—the services that individuals receive from physicians, nurses, and other medical professionals to treat or prevent

> The social determinants of health are the factors *apart from* health care that influence health and are shaped by social policies and forces; "social" includes economic.

illness. Many people, in fact, presume the role of health/medical care in affecting health to be so predominant that they often use the terms *health* and *health care* interchangeably. Many people would probably also cite behaviors such as diet, exercise, smoking, and use of alcohol or drugs as key influences on health. Although ample evidence supports the importance of both health care and behaviors for health, a compelling body of scientific knowledge now calls for a wider and deeper set of explanations for why some of us experience good health and others do not. This body of knowledge challenges us to think beyond common assumptions about the causes of health and illness, to ask not only "What influences health?" but also "What factors shape those influences?"—that is, "What influences the influences?" This knowledge tells us that to achieve real and lasting improvements in health, we must shift the focus to identifying and addressing the *root or fundamental causes* (Link and Phelan 1995)—the underlying factors that set in motion other factors that may be more easily observed but play a less fundamental role in shaping health. Ethical concerns, furthermore, require us to focus not only on a population's overall or average health but also on health *equity*—whether everyone has a fair and just opportunity to be as healthy as possible, which includes whether the resources, opportunities, and conditions required for good health are distributed equitably within the population (Braveman, Arkin, et al. 2017).

The Social Determinants of Health and Health Disparities. Paula Braveman, Oxford University Press. © Oxford University Press 2023. DOI: 10.1093/oso/9780190624118.003.0001

Until fairly recently, the term "social determinants of health" struck many people, if they had heard of it, as unfamiliar and abstract. During the past ten to twenty years, however, the fields of public health and medicine have increasingly embraced this term. Figure 1.1 illustrates the rapid growth in scientific literature focused on the social determinants of health in the United States and elsewhere. The concept has received increasing attention not only in academic settings but also among public health practitioners, health care providers, health-related nonprofit organizations, and, more recently, public and private health care insurers. This gathering momentum reflects a confluence of several phenomena.

First, a critical mass of knowledge in social and biomedical sciences (some of it described in this volume) has enhanced the scientific credibility of claims about the key role of social factors in shaping health. (Throughout this book, "social" includes economic and other factors that shape our lives and can be influenced by policies.) This body of knowledge has expanded our understanding of the ways in which this influence occurs. For example, the health effects of absolute material deprivation—that is, grossly inadequate food, clothing, shelter, water, and sanitation—have been recognized for centuries (Rosen and Rosen 1993). Until relatively recently, discussions of socioeconomic influences on health have focused primarily on links between absolute poverty and health. These discussions have often tended—implicitly or explicitly—to focus attention on modifying the behaviors of poor people to reduce the health risks associated with being poor or the impact of those risks. A more comprehensive, evidence-based, and nuanced perspective on health determinants—including knowledge about the factors that

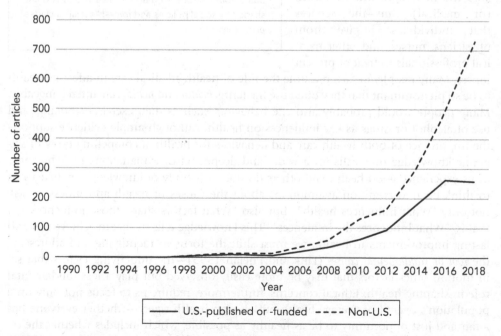

FIGURE 1.1 Increasing number of journal articles on the social determinants of health in the United States and other countries. Results of a PubMed search for "social determinants of health" in the title or abstract. Adapted and updated from Figure 1 in Braveman et al. (2011).

shape people's health-related behaviors—has emerged during recent decades in Europe, Canada, and, more recently, the United States. In contrast with a simple dichotomy between the health of those living in poverty and the health of everyone else, a gradient of incremental improvements in health tied to increasing levels of social advantage has now been observed repeatedly in Europe (Marmot 2017; Marmot et al. 1991; Rose and Marmot 1981), the United States (Braveman et al. 2010; Minkler, Fuller-Thomson, and Guralnik 2006), and developing nations (Gwatkins et al. 2007; J. Williams et al. 2018).

The *socioeconomic gradient in health* demands a different set of explanations than those focused on the health-damaging effects of absolute poverty. Awareness of the socioeconomic gradient has led to greater understanding of how social factors such as income, wealth, and education affect health. By highlighting the relevance of the social determinants of health for "middle-class" as well as poor persons, awareness of the gradient also may have contributed to growing public interest in the social determinants of health. Recognition of widening inequalities in income and accumulated wealth in the United States and globally (Zucman 2019) also has likely contributed to increased interest in the social determinants of health. Evidence of stark racial/ethnic and socioeconomic disparities in rates of COVID-19 infection and deaths (Webb Hooper, Nápoles, and Pérez-Stable 2020) also has brought more attention to this topic.

Second, despite widespread belief that advances in medical care were responsible for the dramatic declines in mortality in the United States and other resource-rich nations during the first half of the twentieth century, a more careful look at the evidence suggests otherwise. For example, in the seminal book, *An Introduction to Social Medicine* (McKeown and Lowe 1974), Scottish physician Thomas McKeown studied mortality rates associated with several different causes from the mid-nineteenth century to the early 1960s in England and Wales (the only nations with acceptably reliable vital statistics dating that far back). McKeown found that mortality from multiple causes had already fallen precipitously and steadily decades *before* the availability of modern medical care modalities such as antibiotics (which were not available until approximately 1940) and intensive care units (which were introduced in the 1960s). The decline in mortality rates had slowed by 1940, when one could arguably say that modern medical therapies first came into use. He attributed the dramatic increases in life expectancy since the nineteenth century primarily to overall improvements in living conditions, including better nutrition, sanitation, housing, and water (McKeown, Record, and Turner 1975). McKeown has been criticized for not giving sufficient credit to the role of public health (Grundy 2005), and some critics have suggested that advances in medical care may have also played a role in extending life expectancy (McKeown et al. 1975; see also Grundy 2005; Mackenbach 1996, 2021; Mackenbach, Stronks, and Kunst 1989). Most scholars, however, agree that nonmedical factors, including conditions within the purview of traditional public health and public health nursing, were probably more important than medical care in the dramatic increase in longevity in the first half of the twentieth century (Goldberg 2017; Grundy 2005; Howse 2007).

Further evidence of the limits of medical care to produce health is the widening of mortality disparities among different socioeconomic groups in the United Kingdom during the decades following the creation in 1948 of the National Health Service, which made medical care universally financially accessible (Black and Whitehead 1988). In addition, Martinson (2012) found that although health overall was better in the United Kingdom than in the United States, which lacks universal health care coverage, disparities in health by income were similar in the two countries, indicating a powerful role for factors other than medical care. Large inequalities in health across different socioeconomic groups have been documented repeatedly in several European countries, even where there is universal financial access to medical care (Mackenbach et al. 1997, 2000, 2008).

Doubts about the primacy of health care as the only or the most important determinant of health also have been raised by clear evidence that, at least among affluent nations, spending on health care has not always been associated with better health. Although current medical care spending in the United States is far higher than in any other nation (reaching nearly $10,000 per person in 2016) (Anderson, Hussey, and Petrosyan 2019), the United States has consistently ranked at or near the bottom among affluent nations on key measures of health, such as life expectancy and infant mortality, and that relative ranking has fallen over time (Organisation for Economic Co-operation and Development 2011). A 2013 report from the National Research Council and Institute of Medicine (now the National Academy of Medicine) that received wide media attention documented the U.S. "health disadvantage" in both morbidity and mortality across most health indicators and in all age groups except those older than age 75 years. This health disadvantage relative to other affluent nations was seen among affluent as well as poor Americans and among non-Latino Whites when considered separately (Woolf and Aron 2013). Another example indicating the limits of health care to shape health is that, although important for maternal health, traditional clinical prenatal care, with few exceptions, has not been shown to improve outcomes in newborns (Alexander and Korenbrot 1995; Alexander and Kotelchuck 2001; Behrman and Butler 2007; Fiscella 1995; Lu and Halfon 2003; Lu et al. 2003).

Apart from the role of social factors, what else could explain the poor U.S. performance in health status relative to other affluent nations despite massive spending on health care? Genetic makeup and the United States' racial/ethnic diversity are unlikely explanations, given that the United States' lower ranking on health persists even when considering only people of European American (White) ancestry in the United States (Banks et al. 2006). Studies have documented higher rates of some important health-damaging behaviors in the United States compared with similar countries; relevant behaviors include physical inactivity and poor dietary practices leading to obesity, which is a strong risk factor for chronic illness in adulthood. Behaviors alone cannot explain the U.S. health disadvantage, however, because America's poor ranking is seen even for illnesses (e.g., many cancers) in which behaviors play a relatively unimportant role (Banks et al. 2006; Martinson 2012; Woolf and Aron 2013).

Systematic efforts at translating the evolving science on the role of the social determinants of health into forms that can reach and be meaningful to wider audiences also have likely played a major role in increasing awareness of the role of social factors in health among the public and decision-makers. Although the growing body of scientific evidence has led to greater recognition within health-related scientific fields of the fundamental importance of nonmedical factors in shaping health, several efforts in recent years have also focused on disseminating that knowledge to broader audiences. Notable initiatives include the World Health Organization (WHO) Commission on the

Social Determinants of Health (2005–2008) (WHO Commission 2008), the MacArthur Foundation Network on Socioeconomic Status and Health (1996–2009) (Adler and Stewart 2010), the Robert Wood Johnson Foundation Commission to Build a Healthier America (2005–2015) (Robert Wood Johnson Foundation 2019b), the Robert Wood Johnson Foundation Culture of Health initiative (2016–present) (Robert Wood Johnson Foundation 2019a), and work of the National Academy of Medicine (especially since 2017) (National Academy of Medicine 2019). The Robert Wood Johnson Foundation's Commission to Build a Healthier America made concerted efforts to communicate the role of social factors in health to a wide audience of decision-makers, philanthropists, and practitioners in health and related sectors nationally. California Newsreel's well-researched four-part PBS film series *Unnatural Causes* (first released in 2008 and circulated widely for several years afterward) reached audiences ranging from churchgoers to medical care practitioners, public health workers, policymakers, and philanthropists in multiple sectors.

1.2. WHAT ARE THE SOCIAL DETERMINANTS OF HEALTH? WHAT ARE HEALTH DISPARITIES? BASIC CONCEPTS

The WHO Commission (2008) defined the social determinants of health as both "the conditions in which people are born, grow, live, work and age" and "the fundamental drivers of these conditions." These factors include a wide array of determinants of health that are often categorized as either *upstream* or *downstream determinants*. The upstream/downstream metaphor refers to how a river flows downward (downstream) from its upstream source. Upstream determinants, the "fundamental drivers" of the conditions that produce health and illness, are more fundamental in that they operate close to or at the source of the river, whereas downstream determinants are located farther away from the source, closer to or at the river's end. Downstream factors are generally more easily observed because they occur closer to the health outcomes in time and space. Interventions that target only downstream factors may have limited effectiveness, however, because upstream factors will continue to trigger the chain of causal events leading to adverse health effects. Focusing on the upstream, fundamental causes thus can often present the most important— yet untapped—opportunities for sustainably improving health and reducing health disparities.

To illustrate the upstream/downstream metaphor, consider people living beside a river who depend on the river for their drinking water. Imagine that many of these people become ill after drinking water contaminated by toxic chemicals released into the river from a factory located upstream. Whereas drinking the contaminated water is the most proximate or downstream cause of illness, the more fundamental (yet potentially less evident, given its temporal and physical distance from those affected and their symptoms) cause is the dumping of toxic chemicals upstream. A downstream remedy might be to recommend that individuals buy bottled water or filters to treat the contaminated water before drinking. Because more affluent individuals could afford to purchase the bottled water or filters, their health might improve, while their poorer neighbors would remain ill or become sicker because they could not afford the recommended options, thus widening disparities in health between more affluent and poor people. An upstream solution would focus on addressing the source of contamination—that is, ending the factory's dumping of pollutants; it would likely have far more equitable impacts on people's health.

Although these concepts make intuitive sense, it is important to note that the causal pathways linking upstream determinants with downstream determinants—and ultimately with health outcomes—are generally complex, often involving multiple intermediate factors along the way, and these intermediate factors may interact with each other in complex ways. In addition, the health effects of upstream factors may not manifest for many decades. Experiences of chronic stress in early childhood, for example, may increase a person's likelihood of heart disease and diabetes in adulthood, with consequent illness, disability, and premature mortality. These adverse health outcomes generally will not be seen, however, until decades later in mid- to late adulthood. It is therefore usually easier to study—and address—downstream determinants of health. By doing so, however, we run the risk of pursuing strategies that—because they do not address the more upstream, fundamental, causes—fail to interrupt the causal chains leading to ill health. (See Link and Phelan's [1995] classic discussion of fundamental causes of health and illness.)

One example of the complexity of the causal pathways leading to health outcomes from the social determinants of health is the repeated observation that compared with their White counterparts, African Americans do not appear to reap the same health benefits of higher socioeconomic status (SES) (generally measured by income and education in the United States and often by occupational class in Europe). Whereas health consistently improves with higher SES among Whites, college-educated or high-income African Americans do not always have appreciably better health outcomes than their African American counterparts of lower SES (Braveman et al. 2015; Braveman, Heck, et al. 2017; Colen et al. 2006, 2018; Collins and Butler 1997; Foster et al. 2000; McGrady et al. 1992; Nuru-Jeter et al. 2009). This phenomenon has been explained by some scholars as reflecting "the hidden costs of upward mobility" for people of color (Cole and Omari 2003; Myers, Lewis, and Dominguez 2003). Because of the barriers posed by racism, people of color may need to work harder and perform better than their White peers to overcome stereotypes (Cole and Omari 2003; Nuru-Jeter et al. 2009). They consequently experience more stress to attain high income, educational, and occupational levels; and even after having achieved a high socioeconomic level, they often confront ongoing discrimination (and an ongoing need to prove themselves against stereotypes). It is biologically plausible that chronic racism-related stress could lead to worse health. Neuroscience has revealed that chronic stress, even at relatively undramatic levels, can set in motion

> In this volume and many contexts, SES refers to both absolute and relative levels (status) of economic resources and opportunities that people have. SES includes absolute levels of income, wealth, and education (educational attainment and schooling). It also encompasses a person's relative social (including economic) status, including a person's relative power based on where their income, wealth, education, and occupational advantage or disadvantage situate them relative to others in a social hierarchy. Both absolute and relative aspects of SES should be measured.

inflammation, dysfunction of the immune system, and adverse vascular mechanisms that, over time, lead to wear and tear on multiple body systems (sometimes referred to as allostatic load [McEwen and Seeman 1999], discussed in Chapter 4).

Figure 1.2 illustrates the general conceptual framework that underlies this volume; minor modifications are made in discussing some of the specific social determinants examined in later chapters. Although in reality the relationships of interest are far more complex than depicted here, this simplified schema is intended to highlight a few important concepts: Power structures (exemplified by laws, policies, and entrenched practices) and values determine who has access to key economic and social resources and opportunities needed to be healthy. Those resources and opportunities then determine who experiences health-promoting or health-harming conditions, which in turn directly trigger the biological mechanisms that ultimately result in good or ill health. The diagram highlights how health is fundamentally and powerfully shaped by the social determinants that are upstream (earlier in a causal chain or pathway) from it, and why, because they are upstream, they are often not obvious. Each subsequent chapter in this book explores a different specific social determinant of health (income and wealth, education, early childhood experiences, racism and other forms of discrimination, work, neighborhoods, housing, stress, and behaviors), discussing the literature linking that social determinant with health.

The box on the left in Figure 1.2 represents the most upstream (fundamental, underlying) social determinants of health: *power and social values*, which determine everything else. Included here are established systems (e.g., the political and economic systems, educational system, medical care system, criminal justice system, and taxation system). Minimum wage laws and unemployment benefits also would be in this category. Also included in this most upstream category are policies, laws, and entrenched practices—for example, minimum wage laws that condemn many people to poverty without chance of escape; those that produce and sustain racial residential segregation; and those that produce disenfranchisement through voter suppression and gerrymandering (the deliberate redrawing of voting districts in ways that favor the party in power, often diminishing the impact of votes by low-income people and people of color). Power structures include *systemic* or *structural racism*—the less visible racism that is deeply embedded in systems and structures (e.g., laws, policies, and entrenched practices)—producing and sustaining racial discrimination in all forms. Systemic racism plays a key upstream role in determining a person's access to power (and, through power, to economic and other social opportunities and resources). Racial residential segregation is an important example of systemic racism; it cuts people off from economic and educational opportunities. Social values and norms include justice, equity, compassion, social inclusion (versus exclusion, embodied in racism and other forms of discrimination), and social cohesion or solidarity (the degree to which people feel connected with and are willing to help each other). Many of the factors within this category influence each other. Values both shape and are shaped by power structures. Power and social values also shape access to the key resources and opportunities needed to experience good health.

Access to the key resources and opportunities needed for good health is represented in the second box from the left in Figure 1.2. These factors also are relatively upstream, although less so than the power structures and social values that determine them. These

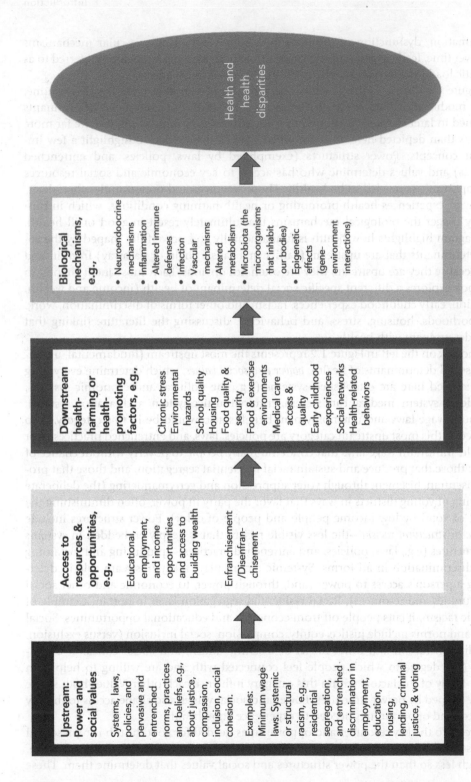

Upstream: Power and social values

Systems, laws, policies, and practices and beliefs, e.g., about justice, compassion, inclusion, social cohesion.

Examples: Minimum wage laws. Systemic or structural racism, e.g., residential segregation; and entrenched discrimination in employment, education, housing, lending, criminal justice, & voting

Access to resources & opportunities, e.g.,

Educational, employment, and income opportunities and access to building wealth

Enfranchisement /Disenfranchisement

Downstream health-harming or health-promoting factors, e.g.,

Chronic stress
Environmental hazards
School quality
Housing
Food quality & security
Food & exercise environments
Medical care access & quality
Early childhood experiences
Social networks
Health-related behaviors

Biological mechanisms, e.g.,

- Neuroendocrine mechanisms
- Inflammation
- Altered immune defenses
- Infection
- Vascular mechanisms
- Altered metabolism
- Microbiota (the microorganisms that inhabit our bodies)
- Epigenetic effects (gene–environment interactions)

Health and health disparities

FIGURE 1.2 What influences health and health disparities? And what influences the influences?

key resources and opportunities include income (earnings from employment, interest, investments, or other sources), wealth (the monetary value of accumulated assets such as a home or other real estate, vehicles, savings, investments, jewelry, etc.), and "education" (educational attainment or schooling [e.g., high school graduate, associate degree, college graduate, or post-graduate degree], which typically and greatly influences income by determining the kind of employment one can obtain; a degree from an elite school generally opens more opportunities than education at a less an improvement institution). A double arrow between the box representing power and social values and the box representing resources and opportunities could have been drawn but is omitted for the sake of readability; such an arrow would signify that these two types of upstream social determinants influence each other in shaping health: Although power and social values influence access to key resources and opportunities needed for optimal health, it is also true that income, wealth, and education can influence access to power and the extent to which an individual or group is valued in society.

The downstream social determinants of health (depicted in the third box from the left in Figure 1.2) are the living and working conditions a person experiences across their entire lifetime, which more or less directly trigger the biological mechanisms (the next box) that result in good or ill health. The downstream social determinants involve exposure to or experience of living/working conditions that may be health-harming or health-promoting. These conditions include the quality of schools to which one has access; toxic environmental exposures such as air pollution, water quality, and proximity to a toxic waste disposal site; whether one's housing has physical hazards including toxic materials, excessive dust, mold, or crowding and excessive heat or cold (see Chapters 7 and 8); and the quality of a person's neighborhood, school, and work environments, both currently and as experienced earlier in life, particularly during early childhood. Although lifelong experiences are important, the health effects of experiences during the first few years of life have been demonstrated to be particularly crucial for health and development across the entire life span (see Chapter 6). In addition, environmental injustice has systematically resulted in the disproportionate location of hazardous waste sites in or near communities of color. Chronic stress, a strong risk factor for chronic disease (e.g., heart disease, stroke, and diabetes) in adulthood, is another health-harming factor thought to play an important role in racial/ethnic and socioeconomic disparities in health. Health-related behaviors (e.g., smoking, diet, and exercise) also are included in the category with health-harming or health-promoting conditions; strictly speaking, they are responses to exposures or experiences rather than exposures or experiences themselves, although they may produce exposures/experiences. It is important to note that within the box representing health-harming or health-promoting conditions (and within all of the boxes), many factors influence each other; for example, stress, food insecurity, and food environments are known to influence behaviors, and housing insecurity and food insecurity are substantial sources of stress.

Some caveats should be stated about Figure 1.2. It is a simplification of what is tremendously complex, presented to highlight certain concepts. Virtually every factor depicted in Figure 1.2 may interact with virtually every other factor in the diagram and with factors not noted in the diagram. Social relationships or networks (a downstream determinant), for example, can influence a person's access to power, income, wealth, education, and many other factors because "who you know" can give a person access to opportunities that influence health. At the same time, those same factors (power, income, wealth, education, etc.) shape social networks and relationships. Health itself also can influence a person's access to power, income, wealth, and education insofar as it makes one physically capable (or incapable) of taking advantage of opportunities. A given factor may play a more or less upstream or downstream role in relation to different health outcomes and/or in different contexts. It should be noted that here are many other conceptual diagrams that also represent the social determinants of health and the pathways through which they influence health (e.g., one developed by the World Health Organization) (Solar and Irwin 2010). Different diagrams can be helpful for different purposes.

A More Specific Example of Likely Causal Pathways Leading from Social Determinants to Health Outcomes: How Education Can Influence Health

Figure 1.3 is a more specific and detailed example of a subset of elements of the general framework depicted in Figure 1.2; it focuses specifically on how one relatively upstream social determinant, educational attainment, may affect health. (The most upstream determinants noted in Figure 1.2—power and the social norms and values that create and sustain power—are not displayed in Figure 1.3.)

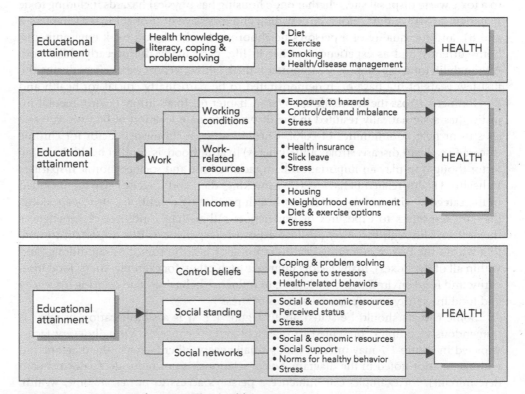

FIGURE 1.3   How can education affect health?

Educational attainment—often referred to simply as "education"—refers to how much formal schooling (as evidenced by degrees or credentials attained, or sometimes years) one has completed. If asked how education could affect health, most people would probably reply that more educated people are more knowledgeable about the factors— such as smoking, diet, and exercise—that influence health, and more knowledge leads to healthier behaviors. Most people would probably readily agree that education also affects health by giving people the coping and problem-solving skills that make them better able to prevent and manage disease in general. All of those beliefs—indicated by the top segment of Figure 1.3—are supported by evidence. It may, however, come as a surprise to many people to learn that education can influence health in other ways, which may be at least as and perhaps more important than its effects on knowledge, skills, and health-related behaviors. For example, as shown in the middle of Figure 1.3, consider how educational attainment determines income, by determining the kind of work a person will have. For anyone who was not born into great wealth, educational attainment is generally the strongest modifiable determinant of the kind of work one obtains. In turn, one's occupation heavily determines one's income and one's ability to accumulate wealth. Education also influences health by influencing work-related resources such as medical insurance and healthy or unhealthy working conditions.

How do income and wealth (accumulated assets such as savings or a home) shape health? The middle segment of Figure 1.3 lists only a few of the many ways in which financial resources shape health. For example, financial resources play a major role in determining who can afford to buy or rent a home that is free of lead, mold, and other hazards (particularly for children) in a neighborhood that is safe (with respect to air and ground pollution, other environmental hazards, and crime), has safe and attractive places for exercise or play, and does not have a high concentration of fast-food outlets or advertisements aiming to attract youth (often, particularly youth of color) to smoke cigarettes and consume alcohol. A healthy diet is typically more expensive than an unhealthy diet. Financial resources also can affect health by determining the levels and chronicity of stress one experiences. For example, those with high incomes and/or substantial wealth do not have to worry about their families going hungry or becoming homeless if they lose a few weeks of work because of illness. Forty-one percent of respondents to a 2017 Federal Reserve Board survey reported that they would struggle to come up with $400 in an emergency (Board of Governors of the Federal Reserve System 2018). Living paycheck to paycheck is now a common experience for middle- and working-class Americans (Walker 2017). The COVID-19 pandemic has underscored the health consequences of lack of wealth. Higher income/wealth can mean being able to afford more convenient transportation to work, versus having to travel two hours each way to and from work, or being able to repair one's automobile when it breaks down. It means that when one's childcare arrangements fall through, one has other childcare options of acceptable quality. Having few financial resources therefore often means being under constant stress due to the strain of coping with daily challenges with inadequate resources. And chronic stress appears to be particularly damaging to health, even in the absence of particularly dramatic but time-limited acute stressors (McEwen 2017).

Still, other pathways from education to health (depicted in the bottom segment of Figure 1.3) also are likely to be important in explaining the strong and pervasive associations between education and health. The bottom segment of Figure 1.3 depicts pathways that involve psychosocial factors, including social networks, one's social standing or prestige, and "control" beliefs—for example, whether you generally feel helpless or able to control what happens to you. All of these have powerful effects on health-related behaviors, and there is evidence that some may potentially also have relatively direct effects on health outcomes, even without involving behaviors.

Based on the literature, all three general pathways from educational attainment to health that are illustrated in Figure 1.3 (and other pathways not illustrated) are likely to be important and may operate at the same time. Note that Figure 1.3, like Figure 1.2, is an oversimplification. For the sake of simplicity and readability, Figure 1.3 does not indicate the extent of likely interactions among the factors shown (and potentially between the factors shown and other factors not displayed). There are, furthermore, numerous steps in many of the pathways that are not shown. Neither Figure 1.2 nor Figure 1.3 indicates how any of the pathways are likely to unfold over time; the health effects of education, which is generally completed by young adulthood, are likely not to manifest until mid- or later adulthood, in the form of chronic disease such as heart disease and diabetes.

The Social Determinants of Health Disparities

This book is not only about the social determinants of health but also about the social determinants of health disparities. Although the term "health disparities" was first introduced in the 1990s to refer specifically to racial or ethnic differences in health that raise concerns about fairness or justice, it evolved rapidly to encompass socioeconomic differences in health and, subsequently, any social difference in health that raises concerns about (but does not necessarily prove the existence of) unfairness or injustice. For example, the term health disparities is now commonly used to refer not only to disparities by racial/ethnic group or SES but also to differences in health among people living with disabilities compared with others, or to health differences among groups defined by sexual orientation, gender identity, religion, or immigration status; all of these characteristics have been associated with being socially disadvantaged. The definitions of terms presented later in this chapter discuss health disparities more fully, but a relatively simple way of thinking about them is that a health disparity entails worse health in a socially disadvantaged (marginalized, excluded, or oppressed) group. This way of defining the concept does not require proving definitively the nature of the upstream causes of a health disparity, which is often very difficult to do, largely because the causal pathways are generally long and complex. It does, however, narrow the possibilities greatly from all health differences to that subset of differences in health in which a socially disadvantaged group has worse health, which should raise concern regarding potential injustice, unless solid evidence exists to the contrary (Braveman, Arkin, et al. 2017).

In most countries outside the United States, the term "health inequalities" is used rather than the term health disparities. Health disparities/inequalities are different from but closely related to the concept of health equity, which has become widely used in public health and medical care circles, although defined in many different ways.

> Health disparities are differences in health among more and less socially advantaged groups of people, which raise concerns about justice.

Disparities/inequalities in health and its key determinants are the metric used to assess progress toward greater health equity; in other words, we measure whether we are moving toward or away from greater health equity by measuring whether the magnitude of disparities in health and its key determinants is decreasing or increasing. Disparities/inequalities (hereafter just "disparities") are not the same as inequities.

Equity means justice, and in the case of health equity, it generally refers to distributive justice—the ethical principle that resources and opportunities should be distributed fairly, particularly when they affect health. There are many ways to define health equity. One very brief definition is that it means that everyone has a fair and just opportunity to be as healthy as possible. (See a more complete definition presented later in this chapter.) Health equity can be thought of as the ethical and human rights principle underlying a commitment to eliminate health disparities (Braveman, Arkin, et al. 2017). Just as disparities/inequalities are not the same as inequities, equity is not the same as equality. "Equality" might lead one to give exactly the same resource—for example, the same-size income supplement to help people meet basic needs such as housing and food during the COVID-19 pandemic—to everyone, regardless of need. By contrast, equity would dictate providing the supplement, or at least a larger supplement, selectively to people who suffer economic hardship. Similarly, low income and/or racial discrimination are likely to take a toll on the health of people experiencing them on a chronic basis (e.g., through the physiologic effects of chronic stress), potentially resulting in a need for more medical care compared to that required by people who do not experience them; equity would dictate providing that additional care and expedited access to those in need, whereas equality might not. Many, but not all, health disparities are inequities. The term health inequity is generally reserved for those health disparities whose causes have been reasonably well identified and judged to be unfair and also when one wants to emphasize the ethical or moral dimension.

Figures 1.2 and 1.3 implicitly suggest how health disparities are created and perpetuated by differences between groups of people in power, resources, and opportunities. These differences then generate differences in exposure to, experience of, or response to health-harming and health-promoting conditions. These conditions are the more proximate (downstream, close to the health outcome) influences on health; they include stress, behaviors, and medical care. Socially disadvantaged groups are those who have been affected by unfavorable upstream determinants of health, such as poverty, racism, and other forms of social exclusion or marginalization. These unfavorable upstream determinants set in motion causal chains leading from unfavorable upstream to unfavorable downstream determinants, culminating in worse health. The social determinants of health are often but not invariably the same as the social determinants of health disparities. To be a determinant of a health disparity, a given risk factor (e.g., low income or low educational attainment) must be more prevalent among the disadvantaged group(s) or have a greater effect on disadvantaged groups compared with more advantaged groups. Thus, for example, it is known that cigarette smoking is a strong risk factor for preterm birth (birth before 37 completed weeks of pregnancy, which is associated with infant mortality, childhood developmental disability, and adult chronic disease). Black women have considerably higher rates of preterm birth than White women. Differences in smoking, however, do not explain the disparity in preterm birth rates between African American (Black) and European American (White) women; Black women smoke less than White women. Although some have suggested that smoking may have a stronger deleterious effect on Black pregnant women than their White counterparts, controlling for smoking does not markedly reduce the racial disparity. Cigarette smoking, therefore, is a cause of preterm birth, but it is not a likely cause of the Black–White disparity in preterm birth (Braveman et al. 2021).

Health disparities arise from disparities in exposure, vulnerability (which is shaped by social advantage/disadvantage), and consequences. Another helpful conceptual framework for understanding the social determinants of health is that developed by Diderichsen (1998). Figure 1.4 is a minor adaptation of a diagram developed by Diderichsen to illustrate how health disparities are caused and perpetuated, not only across an individual's lifetime but also across generations. The Diderichsen diagram captures some of the complexity that Figures 1.2 and 1.3 do not. It explicitly traces out how upstream determinants such as poverty (income) and racism influence not only whether one will experience health-damaging exposures (e.g., to environmental toxins or stressful experiences) but also one's vulnerability to developing ill health once exposed to a potentially harmful condition (e.g., based on one's general health status, nutritional status, ability to pay to have the exposure mitigated or removed, or social support). Figure 1.4 also indicates that upstream determinants ("the social context and the policy context" in Figure 1.4, which correspond in some important ways to power and social values in Figure 1.2) can shape not only exposure and vulnerability to disease if exposed but also the social consequences of ill health. For example, suppose that a university professor and someone whose occupation is housecleaning have an identical

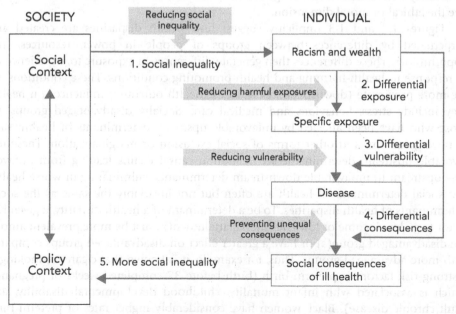

FIGURE 1.4 What produces health disparities across the life course and across generations? Adapted from Diderichsen (1998) [Google Scholar].

injury rendering them permanently unable to walk. Whereas the professor could, after a period of recovery, return to work, the housekeeper could not and would lose her livelihood, with likely severe consequences for herself and her family. Such differential consequences of illness based on social advantage (in this case, occupation) are unjust and would contribute to greater widening of social inequality.

Figure 1.4 also calls attention to how social policies and other aspects of the social context may interrupt the damaging pathways not only by reducing harmful exposures, reducing vulnerability, and creating social programs to buffer against the consequences of ill health but also by reducing social inequality. Reducing social inequality could be accomplished, for example, with policies that reduce economic inequality (e.g., minimum wage laws and tax credits for low-income workers) and/or provide services (e.g., affordable high-quality child care, good public transportation, free and high-quality public schools from kindergarten through college, subsidized housing, and medical care) that enhance health and/or economic opportunity. The literature suggests that social cohesion plays an important role in whether societies make substantial efforts to reduce economic inequality and that high levels of economic inequality in turn reduce social cohesion (Pickett and Wilkinson 2015; Wilkinson and Pickett 2009, 2020).

1.3. CHALLENGES IN ADDRESSING THE SOCIAL DETERMINANTS OF HEALTH AND HEALTH DISPARITIES

A large body of evidence from observational research strongly and repeatedly links multiple upstream social factors with a wide array of health outcomes, and there is growing—albeit still incomplete—understanding of the relevant underlying pathways and biological mechanisms. There is little consensus, however, about effective ways to address upstream social factors to improve health and reduce health disparities—when, where, and how to intervene. Although the lack of consensus to some extent reflects limited knowledge about the precise details of interventions (e.g., ideal teacher to student ratios and teachers' credentials), it largely reflects political and ideological disagreements, reflecting different social values.

Gaps in Knowledge as a Barrier to Action on the Social Determinants of Health

The gaps in knowledge reflect several challenges. As noted previously, often the relationships between upstream and even midstream social factors and health are complex and play out over long periods of time; they often involve multiple intermediate outcomes, each subject to effect modification by characteristics of people and settings along the causal chain. This complexity makes it exceedingly difficult to study the specific pathways through which upstream social factors shape health and to identify priorities for intervention. Addressing the knowledge gaps is also complicated often by our limited ability to measure upstream social factors. Current measures do not fully capture—or permit one to tease out the distinct effects of—many relevant aspects of power, social norms and values, systemic racism, education, occupation, experiences of race-based or other discrimination, or childhood experiences likely to have substantial health effects. Development of better measures of these influences is in its infancy (Braveman et al. 2005; Diez Roux and Mair 2010; Nuru-Jeter et al. 2009; D. Williams and Collins 2016).

Funding for research and programs is another issue. Most U.S. research funding supports studies of single diseases rather than causal or contributory factors with effects that manifest across multiple diseases, putting research on the social determinants of health at a disadvantage. Funding for programs is rarely adequate for a rigorous evaluation; it generally is on too small a scale for an effect to be detected. In addition, conducting randomized controlled trials, the gold standard for establishing effectiveness in health sciences, is particularly challenging for upstream interventions because of the complexity of the causal pathways and the long time periods over which they play out. The health effects of upstream social factors—and interventions to address them—may not manifest for decades or generations. Longitudinal studies can address this but are expensive; access to longitudinal databases with key social information is particularly limited in the United States compared to Canada and some European countries.

Even robust longitudinal data, however, may not provide sufficient information for tracing the effects of an upstream determinant (A) through relevant pathways to its ultimate health outcome (Z), particularly if exposure to A occurs in early childhood and outcome Z only manifests much later—for example, in late adulthood. Attempting to document and quantify the effects of A on Z in a single study represents an important obstacle to understanding how social factors influence health, as well as how to intervene. In addition, at each step on multiple complex causal chains, effects can be modified by features of people and their contexts. Considering all these obstacles, the consistency of existing findings linking upstream social determinants with health outcomes is truly remarkable and suggests that powerful and pervasive forces are indeed at play.

A number of scholars have hypothesized that "reverse causation" (loss of income and/or wealth because of illness) is a more valid explanation of the repeatedly observed relationships between upstream social determinants such as income or wealth and health, rather than income or wealth influencing health (see Chapter 2). Evidence does exist that income/wealth loss due to poor health can occur. The literature on the whole indicates, however, that although reverse causation occurs, and probably accounts for some part of the observed associations, it does not fully account for the observed associations between income/wealth and health, which remain strong and consistent even after considering reverse causation (Kawachi, Adler, and Dow 2010; Muennig 2008). Longitudinal studies can help distinguish chronologically between cause and effect, and thus could reveal reverse causation if it were present. Longitudinal studies have shown that economic resources such as income predict health or its proximate determinants, even after adjustment for many relevant variables, such as education (Avendano and Glymour 2008; Duncan et al. 2002; Herd, Goesling, and House 2007), although education is a stronger predictor for other outcomes (Herd et al. 2007) and both are likely to matter (Braveman et al. 2005; Kawachi et al. 2010). Positive health effects of raising income have been observed in randomized and natural experiments (Kawachi et al. 2010).

The Need for More Translation of Existing Knowledge into Policy and Programs

Although much is unknown, existing knowledge could inform policymaking if more and better efforts were made at translation. Often, the rate-limiting step may not be insufficiently detailed knowledge of causal pathways but, rather, lack of solid evidence about what specifically and concretely works best in different settings to reduce social inequalities in health. For example, although there is convincing evidence that educational attainment and quality powerfully influence health through multiple pathways, lack of consensus about interventions is often invoked to justify inaction. Knowledge of pathways can point to promising or at least plausible approaches but generally cannot indicate which actions will be most effective and efficient under different conditions; that knowledge can only come from well-designed intervention research, including both randomized experiments (when possible and appropriate) and nonrandomized studies with rigorous attention to considering comparability and reducing bias.

The field of social determinants of health has come of age in many ways with respect to accumulating knowledge of pathways and biological mechanisms, documentation of strong and pervasive links between social and economic factors and health, and increased attention within and beyond academia. Although strong associations between social factors and health are no longer in question, we have much to learn—both about the underlying processes linking upstream social determinants and many health outcomes and about effective ways to intervene. Lack of evidence, however, is not always the major barrier to action.

The Key Obstacle to Action Is Often Entrenched Power Rather Than Lack of Knowledge

The rate-limiting step in efforts to eliminate health disparities is often lack of political will to allocate the necessary resources and overcome the many obstacles to coordinated action across different sectors, such as health, housing, education, and early childhood development. This lack of political will often reflects a lack of commitment to justice and inclusion and a lack of compassion and willingness to improve the lives of everyone, particularly those who have been disenfranchised, excluded, or marginalized. Addressing the upstream social determinants of health requires being strategic in addressing not only the research challenges but also the systems of power and the social values that are the fundamental causes at the beginning of the causal chains leading to good or ill health and health disparities.

Comments on Subsequent Chapters

Each subsequent chapter of this book examines how a different social determinant of health—income and wealth (Chapter 2), education (Chapter 3), stress (Chapter 4), racism (Chapter 5), early childhood experiences (Chapter 6), neighborhood context (Chapter 7), housing (Chapter 8), work (Chapter 9), and behaviors (Chapter 10)—is influenced by more upstream social factors and how it in turn comes to influence health and health disparities through complex pathways. The order of presentation of the chapters does not reflect relative importance; all are crucial.

Chapter 5 discusses racism's most upstream form—that is, systemic (or structural) racism—as a fundamental, underlying power structure that creates and perpetuates social inequality; and the role of power, in the form of policies, is acknowledged in all chapters. There is, however, no chapter devoted exclusively to power and the social values that sustain it, where all the causal pathways begin. This important topic requires volumes, not a chapter, to address it, and it is beyond the scope of this book and this author.

1.4. TERMS USED THROUGHOUT THE BOOK

Discrimination is unfair treatment based on belonging to (or being perceived as belonging to) a particular social group. It is a type of social exclusion or marginalization in which members of particular social groups receive prejudicial treatment and their access to key resources and opportunities is blocked. Such treatment can be based on a wide range of characteristics, including racial, ethnic, or religious group; low income; disability; LGBTQ status; national origin; and gender. Discrimination is a broad term that includes, but is not limited to, race-based discrimination.

Economic or *financial resources* are general terms referring to income or wealth or both, which are among the most powerful social determinants of health. *Wealth* (or accumulated wealth) refers to the monetary value of all possessions or assets—such as a home, other real estate, vehicles, savings, and investments—that a person or household has accumulated over time. Wealth is generally measured by *net worth*—the monetary value of accumulated assets after subtracting debts. By contrast, *income* measures only earnings during a specified time period, making it a less comprehensive representation of the economic resources available to a person or household over a longer period of time. Economic resources also include nonmonetary assets, such as education and social networks, which can also provide access to economic opportunities. This volume, however, focuses on monetary resources. Although more income generally allows individuals to accumulate more financial assets, people with similar incomes may have vastly different levels of wealth. Historical and ongoing racial injustices have been documented in bank and government lending practices, housing, racial residential segregation, education, employment, and other domains affecting the ability to accumulate wealth (Rothstein 2017). (See text later in this chapter and also Chapter 5.) Because of this, income markedly underestimates racial or ethnic differences in wealth (Pollack et al. 2007). Because wealth is more difficult to measure than income, however, it is less frequently used in health research.

Excluded, marginalized, or *disadvantaged groups* are groups of people who historically have suffered and continue to suffer discrimination, whether the discrimination is currently intentional or not. These groups have been disenfranchised or marginalized—pushed to the margins of society and the health-promoting resources it has to offer. They have had inadequate access to key opportunities to be healthy (WHO Commission 2008; D. Williams and Mohammed 2009). They are socially disadvantaged (United Nations Human Rights Office of the High Commissioner 2019) in general and often economically disadvantaged in particular. Examples of historically disenfranchised, excluded/

marginalized, or disadvantaged groups include, but are not limited to, people of color (D. Williams and Mohammed 2013); people living in poverty, particularly across generations (Cheng, Johnson, and Goodman 2016; Reeves, Rodrigue, and Keebone 2016; Wagmiller and Adelman 2009); religious minorities; people living with physical or mental disabilities (HealthyPeople.gov 2019b); LGBTQ persons (Meyer and Northridge 2007; Ward et al. 2014); and women (Moss 2002; Quffa 2016). Excluded groups are not always economically disadvantaged; for example, because of racial residential segregation, African Americans and Latinos of all income levels are more likely than Whites with similar incomes to live in neighborhoods with concentrated disadvantage (Reardon, Fox, and Townsend 2015; Sharkey 2014), and they may experience discrimination at work, while shopping, and while interacting with public and private institutions (Assari and Lankarani 2018; Braveman, Heck, et al. 2017; Colen et al. 2018; Myers et al. 2003; Nuru-Jeter et al. 2009).

For the definition of *exclusion*, see the definitions for social inclusion, exclusion, and marginalization; and excluded, marginalized, or disadvantaged groups.

Health refers to physical or mental health status, health outcomes, or well-being. By contrast, *health care* (used interchangeably with *medical care* or *health/medical services*) refers to the services intended to prevent or treat illness that are delivered by physicians, nurses, pharmacists, dentists, clinical psychologists, physical therapists, and other trained health care providers, their assistants, or ancillary personnel.

The concepts of *health equity* and *health disparities* are closely related but not the same. HealthyPeople.gov (2019a) defines health disparities as

> differences in health that adversely affect groups of people who historically have been excluded or marginalized (for example, people of color, people living in poverty, people with disabilities, LGBTQ persons, and girls/women). Health disparities are used to measure progress towards health equity.

HealthyPeople.gov (2019b) further defines a *health disparity* as

> a particular type of health difference that is closely linked with social, economic, and/or environmental disadvantage. Health disparities adversely affect groups of people who have systematically experienced greater obstacles to health based on their racial or ethnic group; religion; socioeconomic status; gender; age; mental health; cognitive, sensory, or physical disability; sexual orientation or gender identity; geographic location; or other characteristics historically linked to discrimination or exclusion.

Equity means justice and fairness. Braveman, Arkin, and colleagues from the Robert Wood Johnson Foundation (2017) define health equity as follows:

> Health equity means that everyone has a fair and just opportunity to be as healthy as possible. This requires removing obstacles to health such as poverty, discrimination, powerlessness, and their consequences, including lack of access to good jobs with fair pay; quality education, housing, and health care; and safe environments. For the purposes of measurement, health equity means reducing and ultimately eliminating disparities in health and its determinants that adversely affect excluded or marginalized groups.

HealthyPeople.gov (2019a) defines health equity as the

> attainment of the highest level of health for all people. Achieving health equity requires valuing everyone equally with focused and ongoing societal efforts to address avoidable inequalities, historical and contemporary injustices, and the elimination of health and health care disparities.

For the definition of *inclusion*, see "social inclusion."

Race or *racial group* generally refers to a group of people who share a common ancestry from a particular continent or region of the world, which may be associated with superficial secondary characteristics such as skin color and hair texture. Superficial secondary characteristics do not reflect underlying biological differences. Most scientific experts agree that given the extent of intermixing of racial groups that has occurred over millennia, race is primarily a social rather than a biological construct. It is sometimes used interchangeably with the terms *ethnic group* or *ethnicity*, which tend to refer to groups of people who share a common ancestry in a large region of the world along with common history and sometimes traditions, beliefs, and practices.

Racism is a system of power relationships and the beliefs that sustain those relationships. It relegates people of color to inferior status and treatment, denying them access to society's benefits and justifying this with beliefs about their innate inferiority. Racism unfairly puts a group or groups of people at an advantage and others at a disadvantage, based on their ancestral origin (e.g., African American, American Indian, Latino, Asian American, and Middle Eastern). Racism is not always conscious or intentional; often it is *systemic* or *structural*—that is, built into laws, policies, systems, institutional practices, beliefs, and attitudes that produce and perpetuate unfair treatment. Racism produces *racial discrimination*, unfair treatment based on race. (See the definition for systemic or structural racism.)

When considering the relationship between health and income, *reverse causation* refers to ways in which ill health may lead to lower income—for example, when sickness causes a loss of income and/or medical care costs deplete one's wealth. Reverse causation—the ways in which health can influence economic resources—is contrasted with the ways in which economic resources can influence health.

Social means "of or relating to human society" (Merriam-Webster 2019). Generally, this term refers to factors apart from medical care that can be influenced by societal forces or policies. Unless otherwise indicated, "social" encompasses economic factors. Social factors may be distinguished from biological factors (e.g., genetic makeup) or certain features of the physical environment (e.g., altitude or climate). It must be kept in mind, however, that both biological and environmental characteristics are often heavily influenced by social factors, including human behavior. For example the health consequences of genetic makeup are often subject to social influence through gene–environment interactions. For example, a gene (e.g., one that conveys higher risk for a certain kind of cancer or heart disease) may only be expressed (i.e., actually have its potential effect on health) under certain environmental and social conditions, including exposure to toxic chemicals and chronic stress; and many features of the physical environment, including air and ground pollution, are results of racism (environmental injustice) and as such reflect social factors.

The term *social advantage or disadvantage* refers to having more or less power, wealth, prestige, and/or acceptance relative to others in society.

The term *social determinants of health* generally refers to factors apart from health care that influence health and that are influenced by social policies or forces. The notable exception is that the 2007 WHO Commission on the Social Determinants of Health treated health care as a social determinant. The term social determinants of health, however, was coined—and is generally used—to refer to the nonmedical factors that influence health. "Social" includes economic.

Inclusion or *social inclusion* is having access to full participation in society and the accompanying benefits, including health-promoting opportunities and resources. In contrast, *exclusion* or *social exclusion* and *marginalization* impose obstacles to full participation in society and its benefits, pushing some people to the margins of society and limiting their access to opportunities and resources. Examples of historically excluded or marginalized groups include, but are not limited to, people of color, people living in poverty (particularly in poverty that has spanned generations), members of persecuted religious or sexual minority groups, people with physical or mental disabilities, and women.

Socioeconomic (or *economic*) *factors* are a subset of social factors that are either directly (like income and wealth) or closely (like education) linked with economic resources and economic opportunity.

Socioeconomic status (SES) refers to a person's absolute and relative ranking in a hierarchy determined by socioeconomic factors; income or poverty level and educational attainment are the most frequently used indicators of SES in the United States. Occupational rank is often used in Europe. Some researchers prefer to use the term *socioeconomic position* rather than SES because they believe that "position" better captures the relative dimension of socioeconomic characteristics—that is, the existence of social hierarchies according to relative socioeconomic advantage or disadvantage. Others (including the author of this book) believe that "status" conveys very well, probably better than "position," the connotation of a relative dimension; and social status explicitly refers to relative social standing. Socioeconomic status is, furthermore, a familiar term to many people, whereas "socioeconomic position" is not.

Systemic or *structural racism* is racism that is so embedded in systems and structures that it may be difficult to recognize. It is racism that is pervasively and deeply embedded in systems, laws, written and unwritten policies, established practices, beliefs, and attitudes that produce, condone, and perpetuate widespread unfair treatment of people of color. It reflects both historical and ongoing injustices. Systemic racism refers to racism embedded within whole systems, such as the criminal justice, education, health care, or political systems. Structural racism refers to racism embedded in structures—e.g., laws, policies, and entrenched practices—that are the scaffolding of systems. Although systemic racism often has its historical origins in deliberate intention to discriminate against people of color, it is so deeply embedded in systems and structures that it can persist even in the absence of current discriminatory intent. Racial residential segregation, environmental racism, and biased policing and sentencing of men and boys of color are examples of systemic and structural racism. Systemic racism may inflict its harm by promoting, justifying, or expressing itself at the individual level as *interpersonal racism*—racially discriminatory actions perpetrated by one or more individuals against one or more other individuals—whether consciously or intentionally discriminatory. It is likely that far greater harm, however, is inflicted by the ways that systemic and structural racism deny people of color access to resources and opportunities needed for optimal health.

The term *upstream* literally refers to the source or origin of a stream of water flowing downstream. *Upstream determinants* include the most fundamental causes of good or bad health operating at the beginning of a causal chain. Invoking different metaphors than upstream/downstream, they are underlying or root causes. *Downstream determinants* include the often more easily recognized factors that occur later in the causal chain and more proximally to the health outcome of interest and therefore are often easier to observe and modify. If upstream factors are not addressed, however, addressing only downstream factors will not remedy the underlying problem, which will continue to set in motion the causal chains leading to disease.

The term *vulnerability* is used at times in this book to denote whether a person/group is at high risk of illness, with the understanding that the most powerful determinants of vulnerability are the social determinants of health.

Wealth refers to accumulated assets, the monetary value of everything owned by an individual or household, including a home, other real estate, vehicles, savings, jewelry and other valuables. Wealth is more likely than income (earnings during a specified period of time, typically a year or a month) to reflect one's financial resources over a long period of time and, because it may reflect inheritance, to reflect one's childhood socioeconomic circumstances.

1.5. KEY POINTS

- A critical mass of knowledge on the social determinants of health has accumulated, documenting associations, exploring causal pathways and biological mechanisms, and providing a previously unavailable scientific foundation for appreciating the fundamental role of social factors in health.
- The questions are no longer about whether social factors are important influences on health but, rather, about how social factors operate and particularly about how to most effectively and efficiently intervene to activate health-promoting pathways and interrupt health-damaging ones.
- Health disparities are the products of disparities in exposure to health-harming and health-promoting conditions, which themselves are the products of disparities in access to key resources and opportunities. These in turn are the products of social values and disparities in power, as reflected, for example, by systemic or structural racism.
- Too little attention in research and policy has been given to the upstream (i.e., fundamental) social determinants of health, such as the laws, policies, and other power structures and systems that are at the beginning of causal chains that lead ultimately to health outcomes. Most research has focused on the more easily studied downstream factors that occur closest to health outcomes and so are more visible. The upstream determinants, however, represent fundamental or root causes in causal pathways influencing the downstream factors that ultimately produce good or ill health effects. Addressing only downstream factors may not be effective because upstream causes will continue to set in motion causal chains leading to ill health.

1.6. QUESTIONS FOR DISCUSSION

1. What are "social determinants of health"? The WHO Commission on the Social Determinants of Health treated health care as a social determinant of health, whereas the term "social determinants of health" was coined expressly (and is generally used) to differentiate nonmedical determinants from medical care. Why do you think the WHO Commission included health care as a social determinant? What are the advantages/disadvantages of including health care as a social determinant of health?

2. It is challenging to study the social determinants of health because of the complexity of the causal chains through which they affect health and the often long time periods before the effects manifest. Does this mean the standards for research on the social determinants of health should be less rigorous? For further reading on this, see Adler, Bush, and Pantell (2012) and Braveman et al. (2011).

ACKNOWLEDGMENT

This chapter builds on material published in Braveman, Egerter, and Williams (2011).

REFERENCES

Adler, N., N. R. Bush, and M. S. Pantell. 2012. "Rigor, vigor, and the study of health disparities." *Proc Natl Acad Sci USA* 109(Suppl 2): 17154–17159.

Adler, N. E., and J. Stewart. 2010. "Using team science to address health disparities: MacArthur network as a case example." *Ann N Y Acad Sci* 1186(1): 252–260.

Alexander, G. R., and C. C. Korenbrot. 1995. "The role of prenatal care in preventing low birth weight." *Future Child* 5(1): 103–120.

Alexander, G. R., and M. Kotelchuck. 2001. "Assessing the role and effectiveness of prenatal care: History, challenges, and directions for future research." *Public Health Rep* 116(4): 306–316. doi:10.1093/phr/116.4.306.

Anderson, G. F., P. Hussey, and V. Petrosyan. 2019. "It's still the prices, stupid: Why the US spends so much on health care, and a tribute to Uwe Reinhardt." *Health Aff* 38(1): 87–95. doi:10.1377/hlthaff.2018.05144.

Assari, S., and M. M. Lankarani. 2018. "Workplace racial composition explains high perceived discrimination of high socioeconomic status African American men." *Brain Sci* 8(8): 139. doi:10.3390/brainsci8080139.

Avendano, M., and M. M. Glymour. 2008. "Stroke disparities in older Americans: Is wealth a more powerful indicator of risk than income and education?" *Stroke* 39(5): 1533–1540.

Banks, J., M. Marmot, Z. Oldfield, and J. P. Smith. 2006. "Disease and disadvantage in the United States and in England." *JAMA* 295(17): 2037–2045. doi:10.1001/jama.295.17.2037.

Behrman, R. E., and A. S. Butler. 2007. *Preterm Birth: Causes, Consequences, and Prevention*. Washington, DC: National Academies Press.

Black, D., and M. Whitehead. 1988. *Inequalities in Health: The Black Report the Health Divide*. London: Penguin.

Board of Governors of the Federal Reserve System. 2018. *Report on the Economic Well-Being of U.S. Households in 2017*. Washington, DC: Board of Governors of the Federal Reserve System.

Braveman, P. A., E. Arkin, T. Orleans, D. Proctor, and A. Plough. 2017. *What Is Health Equity? And What Differences Does a Definition Make?* Princeton, NJ: Robert Wood Johnson Foundation.

Braveman, P. A., C. Cubbin, S. Egerter, S. Chideya, K. S. Marchi, M. Metzler, and S.

Posner. 2005. "Socioeconomic status in health research: One size does not fit all." *JAMA* 294(22): 2879–2888. doi:10.1001/jama.294.22.2879.

Braveman, P. A., C. Cubbin, S. Egerter, D. R. Williams, and E. Pamuk. 2010. "Socioeconomic disparities in health in the United States: What the patterns tell us." *Am J Public Health* 100(Suppl 1): S186–S196. doi:10.2105/AJPH.2009.166082.

Braveman, P. A., T. P. Dominguez, W. Burke, et al. 2021. "Explaining the Black–White disparity in pre-term birth: A consensus statement from a multi-disciplinary scientific work group convened by the March of Dimes." *Front Reprod Health* 3: 684207.

Braveman, P. A., S. Egerter, and D. R. Williams. 2011. "The social determinants of health: Coming of age." *Annu Rev Public Health* 32: 381–398.

Braveman, P. A., S. A. Egerter, S. H. Woolf, and J. S. Marks. 2011. "When do we know enough to recommend action on the social determinants of health?" *Am J Prev Med* 40(1 Suppl 1): S58–S66.

Braveman, P. A., K. Heck, S. Egerter, T. P. Dominguez, C. Rinki, K. S. Marchi, and M. Curtis. 2017. "Worry about racial discrimination: A missing piece of the puzzle of Black–White disparities in preterm birth?" *PLoS One* 12(10): e0186151.

Braveman, P. A., K. Heck, S. Egerter, K. S. Marchi, T. P. Dominguez, C. Cubbin, C. Fingar, J. A. Pearson, and M. Curtis. 2015. "The role of socioeconomic factors in Black–White disparities in preterm birth." *Am J Public Health* 105(4): 694–702.

Cheng, T. L., S. B. Johnson, and E. Goodman. 2016. "Breaking the intergenerational cycle of disadvantage: The three generation approach." *Pediatrics* 137(6): e20152467. doi:10.1542/peds.2015-2467.

Cole, E. R., and S. R. Omari. 2003. "Race, class and the dilemmas of upward mobility for African Americans." *J Soc Issues* 59(4): 785–802.

Colen, C. G., A. T. Geronimus, J. Bound, and S. A. James. 2006. "Maternal upward socioeconomic mobility and Black–White disparities in infant birthweight." *Am J Public Health* 96(11): 2032–2039.

Colen, C. G., D. M. Ramey, E. C. Cooksey, and D. R Williams. 2018. "Racial disparities in health among nonpoor African Americans and Hispanics: The role of acute and chronic discrimination." *Soc Sci Med* 199: 167–180.

Collins, J. W., Jr., and A. G. Butler. 1997. "Racial differences in the prevalence of small-for-dates infants among college-educated women." *Epidemiology* 8(3): 315–317.

Diderichsen, F. 1998. "Understanding health equity in populations—Some theoretical and methodological considerations." In *Promoting Research on Inequality in Health*, edited by B. Arve-Parès, 203–218. Stockholm, Sweden: Swedish Council for Social Research.

Diez Roux, A. V., and C. Mair. 2010. "Neighborhoods and health." *Ann N Y Acad Sci* 1186(1): 125–145.

Duncan, G. J., M. C. Daly, P. McDonough, and D. R. Williams. 2002. "Optimal indicators of socioeconomic status for health research." *Am J Public Health* 92(7): 1151–1157.

Fiscella, K. 1995. "Does prenatal care improve birth outcomes? A critical review." *Obstet Gynecol* 85(3): 468–479. doi:10.1016/0029-7844(94)00408-6.

Foster, H. W., L. Wu, M. B. Bracken, K. Semenya, J. Thomas, and J. Thomas. 2000. "Intergenerational effects of high socioeconomic status on low birthweight and preterm birth in African Americans." *J Natl Med Assoc* 92(5): 213.

Goldberg, D. S. 2017. "Introduction." In *Public Health Ethics and the Social Determinants of Health*, edited by D. S. Goldberg. Cham, Switzerland: Springer, pp. 1–5.

Grundy, E. 2005. "Commentary: The McKeown debate: Time for burial." *Int J Epidemiol* 34(3): 529–533. doi:10.1093/ije/dyh272.

Gwatkins, D. K., S. Rutstein, K. Johnson, E. Suliman, A. Wagstaff, and A. Amouzou. 2007. *Socio-economic Differences in Health, Nutrition, and Population Within Developing Countries*. Washington, DC: World Bank.

HealthyPeople.gov. 2019a. "Disparities." U.S. Department of Health & Human Services, Office of Disease Prevention and Health Promotion. Retrieved August 14, 2019, from https://www.healthypeople.gov/2020/about/foundation-health-measures/Disparities#5.

HealthyPeople.gov. 2019b. "Disability and health." U.S. Department of Health & Human Services, Office of Disease Prevention and Health Promotion. Retrieved August 6, 2019, from https://www.healthypeople.gov/2020/topics-objectives/topic/disability-and-health.

Herd, P., B. Goesling, and J. S. House. 2007. "Socioeconomic position and health: The differential effects of education versus income on the onset versus progression of health problems." *J Health Soc Behav* 48(3): 223–238.

Howse, C. 2007. "'The ultimate destination of all nursing': The development of district nursing in England, 1880–1925." *Nurs Hist Rev* 15: 65–94.

Kawachi, I., N. E. Adler, and W. H. Dow. 2010. "Money, schooling, and health: fCoMechanisms and causal evidence." *Ann N Y Acad Sci* 1186: 56–68. doi:10.1111/j.1749-6632.2009.05340.x.

Link, B. G., and J. Phelan. 1995. "Social conditions as fundamental causes of disease." *J Health Soc Behav* Spec No: 80–94.

Lu, M. C., and N. Halfon. 2003. "Racial and ethnic disparities in birth outcomes: A life-course perspective." *Matern Child Health J* 7(1): 13–30.

Lu, M. C., V. Tache, G. R. Alexander, M. Kotelchuck, and N. Halfon. 2003. "Preventing low birth weight: Is prenatal care the answer?" *J Matern Fetal Neonatal Med* 13(6): 362–380. doi:10.1080/jmf.13.6.362.380.

Mackenbach, J. P. 1996. "The contribution of medical care to mortality decline: McKeown revisited." *J Clin Epidemiol* 49(11): 1207–1213.

Mackenbach, J. P. 2021. "The rise and fall of diseases: Reflections on the history of population health in Europe since ca. 1700." *Eur J Epidemiol* 36: 1199–1205. doi:10.1007/s10654-021-00719-7.

Mackenbach, J. P., A. E. Cavelaars, A. E. Kunst, and F. Groenhof. 2000. "Socioeconomic inequalities in cardiovascular disease mortality: An international study." *Eur Heart J* 21(14): 1141–1151. doi:10.1053/euhj.1999.1990.

Mackenbach, J. P., A. E. Kunst, A. E. Cavelaars, F. Groenhof, and J. J. Geurts. 1997. "Socioeconomic inequalities in morbidity and mortality in western Europe: The EU Working Group on Socioeconomic Inequalities in Health." *Lancet* 349(9066): 1655–1659. doi:10.1016/s0140-6736(96)07226-1.

Mackenbach, J. P., I. Stirbu, A. J. Roskam, M. M. Schaap, G. Menvielle, M. Leinsalu, and A. E. Kunst. 2008. "Socioeconomic inequalities in health in 22 European countries." *N Engl J Med* 358(23): 2468–2481. doi:10.1056/NEJMsa0707519.

Mackenbach, J. P., K. Stronks, and A. E. Kunst. 1989. "The contribution of medical care to inequalities in health: Differences between socio-economic groups in decline of mortality from conditions amenable to medical intervention." *Soc Sci Med* 29(3): 369–376. doi:10.1016/0277-9536(89)90285-2.

Marmot, M. G. 2017. "Social justice, epidemiology and health inequalities." *Eur J Epidemiol* 32(7): 537–546. doi:10.1007/s10654-017-0286-3.

Marmot, M. G., S. Stansfeld, C. Patel, F. North, J. Head, I. White, E. Brunner, A. Feeney, M. G. Marmot, and G. Davey Smith. 1991. "Health inequalities among British civil servants: The Whitehall II study." *Lancet* 337(8754): 1387–1393. doi:10.1016/0140-6736(91)93068-K.

Martinson, M. L. 2012. "Income inequality in health at all ages: A comparison of the United States and England." *Am J Public Health* 102(11): 2049–2056. doi:10.2105/ajph.2012.300929.

McEwen, B. S. 2017. "Neurobiological and systemic effects of chronic stress." *Chronic Stress* 1: 2470547017692328. doi:10.1177/2470547017692328.

McEwen, B. S., and T. Seeman. 1999. "Protective and damaging effects of mediators of stress: Elaborating and testing the concepts of allostasis and allostatic load." *Ann N Y Acad Sci* 896(1): 30–47. doi:10.1111/j.1749-6632.1999.tb08103.x.

McGrady, G. A., J. F. C. Sung, D. L. Rowley, and Carol. J. R. Hogue. 1992. "Preterm delivery and low birth weight among first-born infants of Black and White college graduates." *Am J Epidemiol* 136(3): 266–276.

McKeown, T., and C. R. Lowe. 1974. *An Introduction to Social Medicine*: Oxford, UK: Blackwell.

McKeown, T., R. G. Record, and R. D. Turner. 1975. "An interpretation of the decline of mortality in England and Wales during the twentieth century." *Popul Stud* 29(3): 391–422.

Merriam-Webster. 2019. "Social." Retrieved August 14, 2019, from https://www.merriam-webster.com/dictionary/social.

Meyer, I. H., and M. E. Northridge, eds. 2007. *The Health of Sexual Minorities: Public Health Perspectives on Lesbian, Gay, Bisexual and Transgender Populations*. New York: Springer.

Minkler, M., E. Fuller-Thomson, and J. M. Guralnik. 2006. "Gradient of disability across the socioeconomic spectrum in the United States." *N Engl J Med* 355(7): 695–703. doi:10.1056/NEJMsa044316.

Moss, N. E. 2002. "Gender equity and socioeconomic inequality: A framework for the patterning of women's health." *Soc Sci Med* 54(5): 649–661. doi:10.1016/s0277-9536(01)00115-0.

Muennig, P. 2008. "Health selection vs. causation in the income gradient: What can we learn from graphical trends?" *J Health Care Poor Underserved* 19(2): 574–579. doi:10.1353/hpu.0.0018.

Myers, H. F., T. T. Lewis, and T. P. Dominguez. 2003. "Stress, coping and minority health." In *Handbook of Racial and Ethnic Minority Psychology*, edited by G. Bernal, J. E. Trimble, A. K. Burlew, and F. T. L. Leong. Thousand Oaks, CA: Sage, pp. 377–400.

National Academy of Medicine. 2019. Retrieved August 14, 2019, from https://nam.edu.

Nuru-Jeter, A., T. P. Dominguez, W. P. Hammond, J. Leu, M. Skaff, S. Egerter, C. P. Jones, and P. Braveman. 2009a. "'It's the skin you're in': African-American women talk about their experiences of racism. An exploratory study to develop measures of racism for birth outcome studies." *Matern Child Health J* 13(1): 29–39. doi:10.1007/s10995-008-0357-x.

Organisation for Economic Co-operation and Development. 2011. *OECD Factbook 2011–2012: Economic, Environmental And Social Statistics: Life Expectancy*. Paris, France: OECD Publishing.

Pickett, K. E., and R. G. Wilkinson. 2015. "Income inequality and health: A causal review." *Social Science & Medicine* 128: 316–326. doi:10.1016/j.socscimed.2014.12.031.

Pollack, C. E., S. Chideya, C. Cubbin, B. Williams, M. Dekker, and P. Braveman. 2007. "Should health studies measure wealth? A systematic review." *Am J Prev Med* 33(3): 250–264. doi:10.1016/j.amepre.2007.04.033.

Quffa, W. A. 2016. "A review of the history of gender equality in the United States of America." *Soc Sci Educ Res Rev* 3(2): 143–149.

Reardon, S. F., L. Fox, and J. Townsend. 2015. "Neighborhood income composition by household race and income, 1990–2009." *Ann Am Acad Political Soc Sci* 660(1): 78–97.

Reeves, R., E. Rodrigue, and E. Keebone. 2016. *Five Evils: Multidimensional Poverty and Race in America*. Washington, DC: Brookings Institution.

Robert Wood Johnson Foundation. "Building a culture of health." Retrieved August 14, 2019, from https://www.rwjf.org/en/how-we-work/building-a-culture-of-health.html.

Robert Wood Johnson Foundation. 2019b. "Looking outside the health care system for ways to improve health for all." Robert Wood Johnson Foundation Commission to Build a Healthier America. Retrieved August 14, 2019, from https://www.rwjf.org/en/how-we-work/grants-explorer/featured-programs/rwjf-commission-to-build-a-healthier-america.html.

Rose, G., and M. G. Marmot. 1981. "Social class and coronary heart disease." *Heart* 45(1): 13–19. doi:10.1136/hrt.45.1.13.

Rosen, G., and G. Rosen. 1993. *A History of Public Health*. Baltimore, MD: Johns Hopkins University Press.

Rothstein, R. 2017. *The Color of Law: A Forgotten History of How Our Government Segregated America*. New York, NY: Liveright.

Sharkey, P. 2014. "Spatial segmentation and the Black middle class." *Am J Sociol* 119(4): 903–954.

Solar, O., and A. Irwin. 2010. *A Conceptual Framework for Action on the Social Determinants of Health*. Geneva, Switzerland: World Health Organization.

United Nations Human Rights Office of the High Commissioner. 2019. "United Nations International Covenant on Economic, Social, and Cultural Rights." Retrieved August 6, 2019, from https://www.ohchr.org/en/professionalinterest/pages/cescr.aspx.

Wagmiller, R. L., and R. M. Adelman. 2009. *Childhood and Intergenerational Poverty: The Long-Term Consequences of Growing up Poor.* New York, NY: National Center for Children in Poverty.

Walker, R. 2017. "How to trick people into saving money: Inside Walmart's curious, possibly ingenious effort to get customers to build up their savings accounts." *The Atlantic,* May. https://www.theatlantic.com/magazine/archive/2017/05/how-to-trick-people-into-saving-money/521421.

Ward, B. W., J. M. Dahlhamer, A. M. Galinsky, and S. S. Joestl. 2014. "Sexual orientation and health among U.S. adults: National Health Interview Survey, 2013." *Natl Health Stat Rep* (77): 1–10.

Webb Hooper, M., A. M. Nápoles, and E. J. Pérez-Stable. 2020. "COVID-19 and racial/ethnic disparities." *JAMA* 323(24): 2466–2467. doi:10.1001/jama.2020.8598.

Wilkinson, R. G., and K. Pickett. 2009. The Spirit Level: Why More Equal Societies Almost Always Do Better. London: Lane.

Wilkinson, R. G., and K. Pickett. 2020. *The Inner Level: How More Equal Societies Reduce Stress, Restore Sanity and Improve Everyone's Well-Being.* New York: Penguin.

Williams, D. R., and C. Collins. 2016. "Racial residential segregation: A fundamental cause of racial disparities in health." *Public Health Rep* 116(5): 404–416.

Williams, D. R., and S. A. Mohammed. 2009. "Discrimination and racial disparities in health: Evidence and needed research." *J Behav Med* 32(1): 20–47. doi:10.1007/s10865-008-9185-0.

Williams, D. R., and S. A. Mohammed. 2013. "Racism and health I: Pathways and scientific evidence." *Am Behav Sci* 57(8). doi:10.1177/0002764213487340.

Williams, J., L. Allen, K. Wickramasinghe, B. Mikkelsen, N. Roberts, and N. Townsend. 2018. "A systematic review of associations between non-communicable diseases and socioeconomic status within low- and lower-middle-income countries." *J Global Health* 8(2): 020409. doi:10.7189/jogh.08.020409.

Woolf, S. H., and L. Aron, eds. 2013. *US Health in International Perspective: Shorter Lives, Poorer Health.* Washington, DC: National Academies Press.

World Health Organization Commission on the Social Determinants of Health. 2008. *Final Report: Closing the Gap in a Generation: Health Equity Through Action on the Social Determinants of Health.* Geneva, Switzerland: World Health Organization. Retrieved June 21, 2022, from https://www.who.int/publications/i/item/WHO-IER-CSDH-08.1.

Zucman, G. 2019. "Global wealth inequality." *Annu Rev Econ* 11(1): 109–138. doi:10.1146/annurev-economics-080218-025852.

CHAPTER 2

Income and Wealth Shape Health and Health Disparities in Many Ways

2.1. INTRODUCTION

Few people would doubt that there are many advantages of having more income or wealth (the monetary value of accumulated assets minus debts). Nevertheless, the influence of economic resources on health—apart from how greater income and wealth make medical care more affordable—has received little attention from the general public or policymakers. A large body of scientific evidence, however, reveals that both income and wealth influence individual- and population-level health in many powerful and often complex ways. Research also shows that these relationships reflect not just how economic resources affect access to medical care but also how they enable people to live in safer, less polluted homes and neighborhoods; better educate their children; buy healthier food; have more opportunities for health-promoting physical activity; and experience less health-harming stress.

Understanding the links between income, wealth, and health is important for informing policies aimed at both achieving better health for virtually everyone and reducing social disparities (inequalities) in health. This chapter summarizes the evidence that health varies with both income and accumulated wealth, provides an overview of current knowledge of the pathways and biological mechanisms thought to explain the links between economic resources and health, and discusses implications for policy.

2.2. ECONOMIC RESOURCES: INCOME AND WEALTH

"Economic" or "financial" resources are general terms referring to income or wealth or both. *Wealth* (or *accumulated wealth*) refers to the monetary value of all possessions or assets—such as a home, other real estate, vehicles, savings, and investments—that a person or household has accumulated over time. By contrast, *income* measures only

The Social Determinants of Health and Health Disparities. Paula Braveman, Oxford University Press. © Oxford University Press 2023.
DOI: 10.1093/oso/9780190624118.003.0002

earnings during a specified time period, typically two weeks or a year, making it a less comprehensive representation of the economic resources available to a person or household over a longer period of time. Wealth is generally measured by *net worth*—the monetary value of accumulated assets after subtracting debts. It is arguable that economic resources also include nonmonetary assets, such as education and social networks, which can provide access to economic opportunities. This chapter, however, focuses on monetary resources. Although more income generally allows individuals to accumulate more financial assets, people with similar incomes may have vastly different levels of wealth. Historical and ongoing racial injustices have been documented in bank and government lending practices, housing, racial residential segregation, education, employment, and other domains affecting the ability of people of color to accumulate wealth (Rothstein 2017). (See discussion later in this chapter and also see Chapter 5.) Because of this, income markedly underestimates racial or ethnic differences in wealth (Pollack et al. 2007). Because wealth is more difficult to measure than income, however, it is less frequently used in health research. See Box 2.1 for a more detailed discussion of the distinction between income and wealth.

2.3. HOW ARE INCOME AND WEALTH DISTRIBUTED? AND HOW HAVE THE DISTRIBUTIONS CHANGED OVER TIME?

The distribution of income has become increasingly concentrated among a smaller portion of the population during the past several decades in the United States and globally. For example, in 1969, the highest earning 20% of U.S. households had an average income more than 10 times higher than that of the lowest earning 20%; 50 years later, the difference was more than 16-fold (U.S. Census Bureau 2018). Wealth is even more unequally distributed than income, and increasingly so: While the median net worth of the wealthiest 10% of U.S. households nearly doubled between 1989 and 2016, from approximately $1.3 to $2.4 million (Figure 2.1), the median net worth of the least wealthy 25% decreased from $200 to $100 during that period (Board of Governors of the Federal Reserve System 2017). Figure 2.1 displays the median net worth and the share of all U.S. wealth held by the wealthiest 10% of households and how these have increased over time.

An increasing number of U.S. families have no cushion of wealth to fall back on if faced with job loss (e.g., due to the COVID-19 pandemic) or unexpected major expenses. The percentage of U.S. households with no wealth or negative wealth (debts exceeding assets) increased from 15.5% in 1983 to 21.2% in 2016 (Woff 2017). Forty-one percent of respondents to a 2017 Federal Reserve Board survey reported that they would struggle to come up with $400 in an emergency (Board of Governors of the Federal Reserve System 2018); living paycheck to paycheck is now a common experience for middle- and working-class Americans (Walker 2017). This was true before the 2020–2021 COVID-19 pandemic, and the pandemic has dramatically exacerbated it.

While the shifts in the overall distributions of income and wealth over time have been dramatic, disparities in income and wealth are even more dramatic when comparing subgroups defined by characteristics including race/ethnicity, gender, disability, and age.

BOX 2.1	Income And Wealth

Income

Income—the most commonly used measure of economic resources in U.S. health research—may come from a variety of sources, including employment, government assistance, retirement plans and pension payments, and interest or dividends from investments or other assets. Income can fluctuate considerably from year to year and over a person's lifetime, with dramatic decreases due to unemployment, disability, or retirement. Thus, income measured at a single point in time may provide only limited information about lifetime economic advantage or disadvantage, which could have a greater influence on a person's health (Bond Huie et al. 2003; Makaroun et al. 2017; Smith et al. 1997).

In the United States, income is often reported as a percentage of the Federal Poverty Guidelines (FPG), more widely known as federal poverty levels (FPL) or federal poverty thresholds. The FPG/FPL has been defined as the amount of income needed to provide a bare minimum of food, clothing, transportation, shelter, and other necessities. Taking family size and age of family members into account, a household is assigned to a poverty category/level based on total before-tax income from all cash sources. Originally devised in the mid-1960s by the Social Security Administration to reflect a minimally adequate standard of living, the thresholds have been adjusted annually for inflation using the Consumer Price Index (Fisher 1992). This method of defining poverty has been widely criticized for not reflecting changes over time in prevailing perceptions of what constitutes a minimally acceptable standard of living. In addition, many experts believe that the official FPL-based thresholds are too low, especially in regions with high costs of living (Haveman et al. 2015; National Research Council 1995). Based on the 2021 FPG, a simplified version of the thresholds used to determine eligibility for programs, a family of four living in the 48 contiguous states or District of Columbia is considered to be "poor" with an income of $26,500 or less (U.S. Department of Health and Human Services 2021); a family whose income is below 200% (or, for some programs, 250%) of FPG is often considered to be "low-income"(Koball and Jiang 2018).

Wealth

Wealth—or more precisely, accumulated wealth—is less commonly measured in health studies than income. This is because it may be more difficult for respondents to estimate without consulting records, and it is thought to be more intrusive (Pollack et al. 2007). The most common standard for measuring wealth involves subtracting outstanding debts and liabilities from the cash value of currently owned assets—such as houses, land, vehicles, savings accounts, pension plans, stocks and other financial investments, and businesses. Although families with higher earnings typically tend to accumulate more assets, families with the same income level may have dramatically different levels of wealth (Braveman et al. 2005; Kochhar and Fry 2014). Compared with income, which is measured for a single period of time (typically a month or a year), accumulated assets provide more complete information about a person's *cumulative* lifetime economic resources—their lifetime earnings and inherited assets—which may have greater health effects. Thus, classifying people based on income alone may provide a misleading picture of their economic resources; this is particularly so for racial comparisons, due to the historical and ongoing legacy of racial discrimination that has systematically limited the ability of people of color to acquire wealth (Rothstein 2017). (See further discussion later in this chapter and in Chapter 5.)

Income and Wealth Vary Markedly Across Racial/Ethnic Groups

Because of historic and ongoing inequities mentioned previously, disparities in income and wealth are particularly striking when comparing White Americans and people of color. In 2016, for example, the median household income was approximately $61,200 among Whites and $35,400 among Black people, a ratio of approximately 1.7 to 1 (Board of Governors of the Federal Reserve System 2017). In the same year, the median net worth of White-headed households was $171,000 compared with $17,150 among Black-headed households, a ratio of almost 10 to 1 (McIntosh et al. 2020). (See Chapter 5, Figures 5.3 and 5.4.) At every level of income,

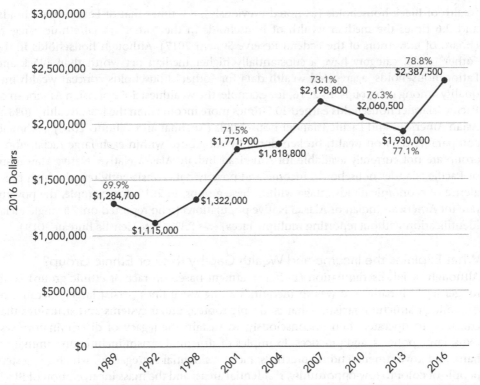

FIGURE 2.1 Median net worth and percentage of U.S. wealth held by the wealthiest 10% of households, 1989–2016. Percents refer to the percentage of all U.S. wealth held by the top 10% of the U.S. population. Share of percentage of wealth is not available for years 1992, 1998, and 2004. *Sources*: Median net worth from Survey of Consumer Finances. Percentage of wealth share from Woff (2017).

moreover, White households are also wealthier than Black households (Orzechowski and Sepielli 2003).

The Black–White wealth gap begins early in life and widens substantially as people age, suggesting that Black people are not only more likely to be born into disadvantage but also more likely to face barriers to homeownership, stable and well-paying employment, and other opportunities crucial for building wealth over the lifecourse (Thomas et al. 2020). This pattern may help explain why the Black–White gap in wealth has not narrowed over time despite the enactment of civil rights laws during the 1960s that made racial discrimination in hiring, pay, and lending illegal. Enforcement has often been weak. Discriminatory policies, practices, and beliefs, furthermore, may be so deeply embedded in social structures that it is difficult to address or sometimes even to identify them.

The "Great Recession" of 2007–2009, for example, exacerbated the already large racial or ethnic gaps in wealth that had been growing steadily for years. Although that recession led to steep declines in wealth in every racial and ethnic group, people of color were disproportionately affected (Kochhar and Fry 2014). That trend has continued; in 2016, for example, the median wealth of White households was nearly 10 times the median wealth of Black households (as noted previously), 8.3 times that of Latino households, and 2.6 times the median wealth of households in the "other" racial/ethnic category (Board of Governors of the Federal Reserve System 2017). Although households in the "other" racial category have a substantially higher median net worth than Black and Latino households, aggregated wealth data for "other" households conceal wealth inequality among subgroups. In 2016, for example, the wealthiest 10% of Asian American or Pacific Islander households earned 10.7 times more income than the least wealthy 10% of Asian American and Pacific Islander households (Kochhar and Cilluffo 2018). Although comparable data on wealth broken down by subgroups within each large racial/ethnic group are not currently available for American Indian, Alaska Native, Native Hawaiian, or Pacific Islander households, income and poverty data consistently reveal a high prevalence of economic disadvantage within these groups; in 2019, for example, the poverty rate for American Indian or Alaska Native populations (who reported only a single racial identification without reporting multiple races) was 23% (U.S. Census Bureau 2019).

What Explains the Income and Wealth Gap by Race or Ethnic Group?

Although racial discrimination (unfair treatment based on race or ethnic group) is no longer legal, income and wealth inequities along racial lines persist largely because of systemic or structural racism—that is, deeply rooted, unfair systems and structures that continue to operate, often unconsciously, to sustain the legacy of discriminatory systems, laws, policies, and practices. Examples of structural racism include discriminatory bank and government lending practices; racial residential segregation, which sequesters people of color to low-opportunity, residential areas; and the mass incarceration of Black and Latino men.

Striking disparities in income—and especially in wealth—between different racial and ethnic groups reflect a long history of discriminatory practices that once were intentionally built into policies and laws. Enslaved people had no rights, including rights to compensation for their labor, property rights, or the right to control their own bodies (vs. being tortured by whipping or other means or coercively and cruelly experimented upon) (Savitt 1982). The end of outright slavery was followed by nearly 100 years of "Jim Crow" laws in formerly Confederate states. These laws, enforced by terror, notably by the Ku Klux Klan, systematically and explicitly supported and perpetuated racial segregation and discrimination against Black, Asian, and Latino people across all domains, limiting their opportunities for education, employment, and building wealth (Rothstein 2017). Immigrants from Latin America, both documented and undocumented, are often deterred from seeking services that might help them advance economically due to fear of discriminatory treatment (Bailliard 2013). American Indians who survived genocide were forcibly moved from their expropriated ancestral lands to "reservations" on lands with generally unfavorable conditions; this has severely limited their economic opportunities (Walters et al. 2011).

Homeownership is the principal form of wealth for most White people of modest means. Although the G.I. Bill, which passed in 1944, allowed many White people to become homeowners, flagrant discrimination in its implementation denied most racial and ethnic minorities that same opportunity. Fewer than 100 of the first 67,000 mortgages insured by the G.I. Bill in New York and northern New Jersey (an area from which records were available) were issued to people who were not White (Katznelson 2005). Similarly, whereas low-interest Federal Housing Authority loans made available by the National Housing Act in 1934 enabled many White people to accumulate wealth in the form of homeownership, racial discrimination often denied that opportunity to people of color. Although the passage of the Civil Rights Act of 1964, the Voting Rights Act of 1965, and the Fair Housing Act of 1968 made discrimination based on race illegal in multiple domains, the path between enactment and enforcement of these laws has been long and many obstacles remain.

Racial residential segregation continues to play a major role in income and wealth inequality. Segregated urban neighborhoods and Indian reservations are more likely to have concentrated poverty and limited opportunity for upward mobility because they tend to lack good land, schools, jobs, and services. "Redlining" refers to a practice of banks involving drawing red lines on maps around urban neighborhoods where people of color reside. Redlining was used to define where loans would and would not be given to purchase homes or start businesses. It began as an effort by the government-sponsored Home Owners' Loan Corporation (HOLC) to stabilize housing markets after the Great Depression. The areas categorized by HOLC as riskiest for lending generally corresponded to areas with high concentrations of African Americans; evidence was not provided to justify this practice. Comparing maps created by HOLC during the 1930s with current information for more than 200 cities, economists at the Federal Reserve Bank of Chicago found that disparities in homeownership, home values, and credit scores in originally redlined neighborhoods remain apparent today (Aaronson, Hartley, and Mazumder 2019).

Employment discrimination also has serious implications for a person's income and ability to accumulate wealth. Although now illegal, racial discrimination in hiring, pay, and promotions persists (Quillian et al. 2017; Lewis, Boyd, and Pathak 2018; Byron 2010); much of it may reflect unconscious or "implicit" bias—that is, prejudicial beliefs one has without being aware of them (Greenwald et al. 2009; Pager and Shepherd 2008). In addition, communities of color are disproportionately targeted by predatory financial services—such as payday lenders, check-cashing services, and pawn shops—that tend to charge excessive fees and usurious interest rates; one study found that from 2004 to 2007, Black and Latino individuals were 103% and 78%, respectively, more likely than White individuals to have high-cost home mortgages, regardless of credit histories and other important risk factors (Bayer, Ferreira, and Ross 2017). Discriminatory policing and sentencing practices have also contributed to racial disparities in income and wealth through mass incarceration. A history of incarceration permanently stigmatizes young people even after release, denying them opportunities to obtain employment and permanently closing off their economic options; Black, Latino, and American Indian youth are approximately 5 (The Sentencing Project 2017a), 1.7 (The Sentencing Project 2017b), and 3 (The Sentencing Project 2017c) times, respectively, more likely than White youth to be incarcerated. Once having been incarcerated, it is very difficult to find employment. The stigma of having been incarcerated follows people throughout their lives, with severe lifelong economic consequences not only for the former prisoners but also for their families (who need their contributions to household expenses) and communities as well.

Income and Wealth Also Vary by Gender, Disability, and Age

Despite increasingly more women joining the workforce, *gender-based disparities* in pay and advancement persist, limiting women's opportunities to generate income and build wealth. Women of color face compound disadvantage based on both gender and race, with less wealth and income compared both with men of the same racial group and with White women (Sullivan and Meschede 2016). In 2007, for example, the median wealth levels for single Black, Latino, and White women were $100, $120, and $41,500, respectively; the median wealth levels for single Black, Latino, and White men were $7,900, $9,730, and $43,800, respectively (Chang 2010).

Even among married and cohabiting couples, most caregiving is done by women, which can limit women's opportunities to earn income and build wealth; this happens because caregiving can reduce both paid work hours and job-related pensions or retirement accounts. Compared with men, women suffer more financially following household changes such as divorce and separation (Loya et al. 2015). Although women of all racial/ethnic groups face financial adversity from changes in household composition, White women as a group are better positioned to handle the economic strain of relationship dissolution, even after taking educational attainment into account. Based on 2013 data for women with bachelor's degrees, the median wealth levels of Black and White women, respectively, were $45,000 and $260,000 for married women and $5,000 and $35,000 for single women (Zaw et al. 2017).

People living with disabilities also often face obstacles to earning income and building wealth. In 2018, only approximately 20% of working-age adults with disabilities, compared to approximately 70% of those without disabilities, were in the labor force (U.S. Department of Labor 2019). Adults living with a disability were more than twice as likely to live in poverty as those with no disability (Goodman et al. 2017). People living with disabilities are 2.6 times less likely to have a bank account, further limiting their opportunities to build credit and savings (Goodman and Morris 2017). Within every age group, Black people are more likely than White or Latino people to have a disability (Goodman et al. 2017).

Wealth disparities across age groups have widened during the past quarter-century—in favor of older people. Between 1989 and 2013, the median wealth of families headed by someone at least 62 years of age increased by 40%, from approximately $150,000 to $210,000. At the same time, the median wealth of families headed by someone aged 40–61 years and by someone younger than age 40 years dropped by 31% and 28%, respectively (Boshara, Emmons, and Noeth 2015). Not all older people have greater wealth, however; according to a 2010 report, 91% of Black and Latino seniors lack the financial resources needed to meet their projected lifetime expenses (Meschede et al. 2010). Even college-graduate, single Black women older than age 60 years are ill-positioned for retirement, with a median wealth of only $11,000 (Zaw et al. 2017).

Many individuals—for example, elderly Black women and disabled Latino men—face multiple disadvantages. The effects of multiple disadvantages (economic and other) may not be simply additive but could interact with each other to generate particularly profound deprivation. This is sometimes referred to as *intersectionality*. Limited information is available on income or wealth differences according to LGBTQ status. Lesbian households (but not gay male households) have lower incomes than otherwise similar heterosexual households.

2.4. SUBSTANTIAL EVIDENCE LINKS BOTH INCOME AND WEALTH WITH HEALTH AND HEALTH DISPARITIES

The Associations Between Income and Health Are Well-Documented

A large body of research documents the links between income and a wide array of health indicators across the life span, beginning even before birth. Figures 2.2–2.5 present a few of many examples of findings linking income with health. Although the data displayed in these figures are mostly cross-sectional, longitudinal studies have also documented strong associations between income and multiple health indicators across the life span (Chetty et al. 2016; Daly et al. 2002; Lantz et al. 1998; McDonough et al. 1997). (The likelihood that these widely observed associations reflect causal relationships rather than mere associations and specifically whether they indicate that income influences health, distinguished from health's influence on income, are discussed later.) Figure 2.2, for example, based on data from Chetty et al. (2016), shows that men in the top household income quartile are likely to live more than 8 years longer than those in the bottom income quartile; for women, the difference is approximately 5 years. (These estimates reflect life expectancy at birth.)

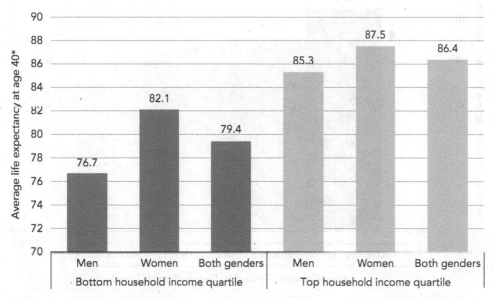

FIGURE 2.2   Higher income, longer life expectancy for both men and women. *Data for years 2001–2014. *Source*: Chart created using data from Appendix eTable7 of Chetty et al. (2016).

Effects of income on health begin early in life. Rates of low birth weight (weighing less than 2500 g at birth)—which is associated with infant mortality, childhood developmental disability, and chronic disease later in life—are highest among infants born to low-income mothers (Blumenshine et al. 2010; Martinson and Reichman 2016). As shown in Figure 2.3, children in poor families (those with incomes at or below 100% of the Federal Poverty Guidelines [FPG]) are 1.5 times as likely to have asthma as children in families with incomes at or above 400% of the FPG. Other research (not shown) demonstrates that lower income children also experience higher rates of heart conditions, hearing problems, digestive disorders, and elevated blood lead levels (Case, Lubotsky, and Paxson 2002; Centers for Disease Control and Prevention 2013).

As seen in Figures 2.4 and 2.5, poor adults (persons 18 years of age or older with incomes at or below the FPG) are more than twice as likely to have four or more chronic conditions (Figure 2.4) and nearly 1.5 times as likely to have activity limitations as adults with family incomes at or above 400% of the FPG (Figure 2.5).

The Associations Between Accumulated Wealth and Health Also Are Well-Documented

Although the relationship between accumulated wealth and health has been studied less frequently than in the case of income, the available evidence indicates that greater levels

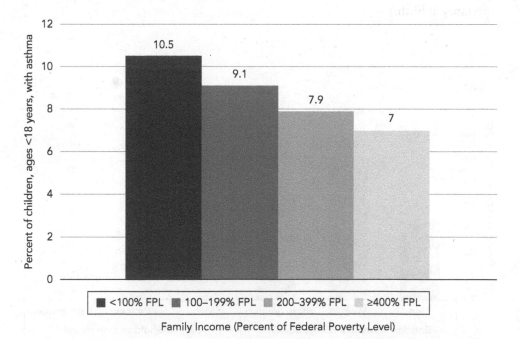

FIGURE 2.3   Higher family income, less childhood asthma. *Age-adjusted; data for years 2014–2016. FPL, federal poverty level. *Source*: National Center for Health Statistics. Percentage of children under age 18 years with asthma, United States, 2014-2016. National Health Interview Survey. Access date 2018.

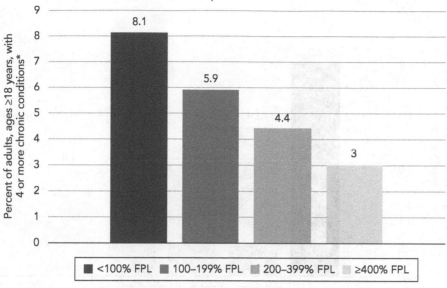

FIGURE 2.4 Higher income, healthier adults. *Age-adjusted; data for year 2016. FPL, federal poverty level. *Source*: National Center for Health Statistics (2018).

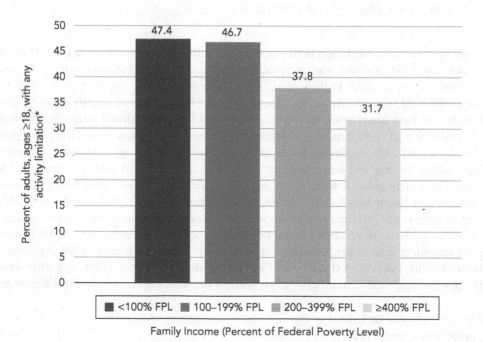

FIGURE 2.5 Higher income, less limitation in activities. *Age-adjusted; data for year 2016. FPL, federal poverty level. *Source*: National Center for Health Statistics (2018).

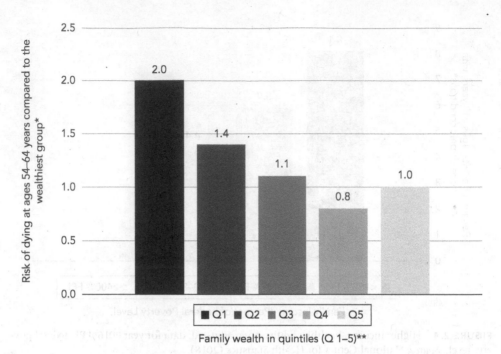

FIGURE 2.6   Greater wealth, lower risk of dying, even after considering income and education. *Adjusted for age, income quintile, race, sex, and education; data for years 2002–2012. **Average wealth per quintile: Q1, $6,511; Q2, $79,312; Q3, $184,332; Q4, $388,466; Q5, $1,503,780. *Source*: Makaroun et al. (2017; Table 2).

of wealth are also linked with better health—including lower mortality, better self-rated health, lower risk of stroke, and lower rates of obesity and other cardiovascular risk factors (Demakakos et al. 2016; Pollack et al. 2013; Hajat et al. 2010a, 2010b; Makaroun et al. 2017). In 2007, a systematic review found that people with greater wealth generally live longer and have lower rates of chronic disease and better functional status throughout life (Pollack et al. 2007). As seen in Figure 2.6, for example, a study found that mortality risk decreased with increasing levels of wealth among adults aged 54–64 years, even after taking income and education into account (Makaroun et al. 2017). A study of 16 countries concluded that wealth was associated with health even after taking income into account (Semyonov, Lewin-Epstein, and Maskileyson 2013). Presumably for wealth and income both, there may be an upper limit beyond which no further improvements in health are seen; those upper limits, however, if they exist, are unknown. It also is possible that there is no upper limit beyond which more economic resources fail to produce better health, because of the health effects of relative differences—that is, having relatively more resources than others—distinguished from the effects of absolute differences.

Neighborhood or Community Economic Resources Also Are Associated with Health

Although much of the research on economic resources and health has focused on income or wealth measured at the individual or household level, increasing attention has been paid to how a person's health may be influenced by economic resources in the neighborhood, community, or area in which they live. A pervasive challenge has been that many studies of area-level economic effects on health have lacked individual-level data, raising questions about whether the findings are due to unmeasured individual-level factors. Many (but not all) studies that have included both area- and individual-level measures of economic resources, however, have found significant associations of area-level factors with illness and mortality independent of individual-level economic measures (Meijer et al. 2012; Diez Roux and Mair 2010; Pickett and Pearl 2001; Hastert et al. 2015). Examining the health effects of area-level factors while adjusting for individual-level factors may be inherently problematic, however, because the individual-level factors may be mediators of the area-level effects—that is, the area-level factors may exert their influence by influencing the individual-level factors; if that is so, then controlling for the individual-level factors amounts to controlling for and therefore eliminating relevant area-level effects from consideration as causal factors.

Economic Inequality Is Associated with Population-Level Health

Up to now, this chapter has focused on the health of individuals. Many studies, however, have also shown associations between a society's health overall and the extent of economic inequality within that society. This is often measured by a statistic called the *Gini coefficient* (R. Wilkinson and Pickett 2006; Pickett and Wilkinson 2015). Although the nature of this association remains controversial (J. Lynch et al. 2004; Kondo et al. 2009; Truesdale and Jencks 2016; Pickett and Wilkinson 2015), the consistency of the findings has been striking.

Countries that have less inequality in income and wealth are generally healthier. It has often been observed that people in rich countries generally have better health than people in poor countries. Newer research, however, shows that overall or average levels of wealth in a country are not the only important factor tied to population health: *How wealth is distributed within a population* also appears to matter. At the national level (and, within the United States, at the state and county levels as well), better overall health has been shown to correspond with less inequality in wealth or income (Pickett and Wilkinson 2015; Nowatzki 2012; Dewan et al. 2019; Johns, Cowling, and Gakidou 2013). Health has been measured in these studies, for example, by average life expectancy or rates of infant mortality, obesity, multiple causes of mortality, and other health indicators. Although the United States is one of the most affluent nations in the world by overall measures, it also has the greatest economic inequality. It has been widely hypothesized that this may help explain why residents of the United States as a whole have generally worse health outcomes than people living in other rich countries, including many countries with lower levels of overall economic resources (Woolf and Aron 2013).

Figure 2.7 shows the substantial correlation between greater wealth inequality and health, measured as life expectancy, at the national level. For infants born in 14 affluent countries during the year

> The Gini coefficient is the most widely used measure of how equally or unequally wealth is distributed within a country's population. It ranges from 0 (corresponding to perfect equality, where everyone has the same amount of economic resources) to 1 (the most unequal, with all of the country's economic resources held by just one individual or household.

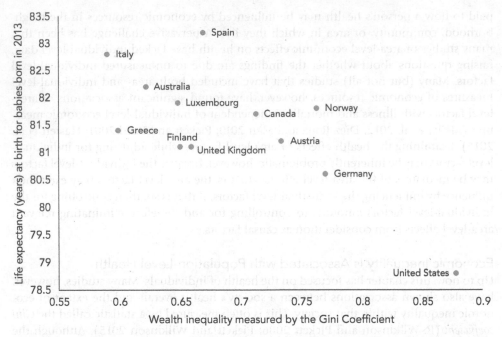

FIGURE 2.7   People in countries with less inequality in wealth generally live longer. Wealth is defined as "disposable net worth"—that is, "the sum of non-financial and financial assets, excluding pension assets and other long-term savings, minus the value of the total liabilities." The unit of analysis is the household. Luxembourg Wealth Study codebook, p. 45 of the following link: https://www.lisdatacenter.org/wp-content/uploads/files/data-lws_codebook.pdf *Sources*: Life expectancy data from the (OECD (2013). Wealth inequality data from the Luxembourg Wealth Study (2013).

2000, the figure illustrates the relationship between a country's average life expectancy at birth—the number of years, on average, that a newborn can be expected to live—and how equally or unequally wealth is distributed in that country. Life expectancy in years is shown along the vertical axis, and wealth inequality—also in the year 2000 and measured using the Gini coefficient—is shown along the horizontal axis. Despite some exceptions, the general pattern is that life expectancy decreases with increasing wealth inequality. Japan has the least wealth inequality and longest life expectancy, whereas the United States and Denmark have the greatest wealth inequality and shortest life expectancies. Similar patterns have been observed repeatedly for other health outcomes, including infant mortality (Nowatzki 2012).

2.5. HOW DO INCOME, WEALTH, AND ECONOMIC INEQUALITY AFFECT HEALTH AND HEALTH DISPARITIES? THE MECHANISMS EXPLAINING THE LINKS

Although there are many unresolved questions, current scientific evidence sheds some light on how—for example, by providing material, psychosocial, and intergenerational benefits—income and wealth can influence health in diverse but overlapping ways. This section discusses several important pathways through which economic resources are thought to influence health at the individual level, including access to health-promoting goods and services; psychological benefits of economic resources, such as protection from stress; and the cumulative effects of economic resources on health over lifetimes and across generations. The pathways through which inequality in income and wealth is thought to influence health at the population level are also discussed.

Wealth and Income Can Promote Health by Providing Access to Health-Promoting Goods and Services, Including Healthier Living Conditions and Access to Health Care

It is obvious that higher income and greater wealth make it easier to pay for medical expenses, including insurance premiums, deductibles, and copayments. Greater wealth, in particular, can preserve access to medical care during times of illness, caregiving, and unemployment, when income is reduced (e.g., during a pandemic). Compared with less affluent families, families with greater wealth are much more likely to have private health insurance, regardless of income and access to employer coverage (Bernard, Banthin, and Encinosa 2009). People with medical and credit card debt are less likely to take medications as prescribed (Kalousova and Burgard 2014). Wealth has been linked with better utilization of dental care (Manski et al. 2012), mammograms (Williams et al. 2008), and receipt of recommended hormonal therapy among women with breast cancer (Hershman et al. 2015).

In addition, greater economic resources also increase people's access to material conditions that help prevent becoming sick in the first place, enabling them to live in safer homes and neighborhoods, eat more nutritious food, and be physically active. Conversely, limited economic resources can mean serious obstacles to good health, limiting a person's opportunities to adopt healthier behaviors. For example, families with more economic resources are better able to buy or rent homes that are free of lead (which can cause lasting neurological damage in young children) and mold or cockroaches, which can trigger asthma attacks. Greater wealth and income permit people to live in neighborhoods with less crime (Friedson and Sharkey 2015), fewer fast-food outlets and liquor stores (N. Larson, Story, and Nelson 2009), and more parks and green spaces to exercise (Gordon-Larsen et al. 2006; Rigolon 2016). Due to environmental injustice, wealthier or higher income neighborhoods also have fewer environmental hazards, such as air pollution and other toxic substances (Hajat et al. 2013). In addition, wealth can protect against the adverse health consequences of job loss; it can prevent homelessness or housing insecurity, food insecurity, and inability to pay for crucial services—such as child care, transportation to/from work, and heat during winter—that can have powerful health effects.

Wealth and Income Can Promote Health by Providing Psychosocial Benefits, Including Protection from Chronic Stress

Advances in neuroscience have provided a better scientific understanding of how persistent stress, even at low levels, can lead to chronic diseases such as heart disease and diabetes. It does so by triggering biological mechanisms, including inflammation and malfunctioning of the immune system (McEwen 2017; Juster, McEwen, and Lupien 2010). Multiple, complex biological processes are involved in the response to stress. One example is the series of bodily processes that results in the secretion of cortisol, a hormone produced by the adrenal glands. When people experience stress, one part of the brain (the hypothalamus) sends a chemical signal, corticotropin-releasing hormone, to another part of the brain (the anterior pituitary gland), which then sends another chemical signal, adrenocorticotropic hormone, to the adrenal glands, causing them to release cortisol into the bloodstream. Occasional short-term release of cortisol apparently is not harmful to health. But persistently high levels of cortisol over time can damage multiple organs and systems in the body, in part by causing inflammation and/or by dysregulating the immune system so that it generates harmful effects rather than performing its proper protective functions. Immune system dysregulation can cause the adrenal glands to produce chronically high levels of cortisol even when a previously chronically stressed person is no longer experiencing chronic stress (McEwen and Seeman 1999).

Higher income and/or greater wealth can protect individuals and families from the stress associated with constant worry about financial hardships. Greater economic resources also can provide protection from the health-damaging psychosocial effects of neighborhood violence or disorder, residential crowding, and constant struggles to meet daily challenges with inadequate resources (Baum, Garofalo, and Yali 1999; Braveman, Marchi, et al. 2010; M. Lynch 2003; Matthews, Gallo, and Taylor 2010). The health effects of economic hardship may occur in part through "stress proliferation," or the compounded negative impacts of financial hardships on family and social relationships, parenting, self-esteem, and other factors that can affect health (Pearlin and Bierman 2013). Higher income and greater wealth also could improve health by providing access to social networks with healthy role models and norms and resources to share (e.g., employment opportunities) (DiMaggio and Garip 2012). In addition, in some studies, health has appeared closely tied not only to individuals' income or education but also to how people view their own social standing relative to others; some studies have found perceived relative social status to be strongly related to health in its own right (Cundiff and Matthews 2017; Tang et al. 2016; Zell, Strickhouser, and Krizan 2018). Income is closely tied to occupation, and the work environment has been a particular focus of research on psychosocial factors affecting health (Watanabe et al. 2018; Theorell et al. 2016). Some researchers, for example, have studied variations in the degree of control that people believe they have over their work and working conditions. They have found that, particularly in the face of high demands being made on them by supervisors, control at work is a major explanation for health differentials across socioeconomic groups—with lower paid workers typically facing higher demands and experiencing lower control (see Chapters 4 and 9; Ravesteijn, van Kippersluis, and van Doorslaer 2013).

Parents' Economic Resources Shape Their Children's Educational, Economic, and Social Opportunities, Which in Turn Shape Their Children's Health Throughout Their Lives

Findings from longitudinal studies indicate that health can be shaped by the *cumulative* effects of economic advantage and disadvantage over a person's lifetime (P. Kim et al. 2018; Johnson-Lawrence, Galea, and Kaplan 2015; Kok et al. 2016; Pollitt, Rose, and

Kaufman 2005; Case, Lubotsky, and Paxson 2002); this is rarely considered in health research. Results of a study that followed residents of Alameda County, California, for more than three decades suggest that combined financial hardships, average income, and changes in income over people's lives affected a range of health-related outcomes, including physical and cognitive functioning, psychological well-being, diabetes, and mortality (Johnson-Lawrence, Galea, and Kaplan 2015; Johnson-Lawrence, Kaplan, and Galea 2013; Kaplan, Shema, and Leite 2008; J. Lynch, Kaplan, and Shema 1997; Maty, James, and Kaplan 2010; Turrell et al. 2007). A nationally representative study of children aged 4 to 14 years found that declines in household income over time predicted children's mental health problems, including depression and antisocial behavior (Strohschein 2005). Other well-known, large, longitudinal studies that have linked economic advantage or disadvantage with health include the Coronary Artery Risk Development in Young Adults Study; the Health and Retirement Study; the National Longitudinal Study of Adolescent Health; and the Whitehall studies in the United Kingdom.

Especially when hardships begin early in life and persist, cumulative economic stress over time can lead to adverse health outcomes later in life, even when financial circumstances improve at some point (Kahn and Pearlin 2006). These outcomes include poorer self-rated health, more chronic disease and depressive symptoms, and reduced functional status. Although economic adversity is not good for one's health at any stage of life, research has revealed that there are certain critical periods of life—for example, during gestation and from birth to age 5 years—when economic adversity and its material and psychosocial consequences can have particularly powerful health effects (Shonkoff, Slopen, and Williams 2021; Boyce and Hertzman 2018). Nobel Laureate economist James Heckman (2008) has called the impact of poverty on a child's future chances "a market failure due to an accident of birth" (p. 314). In addition to its direct effects on health, economic disadvantage—especially in the first 5 years of a child's life—is strongly linked with poor cognitive development and school readiness (Duncan et al. 1998; Votruba-Drzal 2003; Dearing 2008). Predictably adverse consequences have been observed for later educational attainment, employment opportunities, and income, which also are key determinants of adult health. The strong lifelong health effects of adverse childhood experiences, especially during the first 5 years of life (Felitti et al. 1998; Anda et al. 2006), are attributed largely to the sensitivity of a young child's developing brain and other organs (Shonkoff et al. 2012). Cumulative effects over time are consistent with our understanding of the bodily processes likely to be involved in how stress "gets under the skin" to harm health. *Allostatic load* refers to a set of clinical measures that reflect the cumulative wear and tear on the body resulting from chronic stress (Juster, McEwen, and Lupien 2010; McEwen 2017). Adverse childhood experiences are not randomly distributed in populations; their incidence increases with decreasing economic resources of households (Evans 2004; Pelton 1978) (See Chapters 4 and 6).

The Intergenerational Transmission of Wealth and Health

A compelling body of research indicates that children's economic circumstances can influence their health as adults—even when the children's economic circumstances as adults are taken into account (P. Kim et al. 2018; Braveman and Barclay 2009; Duncan et al.

1998). Parents' experiences of chronic financial stress can have adverse consequences for their children's lifelong health (Williams Shanks and Robinson 2013). From birth on, children in families with limited economic resources experience poorer health and are at increased risk of poorer health later in life. Low-income children are more likely to be exposed to hazardous conditions in their homes and neighborhoods, with lasting effects on health; for example, lead poisoning due to unsafe lead levels in housing can result in irreversible neurologic damage with lifelong health consequences (Centers for Disease Control and Prevention 2013). Parents' income has also been linked with nutrition in utero and early childhood, again with potential long-term health effects (Schwarzenberg and Georgieff 2018; Langley-Evans 2015; Gu and Tucker 2016). Low-income children are more likely to be obese (G. Singh 2019), increasing their risks of obesity and related chronic illness as adults (A. Singh et al. 2008; Reilly and Kelly 2011).

Economic circumstances during childhood can shape health later in life in many ways. Parents' income and wealth shape their children's educational, economic, and social opportunities, which in turn shape their children's health throughout life. Parental income has been strongly associated with brain development, apparently through the enrichments, stimulation, and support that economically secure parents are able to give their children. A study of more than 1,000 families with young children found a logarithmic association of parents' income with children's brain surface area. The researchers found that among low-income families, small differences in income were associated with relatively large differences in brain surface area, whereas among higher income families, comparable differences in income were associated with less impressive gains in brain surface area. "These relationships [between socioeconomic status and brain development] were most prominent in [brain] regions supporting language, reading, executive functions and spatial skills; surface area mediated socioeconomic differences in certain neurocognitive abilities" (Noble et al. 2015, p. 773). These relationships likely reflect both parental education and income.

Income differences in brain development may reflect the fact that families struggling to make ends meet are less able to provide their children with cognitive stimulation, enriching materials and experiences, and help with homework (Evans 2004; Bradley and Corwyn 2002; Votruba-Drzal 2003; K. Larson et al. 2015; Chetty et al. 2014). Parents with few or no financial assets who experience the chronic stress associated with low income may have greater obstacles to providing optimal care and attention to their children; they may also adopt unhealthy coping behaviors or develop mental health problems, reducing their ability to work (World Health Organization 2000) or care for their children (Williams Shanks and Robinson 2013). Income-related differences in the cognitive stimulation that parents can provide have implications for academic achievement, educational attainment, and future employment opportunities and earnings. One study found that compared with children in families earning near the median family income (between $35,000 and $49,999 per year at the time of the study), children growing up in families earning less than $15,000 per year were more than 12 times less likely to graduate from high school (Duncan et al. 1998). Among children born in 1986, those from families in the top fifth of the income distribution had a 32% chance of reaching the top income quintile by age 26 years, whereas children from families in the bottom fifth had only a 9% chance.

Although wealth can be passed down directly to subsequent generations through inheritance (and gifts during the older generation's lifetime), research has indicated that these direct transfers may play a smaller role in transmitting wealth across generations than the role played by providing educational and social opportunities (Pfeffer 2015; Pfeffer and Killewald 2017). Parental income and wealth shape the quality of the neighborhood and school contexts in which children grow up and can affect the resources, support, and cognitive stimulation available at home (Evans 2004; K. Larson et al. 2015; Bradley and Corwyn 2002; Votruba-Drzal 2003; Nguyen-Hoang and Yinger 2011; Neuman, Kaefer, and Pinkham 2018).

For the sake of readability, Figure 2.8 omits many important relationships. For example, it does not reflect the notion that both health disadvantage (ill health) and economic disadvantage may accumulate and compound over a person's lifetime, creating increasing obstacles to good health. These obstacles can be transmitted across generations as socioeconomically disadvantaged children become adults and parents who in turn are less able to provide health-promoting social and physical environments for their own children. Stressful experiences associated with socioeconomic disadvantage, moreover, may produce adverse epigenetic effects—interactions between genes and the social or physical environment—that may even be passed on to subsequent generations (McEwen 2017). (Epigenetic effects refer to bodily processes that do not change one's genetic makeup but have powerful effects on whether any given gene is expressed ["turned on"] or suppressed ["turned off"].) Conversely, both good health and socioeconomic advantage tend to accumulate over lifetimes and generations to produce both greater wealth and better health. Together, these patterns act to facilitate or limit social and economic mobility. Without policy interventions, they will increase inequities in both wealth and health over time.

The United States historically has prided itself on being "the land of opportunity," with greater economic mobility than other affluent countries. It is questionable whether this was ever true for people of color; it certainly was not true during the 250 years of slavery followed by nearly a century of Jim Crow laws depriving people of color of their rights. In any case, research has shown that it does not apply currently. Among affluent nations, the United States has the strongest correspondence between parental income and children's later income as adults, reflecting a lack of intergenerational mobility in earnings (Torche 2014). Within every quintile of family wealth (although particularly marked among the highest and lowest wealth quintiles), children are likely to end up with levels of wealth similar to those of their parents (Pfeffer 2015; Pfeffer and Killewald 2017). These general observations may not hold for Black men, however. Examining income mobility, Chetty et al. (2020) found that among adult men who were raised in higher income households, Black men are less likely than White men to be as well-off as their parents. The authors concluded that this reflects a daunting web of race-based disadvantages faced by Black boys and men.

What Could Explain the Links Between Economic Inequality and Population-Level Health?

Based on 30 years of research, Wilkinson and Pickett—and many other scholars—have concluded that health tends to be worse in countries with greater economic

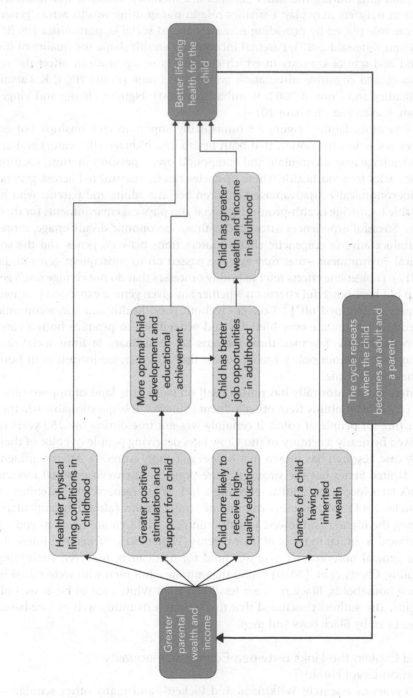

FIGURE 2.8 Both wealth and health are transmitted across generations through material and psychosocial advantages and disadvantages.

inequality in large part because greater economic inequality may make the lives of rich and poor people increasingly separate. This can lead to a lack of empathy or lack of a feeling of connectedness among the "haves" for the "have-nots." This lack of social cohesion or social solidarity can translate into relatively less public spending on policies that benefit the entire society, because the affluent do not feel connected to the poor (L. Wilkinson and Pickett 2010). By undermining social ties and trust, large economic differences between the rich and poor also may exacerbate societal problems associated with poorer health, such as crime and violence (Pickett and Wilkinson 2015). Although economic inequality has repeatedly been correlated with health, the relationship may not be directly causal. There could be some unmeasured factor—such as lack of social solidarity—that produces both economic inequality and worse health. On the other hand, even if one hypothesizes that perhaps a lack of social solidarity, ties, and trust came first, it is plausible that the resultant economic inequality could exacerbate that lack of solidarity, thereby further damaging population health.

Considering Knowledge of Mechanisms as Well as Associations, How Strong Is the Evidence That Income and Wealth Affect Health?

Not everyone is convinced that lower levels of income or wealth lead to poorer health. Despite accumulated evidence, many people still assume that the connections between economic resources and health are explained by access to health care insurance and medical care. And although most economists accept that severe material deprivation due to extreme poverty can play a causal role in poor health outcomes (Subramanian and Kawachi 2006), some question whether income has a major influence on health for those who are not extremely poor. Several economists have noted, with good reason, that poorer health can be the cause of low income rather than the other way around. Associations between economic resources and health could reflect the effects of health on economic resources rather than the effects of economic resources on health (Meer, Miller, and Rosen 2003; Michaud and van Soest 2008; Deaton and Paxson 1998); this is referred to as *reverse causation*. For example, poorer health status could lead to poorer financial status by limiting a person's opportunities to work and earn income while at the same time spending down financial assets for illness-related medical expenses not covered by insurance. (See Box 2.2 and Chapter 9.)

2.6. INTERVENTIONS TO REDUCE ECONOMIC DISADVANTAGE

The idea of enacting policies to lift people out of poverty is not new. What is relatively new, however, is growing awareness of the potential *health* implications of reducing economic disadvantage. Unfortunately, evaluations of economic interventions rarely measure health outcomes. One must therefore in many cases rely on research that "connects the dots" between income or wealth and intermediate outcomes that are known to affect health. Following are a few examples of programs that have tried to improve economic resources for low-income families, particularly those with children. Although none of these programs was designed with health effects as a primary goal, if they are effective in

BOX 2.2	Frequently Asked Questions About the Evidence Base Linking Income/Wealth with Health

Some frequently raised questions about the links between income, wealth, and health are noted here, along with a brief summary of relevant evidence supporting the conclusion that economic resources do in fact shape health (in addition to how they provide access to medical care).

Question 1: Is health care the main issue? Are the links between greater income and wealth and better health explained primarily by the fact that having more money allows a person to obtain medical care (by purchasing medical insurance, paying deductibles and co-payments for insurance, and/or paying out-of-pocket for medical expenses not covered by insurance, and also by lessening barriers to access medical care such as transportation and child care)?

Answer 1: Unlikely. The ability to pay for medical care undoubtedly contributes to health, but the evidence indicates that this does not fully explain the links between economic resources and health-for example:

- Strong and consistent stepwise gradient patterns linking health and socioeconomic advantage—with health improvements seen with every step up the socioeconomic ladder—have been observed in western European countries, including the United Kingdom, France, and the Netherlands, which all have universal financial access to medical care (Avendano et al. 2006; Kunst et al. 1998, 2004; Mackenbach et al. 2000; Marmot et al. 1991).

- Multiple U.S. studies have observed strong associations between income or wealth and different health indicators, even after taking health care insurance/coverage into account (McGrail et al. 2009; Newacheck et al. 2003; Ross and Mirowsky 2000; Sorlie et al. 1994; Sudano and Baker 2006; Szanton et al. 2008; Victorino and Gauthier 2009).

Question 2—Reverse causation: Are the links between income or wealth and health explained by the fact that poorer health leads to reduced income, rather than lower income leading to worse health?

Answer 2: Unlikely.

- Although poor health can certainly influence income and wealth, compelling evidence indicates that this does not fully explain the observed connections between income or wealth and health (Evans and Garthwaite 2014; Fichera and Gathergood 2016; Frech and Damaske 2019; Zagorsky and Smith 2016).

- The causal pathways linking health and economic resources do operate in both directions—income and wealth affect health, and health affects income and wealth. This question arises particularly when studies examine data describing only a single point or short period in people's lives. Results from well-designed longitudinal studies that have followed people over time, however, show that substantial changes in health and important health-related risk factors occur *following* changes in economic resources, which rules out reverse causation (Evans and Garthwaite 2014; Fichera and Gathergood 2016; Frech and Damaske 2019; Zagorsky and Smith 2016).

- Longitudinal studies have also found associations between greater wealth and many favorable health outcomes, including lower mortality; higher life expectancy; slower declines in physical functioning; better self-rated health; and decreased risks of obesity, smoking, hypertension, and asthma (Cai 2009; Hajat et al. 2010a, 2010b; J. Kim and Richardson 2012; Zagorsky and Smith 2016). One prospective study showed that inheriting substantial wealth was followed by a lower risk of asthma, whereas levels of wealth did not decrease after a diagnosis of asthma (Zagorsky and Smith 2016).

Question 3-Scientific (including biological) plausibility: Is it plausible that income and wealth could affect health? Is it consistent with current knowledge of biology?

Answer 3: Yes to both questions.

- Current knowledge of biology and physiology strongly supports a causal role for income and wealth in affecting health along multiple causal pathways and through multiple physiological mechanisms. For example, the harmful biological effects of exposure to lead, mold, air pollution, unsafe traffic conditions, and inadequate nutrition—all more common among impoverished households—are known. Furthermore, current knowledge of the physiology of stress is likely to explain a substantial portion of the income/wealth–health link. Chronically inadequate income or wealth leads to the chronic stress of having to cope with daily challenges (e.g., child care, transportation, and feeding and housing one's family) with inadequate resources. Chronic stress can dysregulate physiological systems, including the hypothalamic–pituitary–adrenal axis and the autonomic nervous system; this dysregulation can set in motion processes that lead to inflammation and depressed immune function, resulting in chronic disease.

Question 4: Is the money–health link likely to be due to other factors that have not been considered, rather than how money affects health? Could the links between income/wealth and health be due to other factors that have not been measured?

Answer 4 overall: Possible but unlikely, given all the evidence. The case supporting the health effects of economic resources is strengthened by evidence from well-done observational studies, including natural experiments and other longitudinal studies, and from several randomized studies. Examples of the evidence include the following:

Answer 4a: Examples of evidence from randomized controlled studies

- In the New Hope Project conducted from 1994 to 1998 in two inner-city areas of Milwaukee, Wisconsin, participants who were willing to work full-time were randomly assigned either to receive a 3-year package of benefits including an earnings supplement to raise their income above the poverty level or to a control group that received no benefits. After 5 years, participants receiving the benefits package reported lower rates of poverty, better physical health, and fewer depressive symptoms compared with the control group. In addition, their children showed improved academic performance compared with children in the control group. After 8 years, children in the benefits group were more engaged and receiving better grades in school, and they were less likely to repeat grades or be placed in special education; they also had more positive social behavior and attitudes about work (Miller et al. 2008). (Most of these outcomes have been linked directly or indirectly with health.)

- An experiment conducted in Gary, Indiana, from 1971 to 1974 randomly assigned participating low-income African American families to one of four income supplement plans (using income tax credits) or a control group. Three years into the study, improvements in birth weight were seen for infants born to women in the highest risk experimental groups relative to the control group; these differences did not appear to be related to prenatal care (Kehrer and Wolin 1979).

Answer 4b: Evidence from natural experiments

- Individuals who received the maximum state Supplementary Security Income (SSI) benefit between 1990 and 2000 were significantly less likely to have mobility limitations compared with those who received lower SSI benefits; the strongest effects were seen among the individuals in the lowest income quartile (Herd, House, and Schoeni 2006).

- A study in Sweden found that each 10% increase in income from lottery winnings was associated with a statistically significant gain in health status, equivalent to an estimated additional 5–8 weeks in life expectancy, on average.(Lindahl 2005)

- Low-income mothers who benefitted from the 1993 Earned Income Tax Credit (EITC) expansion experienced improvements in self-rated health, less inflammation, and lower levels of biomarkers associated with cardiovascular disease and metabolic disorders relative to low-income mothers who did not qualify for the expansion (Evans and Garthwaite 2014).

- Sons of mothers who received Mother's Pension program benefits (administered from 1911 to 1935 in the United States) had lower odds of being underweight, completed more schooling, had higher incomes in adulthood, and lived 1 year longer, on average, than sons of mothers who did not participate in the program (Aizer et al. 2016).

Answer 4c: Evidence of a pervasive stepwise gradient in the relationship between economic resources and health

- The evidence for a causal relationship between economic resources and health is further strengthened by the pervasive finding of a stepwise gradient pattern in that relationship, with greater economic resources generally accompanied by better health, across many, if not most, health indicators. As illustrated in Figures 2.1–2.5, the relationships between economic resources and most, but not all, health outcomes often follow a stepwise gradient pattern: Increases in levels of income or wealth generally correspond with improvements in health, and—although those at the bottom of the economic ladder typically experience the worst health outcomes—even those who would be considered middle class by most standards are less healthy than those who are most affluent (Avendano et al. 2006; Gheorghe et al. 2016; Hoffmann 2011; Kunst et al. 2004; Martinson 2012; Martinson and Reichman 2016). Not surprisingly, the income–health gradient generally has appeared less striking at older ages (Acciai 2018; Hoffmann 2011), when most people are no longer employed and therefore have diminished incomes. As might also be expected, however, the links between accumulated wealth and health appear strong among the elderly (Acciai 2018; Avendano and Glymour 2008). The gradient pattern supports a causal role for economic resources in relation to health because it reflects a dose–response relationship—that is, borrowing a term from the field of medicine, that higher "doses" of income or wealth are accompanied by greater "responses" (improvements in health). A dose–response relationship and other criteria for making a causal inference are discussed later in the chapter.

- The stepwise patterns linking income and wealth with health do not necessarily follow a straight line. For example, although increases in income are generally linked with greater health improvements at the lower end of the income scale, they may not necessarily correspond to better health among the most affluent (Backlund, Sorlie, and Johnson 1996; Braveman, Cubbin, et al. 2010; Dowd et al. 2011; Subramanian and Kawachi 2006). One would not necessarily expect to see a gradient—or a perfectly linear gradient—for all health outcomes in relation to all economic

measures in all populations and contexts. A wide range of pathways and mechanisms are involved, and many different determinants along the pathways can (and often do) interact with other determinants under different circumstances and with different populations in different settings.

Question 5: Does the evidence meet recognized criteria for a causal relationship?

Answer 5: Yes.

- Widely accepted criteria for making a causal inference include that an observed association is of substantial (nontrivial) magnitude, that it is replicable (not merely observed rarely), and that it is chronologically and biologically plausible (i.e., the presumed cause occurs before, not after, the presumed effect, and, for a presumed cause of health effects, that it is plausible in light of current knowledge of biology). All of these criteria are amply met by extensive evidence of associations between economic resources and health, examples of which have been presented previously in this chapter. In addition, observing a dose–response relationship, although not essential, strengthens a causal claim when it is present, as is the case with the stepwise gradient pattern in the relationship between economic resources and many health outcomes.

---

improving economic resources for low-income families, based on the findings reviewed previously in this chapter, they could have major health effects.

Interventions addressing income and/or wealth would be expected to have health implications. Many government entities, nonprofits, and research organizations are working—often in partnership—to provide vulnerable individuals and families with financial education and coaching, subsidized savings accounts, job training, rental and homebuyers assistance, and microloans to start or grow small businesses (Federal Reserve Bank of San Francisco & Corporation for Enterprise Development 2015). Integrating these strategies into existing social services, such as assistance with employment, housing, education, and health care, is a promising approach (Federal Reserve Bank of San Francisco and Low Income Investment Fund 2012). For example, some community health centers offer "financial wellness" or "financial literacy" programs in partnership with financial services providers, and some Head Start centers incorporate financial security counseling into home visits, advertise and promote matched savings accounts, and provide classroom-based financial education to both parents and children (Corporation for Enterprise Development 2013).

Other promising efforts focus more broadly on improving conditions and opportunities at the neighborhood and regional levels that will improve the economic resources of groups that have been excluded or marginalized. Banks and government, community development, nonprofit, and philanthropic organizations are engaged in efforts to increase availability of financial services, safe and affordable housing, employment opportunities, and transportation in economically disadvantaged neighborhoods (Federal Reserve Bank of San Francisco and Low Income Investment Fund 2012). For example, public and private investors are financing "transit-oriented development funds" in Denver, Colorado, and the San Francisco Bay Area in California to develop and maintain affordable housing in close proximity to major bus and rail lines (Srivastava et al. 2010), which are needed for access to employment opportunities.

Existing state and federal policies, e.g., on taxation and minimum wage, play an important role. Child care subsidies and the Earned Income Tax Credit (EITC) have increased employment and earnings among low-income families (County Health Rankings & Roadmaps 2019a, 2019b; Sherman, DeBot, and Huang 2016). Dramatic declines in child poverty have been attributed to strengthened safety nets, including EITC, the Child Tax Credit (part of the 2021 American Rescue Plan), and the Supplemental Nutrition Assistance Program (SNAP) [NBER 2022].

Whereas some strategies have demonstrated positive results for the individuals and communities they serve, others have produced inconsistent results or have been inadequately studied. Many strategies, moreover, represent model efforts in a limited number of places or underfunded national programs. A greater investment in research and evaluation is critical for determining the most effective and efficient approaches, and more strategic support is needed to bring promising models to scale.

The continued exclusion of people of color from opportunities to acquire and build income and wealth must be addressed because it is unfair. In addition, it can be argued that permitting ongoing exclusion of some groups from economic opportunity also comes with high risks for the nation as a whole. These risks include continued, unacceptably high rates of preventable illness and premature death, which in turn generate human and economic costs—not only the suffering and costs associated with health care for illness that could have been prevented but also the consequences of lost economic productivity and prosperity and the lost potential for families and communities to thrive.

Ensuring that all people have access to equitable opportunities to acquire and build wealth will require changes at the systemic and policy levels in states and nationally. Effective policies and programs that assist vulnerable individuals and families with financial stability, provide protection from debt and discriminatory financial practices, and increase access to shelter and other necessities should be expanded. An array of interventions in multiple sectors is needed. For example, awareness of the intergenerational pathways linking wealth and health underscores the need for increased investment in early childhood development, including early care and education and services to strengthen parents' ability to provide health-promoting home environments for their children—both of which are essential for economic opportunity. Experience to date suggests, however, that such services alone are unlikely to overcome some of the most fundamental obstacles—such as systemic racism and entrenched, intergenerational poverty—that undermine the economic well-being of segments of the U.S. population.

Policies and programs need to address the lack of economic opportunity among people of all racial/ethnic backgrounds. The struggles of the approximately 17 million poor White Americans (Fontenot, Semega, and Kollar 2018) must be addressed as an issue of economic equity, without losing sight of the many ways in which their Black, Latino, Indigenous, and some Asian counterparts face additional, daunting obstacles created by centuries of racial injustice.

Although there is much that we do not know, we know that no single strategy will succeed on its own. Enhancing wealth-building opportunities among individuals, families, and communities where such opportunities have been lacking will require strategic coordination across multiple programs and sectors addressing multiple social determinants of health. Despite the lack of certainty, we should build on promising U.S. policies and programs, and we can learn from the experiences of other countries with more equitable income and wealth distributions and better health outcomes, keeping in mind unique features of the U.S. context. Resources will be needed to go to scale with promising strategies to build wealth in communities that have historically been excluded from opportunities, and there will be resistance to covering the necessary costs. We must weigh those costs against the costs of continued inaction—the high stakes for our society of failing to act to improve health for everyone while reducing the gaping chasms in income, wealth, and health between the haves and have-nots.

Examples of Initiatives to Reduce Economic Disadvantage That Can Be Expected to Have Favorable Effects on Health and/or Health Disparities

Following are a number of selected policies, programs, and institutions that are relevant to reducing economic disadvantage, although that has not been the central aim for all. These include programs that have been tried in a number of communities, as well as programs and agencies mandated by national or state policies. The initial strategies are featured on the Robert Wood Johnson Foundation–supported website What Works for Health: County Health Rankings & Roadmaps (https://www.countyhea lthrankings.org/take-action-to-improve-health/what-works-for-health), which provides an evidence-informed menu of policies and programs to improve health by building wealth. Following the strategies featured on What Works are additional initiatives that warrant mention.

Adult financial education programs are facilitated by for- and nonprofit organizations, government entities, and employers and serve low-income individuals one-on-one, in groups, in person, over the phone, or online. Participants are educated on basic budgeting, bank use, and credit management. More specialized programs provide guidance on divorce preparation, bankruptcy, credit building, homeownership, retirement, and other relevant topics.

Child care subsidy programs help working parents and parents attending education/ training programs cover the costs of child care. Eligibility is determined by income; the federal threshold is at or below 85% of state median income, but most states have limits under 200% of the federal poverty line.

Children's saving accounts (CSAs) are designated for a specific child to accumulate savings over time through deposits from family, friends, or the children themselves. Sponsors (e.g., a government, nonprofit, or philanthropic organization) start the account with an initial contribution and may provide ongoing savings incentives, such as matching deposits and financial education. Families may access CSAs through school-based initiatives, citywide public–private partnerships, or statewide programs.

The *Child Tax Credit* (CTC) is a federal tax credit that helps working families offset the costs of raising children. The CTC phases out at higher levels of income than the EITC (see below), helping not only low- and moderate-income but also middle- and upper-middle-income families. The CTC refunds 15% of earnings above $2,500 up to a maximum value of $1,400 for each child younger than age 17 years.

The *Community Development Block Grant Program* (CDBG) provides annual grants to 1,209 qualified localities and states for community development programs, such as affordable housing, infrastructure development, and anti-poverty initiatives. The CDBG was designed to be a "bottom-up" strategy, in that applicants must identify the most pressing community needs and consult with residents and local organizations on how to address them. The CDBG requires that at least 70% of the funds be used to benefit low- and moderate-income individuals.

Community land trusts (CLTs) are nonprofit, community-based organizations that ensure community control of land in order to secure long-term affordable housing. CLTs acquire land and provide long-term leases to prospective homeowners. Homeowners receive a portion of the increased property value when selling; the CLT retains the remainder to preserve affordability for future homebuyers.

The *Earned Income Tax Credit*(EITC), which refunds federal taxes to low- and moderate-income working families, has been shown to increase employment and lift approximately 6 million people—more than half of them children—out of poverty annually (Hoynes and Rothstein 2016; National Conference of State Legislatures 2019). The refund increases for each additional dollar of earnings until reaching a maximum value. In 2017, 25 million working individuals and families received the EITC. In addition to the federal credit, 29 states and the District of Columbia have established their own EITCs as of 2019.

Full child support pass-through and disregard policies allow custodial parents to receive all state-collected child support payments along with their Temporary Assistance for Needy Families (TANF) benefits. States with full disregard policies disregard child support payments when determining TANF eligibility. As of 2017, half the U.S. states have some form of pass-through and disregard policy; Minnesota is the only state to have a full pass-through policy.

The *HOME Investment Partnership Program* is the largest federal block grant program providing states and localities with funds to build, buy, and/or rehabilitate affordable housing or provide rental and/or homebuyer assistance to low-income households. Communities often collaborate with local nonprofits and are required to fund a 25-cent match for every dollar received.

Housing trust funds (HTFs) develop and maintain low-income housing, subsidize rental housing, and provide support to nonprofit housing developers. Some HTFs provide down payment support, counseling, interest subsidies, or "gap subsidies" to low-income buyers. HTFs are administered by nonprofits and governmental housing finance agencies, and they operate at the city, county, state, and national levels.

Individual development accounts (IDAs) are subsidized bank accounts for low- and moderate-income individuals and families. IDAs typically are sponsored by government agencies and facilitated by partnerships between financial institutions and nonprofits. Sponsors match savings deposited into IDAs, and participants must use withdrawals only for qualified expenditures (e.g., education, small business development, and home purchase) to receive matching funds.

Matched dollar incentives for saving tax refunds are efforts to provide matched dollar incentives for individuals to put some or all of their tax refund into a savings account. Several nonprofit and government organizations have piloted programs offering matching deposits up to 100% of savings from tax refunds. Most programs require a minimum amount placed in savings and a minimum period of time before allowing withdrawals with matching funds.

Microfinance programs provide microloans to economically disadvantaged individuals to start or grow small businesses. Microfinance is usually part of a larger microenterprise program that provides business education and/or credit to businesses with fewer than five employees.

Minimum or living wage ordinances are locally mandated wages that exceed the state or federal minimum wage. The current federal minimum wage for covered nonexempt employees (effective July 24, 2009) is $7.25 per hour—representing a level of income that places many families in poverty. Some ordinances require or encourage companies to provide health care coverage and other benefits. As of 2013, more than 140 U.S. communities have enacted living wage ordinances.

In addition to those listed and ranked by County Health Rankings, a number of other institutions or policies also appear worth considering.

Community development corporations (CDCs) are nonprofit, community-based organizations typically involved in affordable housing, commercial property, and business development in underserved, low-income communities. Many CDCs also aid in neighborhood sanitation, planning, and streetscaping, and they offer education and social services.

Community development financial institutions (CDFIs) bring together government funding and funds from private financial institutions to invest in economically distressed communities and provide responsible, affordable loans to economically disadvantaged individuals. Investments by CDFIs fund community development efforts, such as microenterprise, small businesses, housing, and community service organizations.

The *Community Reinvestment Act* (CRA) requires that U.S. depository institutions (e.g., savings banks, commercial banks, and credit unions) be evaluated periodically by federal financial supervisory agencies for their efforts to meet the credit needs of their communities. CRA performance is particularly dependent on the loans, investments, and services that banks provide to lower income individuals and neighborhoods, and it is taken into consideration when banks apply for deposit facilities.

The *Consumer Financial Protection Bureau* (CFPB) is a U.S. government agency established after the Great Recession to protect consumers from discrimination, abuse, fraud, and other predatory practices by banks, credit unions, payday lenders, and other financial companies operating in the United States. Since its inception in 2011, the CFPB has played a key role in protecting vulnerable communities from financial malfeasance—returning approximately $12 billion to 29 million victims and managing more than 1 million consumer complaints.

Early child development programs of high quality, accompanied by services for families, have repeatedly been demonstrated to lead to higher educational attainment, which is crucial for escaping poverty.

The *Federal Reserve*, the central bank of the United States, was established by Congress in 1913 to advance the health and stability of the U.S. economy. The Federal Reserve promotes wealth-building among vulnerable groups through rigorous research and analysis, oversight and regulation of financial institutions, financial education initiatives, and community economic development and reinvestment.

Job training and job creation programs. Even when jobs are available, low-skilled workers often cannot escape poverty. Many experts have called for greater investment in human capital—for example, training, education, substance abuse and mental health services, help with child and elder care responsibilities that conflict with work, and minimum wage legislation—to help workers achieve a living wage and become fully functional members of the workforce (Acs and Nichols 2007). For example, the TANF Emergency Contingency Fund, created as part of the American Recovery and Reinvestment Act of 2009 and in effect through September 2010, enabled states to create more than 250,000 subsidized jobs (Farrell, Elkin, and Broadus 2011).

The *New Markets Tax Credit Program* provides individuals and corporate investors with a federal tax credit in exchange for investing in Community Development Entities— corporations and partnerships that serve as intermediaries in the provision of investments, loans, or financial counseling in low-income communities. The New Markets Tax Credit Program is supported by the CDFI Fund.

Paid parental leave. Although a 1993 federal law mandated that full-time employees of businesses with more than 50 workers be eligible for 12 weeks of unpaid leave following the birth or adoption of a child, workers in smaller businesses are not covered, and very few states have implemented *paid* family leave benefits as well (Donovan 2019).

Public municipal banks are owned by state or public entities and are designed to collaborate with, rather than compete with, private financial institutions. The Bank of North Dakota (BND) is currently the only state-owned bank in the United States. BND guarantees student and business development loans and also state and municipal bonds.

Unemployment insurance is estimated to have prevented 680,000 unemployed persons from joining the 44.6 million people already living in poverty in 2016 (Cooper and Wolfe 2017). Millions of people who file unemployment claims are denied benefits due to ineligibility (Vroman 2018).

Other safety net programs that make income go further: Housing subsidies, supplemental food assistance programs (e.g., Supplemental Nutrition Assistance Program [formerly food stamps]; Women, Infants and Children program; and school nutrition programs), and free or subsidized health insurance can help a low-income family more adequately cover the basic necessities.

2.7. KEY POINTS

- Both income and wealth (the monetary value of all the accumulated assets an individual or household owns minus their debts) influence health in many ways.

Wealth is more difficult to measure than income but may have even more powerful effects on health.

- Systemic or structural racism—embedded in systems, laws, policies, entrenched practices, and beliefs—has constrained the economic opportunities of people of color, resulting in poorer health. Racial residential segregation continues to be a powerful structure that traps many people of color into economically resource- and opportunity-poor environments, which pose short- and long-term risks to health.
- Racial/ethnic disparities in wealth are even greater than racial/ethnic disparities in income. They reflect hundreds of years of obstacles faced by people of color to the accumulation of wealth.
- A stepwise gradient pattern, with health improving incrementally as income or wealth increases, has been repeatedly observed in Europe, the United States, and developing countries. It sheds light on our understanding of how economic resources affect health.
- The distribution of wealth and income has become increasingly unequal over time in the United States and globally.

2.8. QUESTIONS FOR DISCUSSION

1. What explains the Black–White gap in income and wealth?
2. How does income influence health? Discuss at least five different ways.
3. How can wealth affect health? Are these ways different from how income affects health?
4. What policies could help mitigate the negative health effects of economic disadvantage? What upstream strategies seem most promising to reduce economic inequities themselves?
5. What does the stepwise gradient in health (with health improving incrementally as economic resources increase) tell us about the relationship between upstream determinants such as income or wealth and health? What are the implications of the gradient for policy?

ACKNOWLEDGMENTS

Portions of this chapter build on material from the following sources:

Braveman, P., J. Acker, E. Arkin, D. Proctor, A. Gillman, K. A. McGeary, and G. Mallya. 2018. *Wealth Matters for Health Equity*. Princeton, NJ: Robert Wood Johnson Foundation.

Braveman, P., S. Egerter, and C. Barclay. 2011. *Income, Wealth, and Health*. Princeton, NJ: Robert Wood Johnson Foundation.

REFERENCES

Aaronson, D., D. Hartley, and B. Mazumder. 2019. "The effects of the 1930s HOLC 'redlining' maps." https://papers.ssrn.com/sol3/papers.cfm?abstract_id=3038733

Acciai, F. 2018. "The age pattern of social inequalities in health at older ages: Are common measures of socio-economic status interchangeable?" *Public Health* 157: 135–141. https://doi.org/10.1016/j.puhe.2018.01.002.

Acs, G., and A. Nichols. 2007. *Low-Income Workers and Their Employers: Characteristics and Challenges.* Washington, DC: Urban Institute.

Aizer, A., S. Eli, J. Ferrie, and A. Lleras-Muney. 2016. "The long-run impact of cash transfers to poor families." *Am Econ Rev* 106(4): 935–971.

Anda, R. F., V. J. Felitti, J. D. Bremner, J. D. Walker, C. Whitfield, B. D. Perry, S. R. Dube, and W. H. Giles. 2006. "The enduring effects of abuse and related adverse experiences in childhood." *Eur Arch Psychiatry Clin Neurosci* 256(3): 174–186. https://doi.org/10.1007/s00406-005-0624-4.

Avendano, M., and M. M. Glymour. 2008. "Stroke disparities in older Americans: Is wealth a more powerful indicator of risk than income and education?" *Stroke* 39(5): 1533–1540. https://doi.org/10.1161/strokeaha.107.490383.

Avendano, M., A. E. Kunst, M. Huisman, F. V. Lenthe, M. Bopp, E. Regidor, M. Glickman, et al. 2006. "Socioeconomic status and ischaemic heart disease mortality in 10 western European populations during the 1990s." *Heart* 92(4): 461–467. https://doi.org/10.1136/hrt.2005.065532.

Backlund, E., P. D. Sorlie, and N. J. Johnson. 1996. "The shape of the relationship between income and mortality in the United States—Evidence from the National Longitudinal Mortality Study." *Ann Epidemiol* 6(1): 12–20. https://doi.org/10.1016/1047-2797(95)00090-9.

Bailliard, A. 2013. "Laying low: Fear and injustice for Latino migrants to smalltown, USA." *J Occup Sci* 20(4): 342–356. https://doi.org/10.1080/14427591.2013.799114.

Baum, A., J. P. Garofalo, and A. M. Yali. 1999. "Socioeconomic status and chronic stress. Does stress account for SES effects on health?" *Ann N Y Acad Sci* 896: 131–144.

Bayer, P., F. Ferreira, and S. L. Ross. 2017. "What drives racial and ethnic differences in high-cost mortgages? The role of high-risk lenders." *Rev Financial Stud* 31(1): 175–205. https://doi.org/10.1093/rfs/hhx035.

Bernard, D. M., J. S. Banthin, and W. E. Encinosa. 2009. "Wealth, income, and the affordability of health insurance." *Health Affairs* 28(3): 887–896. https://doi.org/10.1377/hlthaff.28.3.887.

Blumenshine, P., S. Egerter, C. J. Barclay, C. Cubbin, and P. A. Braveman. 2010. "Socioeconomic disparities in adverse birth outcomes: A systematic review." *Am J Prev Med* 39(3): 263–272. https://doi.org/10.1016/j.amepre.2010.05.012.

Board of Governors of the Federal Reserve System. 2017. *Survey of Consumer Finances, Historic Tables and Charts.* Washington, DC: Board of Governors of the Federal Reserve System.

Board of Governors of the Federal Reserve System. 2018. *Report on the Economic Well-Being of U.S. Households in 2017.* Washington, DC: Board of Governors of the Federal Reserve System.

Bond Huie, S. A., P. M. Krueger, R. G. Rogers, and R. A. Hummer. 2003. "Wealth, race, and mortality." *Soc Sci Q* 84(3): 667–684. https://doi.org/10.1111/1540-6237.8403011.

Boshara, R., W. R. Emmons, and B. T. Noeth. 2015. *The Demographics of Wealth: How Age, Education, and Race Separate Thrivers from Strugglers in Today's Economy. Essay No. 3: Age, Birth Year and Wealth.* St. Louis, MO: Federal Reserve Bank.

Boyce, T. W., and C. Hertzman. 2018. "Early childhood health and the life course: The state of the science and proposed research priorities: A background paper for the MCH Life Course Research Network." In *Handbook of Life Course Health Development*, edited by N. Halfon, C. B. Forrest, R. M. Lerner, and E. M. Faustman, 61–93. Cham, Switzerland: Springer.

Bradley, R. H., and R. F. Corwyn. 2002. "Socioeconomic status and child development." *Annu Rev Psychol* 53: 371–399. https://doi.org/10.1146/annurev.psych.53.100901.135233.

Braveman, P., J. Acker, E. Arkin, D. Proctor, A. Gillman, K. A. McGeary, & G. Mallya. 2018. *Wealth Matters for Health Equity.* Princeton, NJ: Robert Wood Johnson Foundation.

Braveman, P., and C. Barclay. 2009. "Health disparities beginning in childhood: A life-course perspective." *Pediatrics* 124(Suppl 3): S163–S175. https://doi.org/10.1542/peds.2009-1100D.

Braveman, P. A., C. Cubbin, S. Egerter, S. Chideya, K. S. Marchi, M. Metzler, and S.

Posner. 2005. "Socioeconomic status in health research: One size does not fit all." *JAMA* 294(22): 2879–2888. https://doi.org/10.1001/jama.294.22.2879.

Braveman, P. A., C. Cubbin, S. Egerter, D. R. Williams, and E. Pamuk. 2010. "Socioeconomic disparities in health in the United States: What the patterns tell us." *Am J Public Health* 100: S186–S196. https://doi.org/10.2105/Ajph.2009.166082.

Braveman, P. A., S. Egerter, & C. Barclay. 2011. *Income, Wealth, and Health*. Princeton, NJ: Robert Wood Johnson Foundation.

Braveman, P. A., K. Marchi, S. Egerter, S. Kim, M. Metzler, T. Stancil, and M. Libet. 2010. "Poverty, near-poverty, and hardship around the time of pregnancy." *Matern Child Health J* 14(1): 20–35. https://doi.org/10.1007/s10995-008-0427-0.

Byron, Reginald A. 2010. "Discrimination, complexity, and the public/private sector question." *Work Occup* 37(4): 435–475. https://doi.org/10.1177/0730888410380152.

Cai, L. X. 2009. "Be wealthy to stay healthy: An analysis of older Australians using the HILDA survey." *J Sociol* 45(1): 55–70. https://doi.org/10.1177/1440783308099986.

Case, A., D. Lubotsky, and C. Paxson. 2002. "Economic status and health in childhood: The origins of the gradient." *Am Econ Rev* 92(5): 1308–1334.

Centers for Disease Control and Prevention. 2013. "Number sampled and estimated percentage of children aged 1–5 years with blood lead levels ≥5 µg/dL, by selected characteristics—United States, National Health and Nutrition Examination Survey, 1999–2002, 2003–2006, and 2007–2010. *Morbid Mortal Wkly Rep* 62(13): 245–248.

Chang, M. 2010. *Lifting as We Climb: Women of Color, Wealth and America's Future*. Oakland, CA: Insight Center.

Chetty, R., N. Hendren, M. R. Jones, and S. R. Porter. 2020. "Race and economic opportunity in the United States: An intergenerational perspective." *Q J Econ* 135(2): 711–783.

Chetty, R., N. Hendren, P. Kline, E. Saez, and N. Turner. 2014. "Is the United States still a land of opportunity? Recent trends in intergenerational mobility." Working Paper 19844. Cambridge, MA: National Bureau of Economic Research.

Chetty, R., M. Stepner, S. Abraham, S. Lin, B, Scuderi, N. Turner, A. Bergeron, and D. Cutler. 2016. "The association between income and life expectancy in the United States, 2001–2014." *JAMA* 315(16): 1750–1766. https://doi.org/10.1001/jama.2016.4226.

Cooper, D., and J. Wolfe. 2017. "Poverty declined modestly in 2016; Government programs continued to keep tens of millions out of poverty" [Blog]. Washington, DC: Economic Policy Institute.

Corporation for Enterprise Development. 2013. *Family* Strengthening Through Integration *and* Scaling *of* Asset-Building Strategies: *The ASSET Initiative Partnership Environmental Field Scan* Report. Washington, DC: Corporation for Enterprise Development.

County Health Rankings & Roadmaps. 2019a. "Child care subsidies." Accessed May 2019. http://www.countyhealthrankings.org/take-action-to-improve-health/what-works-for-health/policies/child-care-subsidies.

County Health Rankings & Roadmaps. 2019b. "Earned Income Tax Credit (EITC)." Accessed May 2019. http://www.countyhealthrankings.org/take-action-to-improve-health/what-works-for-health/policies/earned-income-tax-credit-eitc.

Cundiff, J. M., and K. A. Matthews. 2017. "Is subjective social status a unique correlate of physical health? A meta-analysis." *Health Psychol* 36(12): 1109–1125. https://doi.org/10.1037/hea0000534.

Daly, M. C., G. J. Duncan, P. McDonough, and D. R. Williams. 2002. "Optimal indicators of socioeconomic status for health research." *Am J Public Health* 92(7): 1151–1157. https://doi.org/10.2105/ajph.92.7.1151.

Dearing, E. 2008. "Psychological costs of growing up poor." *Ann N Y Acad Sci* 1136: 324–332. https://doi.org/10.1196/annals.1425.006.

Deaton, A. S., and C. H. Paxson. 1998. "Aging and inequality in income and health." *Demographic Trends Econ Consequences* 88(2): 248–253.

Demakakos, P., J. P. Biddulph, M. Bobak, and M. G. Marmot. 2016. "Wealth and mortality at older ages: A prospective cohort study." *J*

Epidemiol Community Health 70(4): 346–353. https://doi.org/10.1136/jech-2015-206173.

Dewan, P., R. Rørth, P. S. Jhund, J. P. Ferreira, F. Zannad, L. Shen, L. Køber, et al. 2019. "Income inequality and outcomes in heart failure: A global between-country analysis." *JACC: Heart Failure* 7(4): 336–346. https://doi.org/10.1016/j.jchf.2018.11.005.

Diez Roux, A. V, and C. Mair. 2010. "Neighborhoods and health." *Ann N Y Acad Sci* 1186(1): 125–145.

DiMaggio, P., and F. Garip. 2012. "Network effects and social inequality." *Annu Rev Sociol* 38(1): 93–118. https://doi.org/10.1146/annurev.soc.012809.102545.

Donovan, S. A. 2019. *Paid Family Leave in the United States.* Washington, DC: Congressional Research Service.

Dowd, J. B., J. Albright, T. E. Raghunathan, R. F. Schoeni, F. LeClere, and G. A. Kaplan. 2011. "Deeper and wider: Income and mortality in the USA over three decades." *Int J Epidemiol* 40(1): 183–188. https://doi.org/10.1093/ije/dyq189.

Duncan, G. J., W. J. Yeung, J. Brooks-Gunn, and J. R. Smith. 1998. "How much does childhood poverty affect the life chances of children?" *Am Sociol Rev* 63(3): 406–423. https://doi.org/10.2307/2657556.

Evans, G. W. 2004. "The environment of childhood poverty." *Am Psychol* 59(2): 77–92. https://doi.org/10.1037/0003-066x.59.2.77.

Evans, W. N., and C. L. Garthwaite. 2014. "Giving mom a break: The impact of higher EITC payments on maternal health." *Am Econ J Econ Policy* 6(2): 258–290.

Farrell, M., S. Elkin, and J. Broadus. 2011. *Subsidizing Employment Opportunities for Low-Income Families: A Review of State Employment Programs Created Through the TANF Emergency Fund.* Washington, DC: U.S. Department of Health and Human Services.

Federal Reserve Bank of San Francisco and Corporation for Enterprise Development. 2015. *What It's Worth: Strengthening the Financial Future of Families, Communities, and the Nation.* San Francisco, CA: Federal Reserve Bank of San Francisco.

Federal Reserve Bank of San Francisco and Low Income Investment Fund. 2012. *Investing in What Works for America's Communities: Essays on People, Place & Purpose.* San Francisco, CA: Federal Reserve Bank of San Francisco.

Felitti, V. J., R. F. Anda, D. Nordenberg, D. F. Williamson, A. M. Spitz, V. Edwards, M. P. Koss, and J. S. Marks. 1998. "Relationship of childhood abuse and household dysfunction to many of the leading causes of death in adults: The Adverse Childhood Experiences (ACE) study." *Am J Prev Med* 14(4): 245–258.

Fichera, E., and J. Gathergood. 2016. "Do wealth shocks affect health? New evidence from the housing boom." *Health Econ* 25(Suppl 2): 57–69. https://doi.org/10.1002/hec.3431.

Fisher, G. M. 1992. "The development and history of poverty thresholds." *Social Security Bull* 55(4): 3–14.

Fontenot, K., J. Semega, and M. Kollar. 2018. *Current Population Reports: Income and Poverty in the United States: 2017.* Washington, DC: U.S. Census Bureau.

Frech, A., and S. Damaske. 2019. "Men's income trajectories and physical and mental health at midlife." *Am J Sociol* 124(5): 1372–1412. https://doi.org/10.1086/702775.

Friedson, M., and P. Sharkey. 2015. "Violence and neighborhood disadvantage after the crime decline." *Ann Am Acad Pol Soc Sci* 660(1): 341–358. https://doi.org/10.1177/0002716215579825.

Gheorghe, M., P. Wubulihasimu, F. Peters, W. Nusselder, and P. H. M. Van Baal. 2016. "Health inequalities in the Netherlands: Trends in quality-adjusted life expectancy (QALE) by educational level." *Eur J Public Health* 26(5): 794–799. https://doi.org/10.1093/eurpub/ckw043.

Goodman, N., and M. Morris. 2017. *Banking Status and Financial Behaviors of Adults with Disabilities: Findings from the 2015 FDIC National Survey of Unbanked and Underbanked Households.* Washington, DC: National Disability Institute.

Goodman, N., M. Morris, K. Boston, and D. Walton. 2017. *Financial Inequality: Disability, Race, and Poverty in America.* Washington, DC: HCBS Clearinghouse.

Gordon-Larsen, P., M. C. Nelson, P. Page, and B. M. Popkin. 2006. "Inequality in the built environment underlies key health disparities in physical activity and obesity." *Pediatrics* 117(2): 417–424. https://doi.org/10.1542/peds.2005-0058.

Greenwald, A. G., T. A. Poehlman, E. L. Uhlmann, and M. R. Banaji. 2009. "Understanding and using the Implicit Association Test: III. Meta-analysis of predictive validity." *J Pers Soc Psychol* 97(1): 17–41. https://doi.org/10.1037/a0015575.

Gu, X., and K. L. Tucker. 2016. "Dietary quality of the US child and adolescent population: Trends from 1999 to 2012 and associations with the use of federal nutrition assistance programs." *Am J Clin Nutr* 105(1): 194–202. https://doi.org/10.3945/ajcn.116.135095.

Hajat, A., A. V. Diez-Roux, S. D. Adar, A. H. Auchincloss, G. S. Lovasi, M. S. O'Neill, L. Sheppard, and J. D. Kaufman. 2013. "Air pollution and individual and neighborhood socioeconomic status: Evidence from the Multi-Ethnic Study of Atherosclerosis (MESA)." *Environ Health Perspect* 121(11–12): 1325–1333. https://doi.org/10.1289/ehp.1206337.

Hajat, A., J. S. Kaufman, K. M. Rose, A. Siddiqi, and J. C. Thomas. 2010a. "Do the wealthy have a health advantage? Cardiovascular disease risk factors and wealth." *Soc Sci Med* 71(11): 1935–1942. https://doi.org/10.1016/j.socscimed.2010.09.027.

Hajat, A., J. S. Kaufman, K. M. Rose, A. Siddiqi, and J. C. Thomas. 2010b. "Long-term effects of wealth on mortality and self-rated health status." *Am J Epidemiol* 173(2): 192–200. https://doi.org/10.1093/aje/kwq348.

Hastert, T. A., S. A. A. Beresford, L. Sheppard, and E. White. 2015. "Disparities in cancer incidence and mortality by area-level socioeconomic status: A multilevel analysis." *J Epidemiol Community Health* 69(2): 168–176. https://doi.org/10.1136/jech-2014-204417.

Haveman, R., R. Blank, R. Moffitt, T. Smeeding, and G. Wallace. 2015. "The war on poverty: Measurement, trends, and policy." *J Policy Anal Manage* 34(3): 593–638. https://doi.org/10.1002/pam.21846.

Heckman, J. J. 2008. "Role of income and family influence on child outcomes." *Ann N Y Acad Sci* 1136: 307–323. https://doi.org/10.1196/annals.1425.031.

Herd, P., J, House, and R. F. Schoeni. 2006. "Income support policies and health among the elderly." In *Health Effects of Non-Health Policy*. Bethesda, MD: National Poverty Center.

Hershman, D. L., J. Tsui, J. D. Wright, E. J. Coromilas, W. Y. Tsai, and A. I. Neugut. 2015. "Household net worth, racial disparities, and hormonal therapy adherence among women with early-stage breast cancer." *J Clin Oncol* 33(9): 1053.

Hoffmann, R. 2011. "Socioeconomic inequalities in old-age mortality: A comparison of Denmark and the USA." *Soc Sci Med* 72(12): 1986–1992. https://doi.org/10.1016/j.socscimed.2011.04.019.

Hoynes, H., and J. Rothstein. 2016. *Tax Policy Toward Low-Income Families*. Cambridge, MA: National Bureau of Economic Research.

Johns, N. E., K. Cowling, and E. Gakidou. 2013. "The wealth (and health) of nations: A cross-country analysis of the relation between wealth and inequality in disease burden estimation." *Lancet* 381: S66. https://doi.org/10.1016/S0140-6736(13)61320-3.

Johnson-Lawrence, V., S. Galea, and G. Kaplan. 2015. "Cumulative socioeconomic disadvantage and cardiovascular disease mortality in the Alameda County Study 1965 to 2000." *Ann Epidemiol* 25(2): 65–70. https://doi.org/10.1016/j.annepidem.2014.11.018.

Johnson-Lawrence, V., G. Kaplan, and S. Galea. 2013. "Socioeconomic mobility in adulthood and cardiovascular disease mortality." *Ann Epidemiol* 23(4): 167–171. https://doi.org/10.1016/j.annepidem.2013.02.004.

Juster, R.-P., B. S. McEwen, and S. J. Lupien. 2010. "Allostatic load biomarkers of chronic stress and impact on health and cognition." *Neurosci Biobehav Rev* 35(1): 2–16. https://doi.org/10.1016/j.neubiorev.2009.10.002.

Kahn, J. R., and L. I. Pearlin. 2006. "Financial strain over the life course and health among older adults." *J Health Soc Behav* 47(1): 17–31. https://doi.org/10.1177/002214650604700102.

Kalousova, L., and S. A. Burgard. 2014. "Tough choices in tough times: Debt and medication nonadherence." *Health Educ Behav* 41(2), 155–163. https://doi.org/10.1177/1090198113493093.

Kaplan, G. A., S. J. Shema, and C. M. A. Leite. 2008. "Socioeconomic determinants of psychological well-being: The role of income,

income change, and income sources during the course of 29 years." *Ann Epidemiol.* *18*(7): 531–537. https://doi.org/10.1016/j.annepidem.2008.03.006.

Katznelson, I. 2005. *When Affirmative Action Was White: An Untold History of Racial Inequality in Twentieth-Century America.* New York: Norton.

Kehrer, B. H., and C. M. Wolin. 1979. "Impact of income maintenance on low birth weight: Evidence from the Gary Experiment." *J Hum Resour* 14(4): 434–462.

Kim, J., and V. Richardson. 2012. "The impact of socioeconomic inequalities and lack of health insurance on physical functioning among middle-aged and older adults in the United States." *Health Soc Care Community* 20(1): 42–51. https://doi.org/10.1111/j.1365-2524.2011.01012.x.

Kim, P., G. W. Evans, E. Chen, G. Miller, and T. Seeman. 2018. "How socioeconomic disadvantages get under the skin and into the brain to influence health development across the lifespan." In *Handbook of Life Course Health Development*, edited by N. Halfon, C. B. Forrest, R. M. Lerner, and E. M. Faustman, 463–497. Cham, Switzerland: Springer.

Koball, H., and Y. Jiang. 2018. "Basic facts about low-income children: Children under 18 years, 2016." New York, NY: National Center for Children in Poverty.

Kochhar, R., and A. Cilluffo. 2018. "Income inequality in the U.S. is rising most rapidly among Asians." Washington, DC: Pew Research Center.

Kochhar, R., and R. Fry. 2014. "Wealth inequality has widened along racial, ethnic lines since the end of the Great Recession." Washington, DC: Pew Research Center.

Kok, A. A. L., M. J. Aartsen, D. J. H. Deeg, and M. Huisman. 2016. "Socioeconomic inequalities in a 16-year longitudinal measurement of successful ageing." *J Epidemiol Community Health* 70(11): 1106–1113. https://doi.org/10.1136/jech-2015-206938.

Kondo, N., G. Sembajwe, I. Kawachi, R. M. van Dam, S. V. Subramanian, and Z. Yamagata. 2009. "Income inequality, mortality, and self rated health: Meta-analysis of multilevel studies." *BMJ* 339: b4471.

Kunst, A. E, V. Bos, E. Lahelma, M. Bartley, I. Lissau, E. Regidor, A. Mielck, et al. 2004. "Trends in socioeconomic inequalities in self-assessed health in 10 European countries." *Int J Epidemiol* 34(2): 295–305. https://doi.org/10.1093/ije/dyh342.

Kunst, A. E., M. del Rios, F. Groenhof, and J. P. Mackenbach; European Union Working Group on Socioeconomic Inequalities in Health. 1998. "Socioeconomic inequalities in stroke mortality among middle-aged men: An international overview." *Stroke* 29 (11): 2285–2291. https://doi.org/10.1161/01.str.29.11.2285.

Langley-Evans, S. C. 2015. "Nutrition in early life and the programming of adult disease: A review." *J Hum Nutr Diet* 28(Suppl 1): 1–14. https://doi.org/10.1111/jhn.12212.

Lantz, P. M., J. S. House, J. M. Lepkowski, D. R. Williams, R. P. Mero, and J. Chen. 1998. "Socioeconomic factors, health behaviors, and mortality: Results from a nationally representative prospective study of US adults." *JAMA* 279(21): 1703–1708. https://doi.org/10.1001/jama.279.21.1703.

Larson, K., S. A. Russ, B. B. Nelson, L. M. Olson, and N. Halfon. 2015. "Cognitive ability at kindergarten entry and socioeconomic status." *Pediatrics* 135(2): e440–e448. https://doi.org/10.1542/peds.2014-0434.

Larson, N. I., M. T. Story, and M. C. Nelson. 2009. "Neighborhood environments: Disparities in access to healthy foods in the U.S." *Am J Prev Med* 36(1): 74–81.e10. https://doi.org/10.1016/j.amepre.2008.09.025.

Lewis, G. B., J. Boyd, and R. Pathak. 2018. "Progress toward pay equity in state governments?" *Public Admin Rev* 78(3): 386–397. https://doi.org/10.1111/puar.12897.

Lindahl, M. 2005. "Estimating the effect of income on health and mortality using lottery prizes as an exogenous source of variation in income." *J Hum Resour* 40(1): 144–168.

Loya, R., A. Mann, J. Boguslaw, and T. Shapiro. 2015. *Tipping the Scale: How Assets Shape Economic Wellbeing for Women and Families.* Boston, MA: Mel King Institute for Community Building.

Luxembourg Wealth Study. 2013. https://dart.lisdatacenter.org/dart

Lynch, J., G. D. Smith, S. A. M. Harper, M. Hillemeier, N. Ross, G. A. Kaplan, and M. Wolfson. 2004. "Is income inequality a determinant of population health? Part 1. A systematic review." *Milbank Q* 82(1): 5–99.

Lynch, J. W., G. A. Kaplan, and S. J. Shema. 1997. "Cumulative impact of sustained economic hardship on physical, cognitive, psychological, and social functioning." *N Engl J Med* 337(26): 1889–1895. https://doi.org/10.1056/nejm199712253372606.

Lynch, M. 2003. "Consequences of children's exposure to community violence." *Clin Child Fam Psychol Rev* 6(4): 265–274. https://doi.org/10.1023/B:CCFP.0000006293.77143.e1.

Mackenbach, J. P., A. E. Cavelaars, A. E. Kunst, and F. Groenhof. 2000. "Socioeconomic inequalities in cardiovascular disease mortality: An international study." *Eur Heart J* 21(14): 1141–1151. https://doi.org/10.1053/euhj.1999.1990.

Makaroun, L. K., R. T. Brown, L. Grisell Diaz-Ramirez, C. Ahalt, W. J. Boscardin, S. Lang-Brown, and S. Lee. 2017. "Wealth-associated disparities in death and disability in the United States and England." *JAMA Int Med* 177(12): 1745–1753. https://doi.org/10.1001/jamainternmed.2017.3903.

Manski, R. J., J. F. Moeller, H. Chen, P. A. St. Clair, J. Schimmel, and J. V. Pepper. 2012. "Wealth effect and dental care utilization in the United States." *J Public Health Dent* 72(3): 179–189. https://doi.org/10.1111/j.1752-7325.2012.00312.x.

Marmot, M. G., G. D. Smith, S. Stansfeld, C. Patel, F. North, J. Head, I. White, E. Brunner, and A. Feeney. 1991. "Health inequalities among British civil servants: The Whitehall II study." *Lancet* 337(8754): 1387–1393. https://doi.org/10.1016/0140-6736(91)93068-k.

Martinson, M. L. 2012. "Income inequality in health at all ages: A comparison of the United States and England." *Am J Public Health* 102(11): 2049–2056. https://doi.org/10.2105/ajph.2012.300929.

Martinson, M. L., and N. E. Reichman. 2016. "Socioeconomic inequalities in low birth weight in the United States, the United Kingdom, Canada, and Australia." *Am J Public Health* 106(4): 748–754. https://doi.org/10.2105/AJPH.2015.303007.

Matthews, K. A., L. C. Gallo, and S. E. Taylor. 2010. "Are psychosocial factors mediators of socioeconomic status and health connections? A progress report and blueprint for the future." *Ann N Y Acad Sci* 1186:146–173. https://doi.org/10.1111/j.1749-6632.2009.05332.x.

Maty, S. C., S. A. James, and G. A. Kaplan. 2010. "Life-course socioeconomic position and incidence of diabetes mellitus among Blacks and Whites: The Alameda County Study, 1965–1999." *Am J Public Health* 100(1): 137–145. https://doi.org/10.2105/ajph.2008.133892.

McDonough, P., G. J. Duncan, D. Williams, and J. House. 1997. "Income dynamics and adult mortality in the United States, 1972 through 1989." *Am J Public Health* 87(9): 1476–1483.

McEwen, B. S. 2017. "Neurobiological and systemic effects of chronic stress." *Chronic Stress* 1: 2470547017692328. https://doi.org/10.1177/2470547017692328.

McEwen, B. S., and T. Seeman. 1999. "Protective and damaging effects of mediators of stress. Elaborating and testing the concepts of allostasis and allostatic load." *Ann N Y Acad Sci* 896: 30–47. https://doi.org/10.1111/j.1749-6632.1999.tb08103.x.

McGrail, K. M., E. van Doorslaer, N. A. Ross, and C. Sanmartin. 2009. "Income-related health inequalities in Canada and the United States: A decomposition analysis." *Am J Public Health* 99(10): 1856–1863. https://doi.org/10.2105/ajph.2007.129361.

McIntosh, K., E. Moss, R. Nunn, and J. Shambaugh. 2020. *Examining the Black–White Wealth Gap.* Washington, DC: Brookings.

Meer, J., D. L. Miller, and H. S. Rosen. 2003. "Exploring the health–wealth nexus." *J Health Econ* 22(5): 713–730. https://doi.org/10.1016/S0167-6296(03)00059-6.

Meijer, M., J. Röhl, K. Bloomfield, and U. Grittner. 2012. "Do neighborhoods affect individual mortality? A systematic review and meta-analysis of multilevel studies." *Social Sci Med* 74(8): 1204–1212. https://doi.org/10.1016/j.socscimed.2011.11.034.

Meschede, T., T. M. Shapiro, L. Sullivan, and J. S. Wheary. 2010. *Severe Financial Insecurity Among African-American and Latino Seniors.* Waltham, MA: The Institute on Assets and Social Policy at Brandeis University.

Michaud, P. C., and A. van Soest. 2008. "Health and wealth of elderly couples: Causality tests using dynamic panel data models." *J Health*

Econ 27(5): 1312–1325. https://doi.org/10.1016/j.jhealeco.2008.04.002.

Miller, C., A. C. Huston, G. J. Duncan, V. C. McLoyd, and T. S. Weisner. 2008. *New Hope for the Working Poor: Effects After Eight Years for Families and Children*. New York, NY: MDRC.

National Bureau of Economic Research. 2022. Children and the US social safety net: balancing disincentives for adults and benefits for children. https://www.nber.org/papers/w29754

National Conference of State Legislatures. 2019. "Tax credits for working families: Earned Income Tax Credit (EITC)." Accessed May 2019. http://www.ncsl.org/research/labor-and-employment/earned-income-tax-credits-for-working-families.aspx.

National Research Council. 1995. *Measuring Poverty: A New Approach*, edited by C. F. Citro and R. T. Michael. Washington, DC: National Academies Press.

Neuman, S. B., T. Kaefer, and A. M. Pinkham. 2018. "A double dose of disadvantage: Language experiences for low-income children in home and school." *J Educ Psychol* 110(1): 102–118.

Newacheck, P. W., Y. Y. Hung, M. J. Park, C. D. Brindis, and C. E. Irwin, Jr. 2003. "Disparities in adolescent health and health care: Does socioeconomic status matter?" *Health Services Res* 38(5): 1235–1252. https://doi.org/10.1111/1475-6773.00174.

Nguyen-Hoang, P., and J. Yinger. 2011. "The capitalization of school quality into house values: A review." *J Hous Econ* 20(1): 30–48. https://doi.org/10.1016/j.jhe.2011.02.001.

Noble, K. G., S. M. Houston, N. H. Brito, H. Bartsch, E. Kan, J. M. Kuperman, N. Akshoomoff, et al. 2015. "Family income, parental education and brain structure in children and adolescents." *Nature Neurosci* 18(5): 773–778. https://doi.org/10.1038/nn.3983.

Nowatzki, N. R. 2012. "Wealth inequality and health: A political economy perspective." *Int J Health Serv* 42(3): 403–424. https://doi.org/10.2190/HS.42.3.c.

Organisation for Economic Cooperation and Development. 2013. *Health Status: Life Expectancy*. Paris, France: Organisation for Economic Cooperation and Development.

Orzechowski, S., and P. Sepielli. 2003. Current *Population Reports: Net Worth and Asset Ownership of Households: 1998 and 2000*. Washington, DC: U.S. Census Bureau.

Pager, D., and H. Shepherd. 2008. "The sociology of discrimination: Racial discrimination in employment, housing, credit, and consumer markets." *Annu Rev Sociol* 34(1): 181–209. https://doi.org/10.1146/annurev.soc.33.040406.131740.

Pearlin, L. I., and A. Bierman. 2013. "Current issues and future directions in research into the stress process." In *Handbook of the Sociology of Mental Health*, edited by C. S. Aneshensel, J. C. Phelan, and A. Bierman, 325–340. Dordrecht, the Netherlands: Springer.

Pelton, L. H. 1978. "Child abuse and neglect: The myth of classlessness." *Am J Orthopsychiatry* 48(4): 608–617.

Pfeffer, F. T. 2015. *How Rigid Is the Wealth Structure and Why? Inter- and Multigenerational Associations in Family Wealth*. Ann Arbor, MI: Populations Study Center, University of Michigan.

Pfeffer, F. T., and A. Killewald. 2017. "Generations of advantage: Multigenerational correlations in family wealth." *Social Forces* 96(4): 1411–1442. https://doi.org/10.1093/sf/sox086.

Pickett, K. E., and M. Pearl. 2001. "Multilevel analyses of neighbourhood socioeconomic context and health outcomes: A critical review." *J Epidemiol Community Health* 55(2): 111–122. https://doi.org/10.1136/jech.55.2.111.

Pickett, K. E., and R. G. Wilkinson. 2015. "Income inequality and health: A causal review." *Soc Sci Med* 128: 316–326. https://doi.org/10.1016/j.socscimed.2014.12.031.

Pollack, C. E., S. Chideya, C. Cubbin, B. Williams, M. Dekker, and P. Braveman. 2007. "Should health studies measure wealth? A systematic review." *Am J Prev Med* 33(3): 250–264. https://doi.org/10.1016/j.amepre.2007.04.033.

Pollack, C. E., C. Cubbin, A. Sania, M. Hayward, D. Vallone, B. Flaherty, and P. A. Braveman. 2013. "Do wealth disparities contribute to health disparities within racial/ethnic groups?" *J Epidemiol Community Health* 67(5): 439–445.

Pollitt, R. A., K. M. Rose, and J. S. Kaufman. 2005. "Evaluating the evidence for models of life course socioeconomic factors and cardiovascular outcomes: A systematic review."

BMC Public Health 5: 7–7. https://doi.org/ 10.1186/1471-2458-5-7.

Quillian, L., D. Pager, O. Hexel, and A. H. Midtbøen. 2017. "Meta-analysis of field experiments shows no change in racial discrimination in hiring over time." *Proc Natl Acad Sci USA* 114(41): 10870–10875. https:// doi.org/10.1073/pnas.1706255114.

Ravesteijn, B., H. van Kippersluis, and E. van Doorslaer. 2013. "The contribution of occupation to health inequality." *Res Econ Inequal* 21: 311–332. https://doi.org/10.1108/S1049-2585(2013)0000021014.

Reilly, J. J., and J. Kelly. 2011. "Long-term impact of overweight and obesity in childhood and adolescence on morbidity and premature mortality in adulthood: Systematic review." *Int J Obes* 35: 891. https://doi.org/10.1038/ijo.2010.222.

Rigolon, A. 2016. "A complex landscape of inequity in access to urban parks: A literature review." *Landscape and Urban Planning* 153: 160–169. https://doi.org/10.1016/j.landurbplan.2016.05.017.

Ross, C. E., and J. Mirowsky. 2000. "Does medical insurance contribute to socioeconomic differentials in health?" *Milbank Q* 78(2): 291–321. https://doi.org/10.1111/1468-0009.00171.

Rothstein, R. 2017. *The Color of Law: A Forgotten History of How Our Government Segregated America*. New York, NY: Liveright.

Savitt, T. L. 1982. "The use of Blacks for medical experimentation and demonstration in the Old South." *Journal of Southern History* 48(3): 331–348. https://doi.org/10.2307/2207450.

Schwarzenberg, S. J., and M. K. Georgieff. 2018. "Advocacy for improving nutrition in the first 1000 days to support childhood development and adult health." *Pediatrics* 141(2): e20173716. https://doi.org/10.1542/peds.2017-3716.

Semyonov, M., N. Lewin-Epstein, and D. Maskileyson. 2013. "Where wealth matters more for health: The wealth–health gradient in 16 countries." *Social Science & Medicine* 81: 10–17. https://doi.org/10.1016/j.socscimed.2013.01.010.

Sherman, A., B. DeBot, and C.-C. Huang. 2016. "Boosting low-income children's opportunities to succeed through direct income support." *Acad Pediatr* 16(3): S90–S97. https://doi.org/10.1016/j.acap.2016.01.008.

Shonkoff, J. P., A. S. Garner, B. S. Siegel, M. I. Dobbins, M. F. Earls, L. McGuinn, J. Pascoe, D. L Wood; Committee on Psychosocial Aspects of Child and Family Health; Committee on Early Childhood, Adoption, and Dependent Care; and Section on Developmental and Behavioral Pediatrics. 2012. "The lifelong effects of early childhood adversity and toxic stress." *Pediatrics* 129(1): e232–e246.

Shonkoff, J. P., N. Slopen, and D. R. Williams. 2021. "Early childhood adversity, toxic stress, and the impacts of racism on the foundations of health." *Annu Rev Public Health* 42(1): 115–134. https://doi.org/10.1146/annurev-publhealth-090419-101940.

Singh, A. S., C. Mulder, J. W. Twisk, W. van Mechelen, and M. J. Chinapaw. 2008. "Tracking of childhood overweight into adulthood: A systematic review of the literature." *Obes Rev* 9(5): 474–488. https://doi.org/10.1111/j.1467-789X.2008.00475.x.

Singh, G. K. 2019. "Trends and contemporary racial/ethnic and socioeconomic disparities in US childhood obesity." In *Global Perspectives on Childhood Obesity*, edited by D. Bagchi, 79–94. New York, NY: Academic Press.

Smith, G. D., C. Hart, D. Blane, C. Gillis, and V. Hawthorne. 1997. "Lifetime socioeconomic position and mortality: Prospective observational study." *BMJ* 314(7080): 547. https://doi.org/10.1136/bmj.314.7080.547.

Sorlie, P. D., N. J. Johnson, E. Backlund, and D. D. Bradham. 1994. "Mortality in the uninsured compared with that in persons with public and private health insurance." *Arch Intern Med* 154(21): 2409–2416.

Srivastava, S., N. Fogarty, D. Belzer, S. Breznau, and A. Brooks. 2010. *CDFIs and Transit-Oriented Development*. San Francisco, CA: Federal Reserve Bank of San Francisco, Community Development Investment Center.

Strohschein, L. 2005. "Household income histories and child mental health trajectories." *J Health Soc Behav* 46(4): 359–375. https://doi.org/10.1177/002214650504600404.

Subramanian, S. V., and I. Kawachi. 2006. "Being well and doing well: On the importance of income for health." *Int J Social*

Welfare 15(Suppl 1): S13–S22. https://doi.org/10.1111/j.1468-2397.2006.00440.x.

Sudano, J. J., and D. W. Baker. 2006. "Explaining US racial/ethnic disparities in health declines and mortality in late middle age: The roles of socioeconomic status, health behaviors, and health insurance." *Soc Sci Med* 62(4): 909–922. https://doi.org/10.1016/j.socscimed.2005.06.041.

Sullivan, L., and T. Meschede. 2016. "Race, gender, and senior economic well-being: How financial vulnerability over the life course shapes retirement for older women of color." *Public Policy Aging Rep* 26(2): 58–62. https://doi.org/10.1093/ppar/prw001.

Szanton, S. L., J. K. Allen, R. J. Thorpe, Jr., T. Seeman, K. Bandeen-Roche, and L. P. Fried. 2008. "Effect of financial strain on mortality in community-dwelling older women." *J Gerontol B Psychol Sci Soc Sci* 63(6): S369–S374. https://doi.org/10.1093/geronb/63.6.s369.

Tang, K. L., R. Rashid, J. Godley, and W. A. Ghali. 2016. "Association between subjective social status and cardiovascular disease and cardiovascular risk factors: A systematic review and meta-analysis." *BMJ Open* 6(3): e010137. https://doi.org/10.1136/bmjopen-2015-010137.

Theorell, T., K. Jood, L. S. Jarvholm, E. Vingard, J. Perk, P. O. Ostergren, and C. Hall. 2016. "A systematic review of studies in the contributions of the work environment to ischaemic heart disease development." *Eur J Public Health* 26(3): 470–477. https://doi.org/10.1093/eurpub/ckw025.

The Sentencing Project. 2017a. "Black disparities in youth incarceration." Washington, DC: The Sentencing Project.

The Sentencing Project. 2017b. "Latino disparities in youth incarceration." Washington, DC: The Sentencing Project.

The Sentencing Project. 2017c. "Native disparities in youth incarceration." Washington, DC: The Sentencing Project.

Thomas, M., C. Herring, H. D. Horton, M. Semyonov, L. Henderson, and P. L. Mason. 2020. "Race and the accumulation of wealth: Racial differences in net worth over the life course, 1989–2009." *Social Problems* 67(1): 20–39. https://doi.org/10.1093/socpro/spz002.

Torche, F. 2014. "Analyses of intergenerational mobility: An interdisciplinary review." *Annals Am Acad Pol Soc Sci* 657(1): 37–62. https://doi.org/10.1177/0002716214547476.

Truesdale, B. C., and C. Jencks. 2016. "The health effects of income inequality: Averages and disparities." *Annu Rev Public Health* 37: 413–430. https://doi.org/10.1146/annurev-publhealth-032315-021606.

Turrell, G., J. W. Lynch, C. Leite, T. Raghunathan, and G. A. Kaplan. 2007. "Socioeconomic disadvantage in childhood and across the life course and all-cause mortality and physical function in adulthood: Evidence from the Alameda County Study." *J Epidemiol Community Health* 61(8): 723–730. https://doi.org/10.1136/jech.2006.050609.

U.S. Census Bureau. 2018. "Table H-2. Share of aggregate income received by each fifth and top 5 percent of households, all races: 1967 to 2017." Washington, DC: U.S. Census Bureau.

U.S. Census Bureau. 2019. "American Community Survey, selected population profile in the United States Table S0201." Washington, DC: U.S. Census Bureau.

U.S. Department of Health and Human Services. 2021. "HHS poverty guidelines for 2021." https://aspe.hhs.gov/poverty-guidelines.

U.S. Department of Labor. 2019. "Persons with a disability: Labor force characteristics—2018." Washington, DC: U.S. Department of Labor.

Victorino, C. C., and A. H. Gauthier. 2009. "The social determinants of child health: Variations across health outcomes—A population-based cross-sectional analysis." *BMC Pediatr* 9: 53. https://doi.org/10.1186/1471-2431-9-53.

Votruba-Drzal, E. 2003. "Income changes and cognitive stimulation in young children's home learning environments." *J Marriage Fam* 65(2): 341–355. https://doi.org/10.1111/j.1741-3737.2003.00341.x.

Vroman, W. 2018. "Unemployment insurance benefits: Performance since the Great Recession." Washington, DC: Urban Institute.

Walker, R. 2017. "How to trick people into saving money: Inside Walmart's curious, possibly ingenious effort to get customers to build up their savings accounts." *The Atlantic*. https://www.theatlantic.com/magazine/archive/2017/05/how-to-trick-people-into-saving-money/521421.

Walters, K. L., R. Beltran, D. Huh, and T. Evans-Campbell. 2011. "Dis-placement and Disease: Land, place, and health among American Indians and Alaska Natives." In *Communities, Neighborhoods, and Health: Expanding the Boundaries of Place*, edited by L. M. Burton, S. A. Matthews, M. C. Leung, S. P. Kemp, and D. T. Takeuchi, 163–199. New York, NY: Springer.

Watanabe, K., A. Sakuraya, N. Kawakami, K. Imamura, E. Ando, Y. Asai, H. Eguchi, et al. 2018. "Work-related psychosocial factors and metabolic syndrome onset among workers: A systematic review and meta-analysis." *Obes Rev* 19(11): 1557–1568. https://doi.org/10.1111/obr.12725.

Wilkinson, L. R., and K. P. Pickett. 2010. *The Spirit Level: Why Greater Equality Makes Societies Stronger*. New York, NY: Bloomsbury.

Wilkinson, R. G., and K. E. Pickett. 2006. "Income inequality and population health: A review and explanation of the evidence." *Soc Sci Med* 62(7): 1768–1784. https://doi.org/10.1016/j.socscimed.2005.08.036.

Williams, B. A., K. Lindquist, R. L. Sudore, K. E. Covinsky, and L. C. Walter. 2008. "Screening mammography in older women: Effect of wealth and prognosis." *JAMA Intern Med* 168(5): 514–520. https://doi.org/10.1001/archinternmed.2007.103.

Williams Shanks, T. R., and C. Robinson. 2013. "Assets, economic opportunity and toxic stress: A framework for understanding child and educational outcomes." *Econ Educ Rev* 33: 154–170. shttps://doi.org/10.1016/j.econedurev.2012.11.002.

Woff, E. N. 2017. "Deconstructing household wealth trends in the United States, 1983 to 2016." WID World Conference, Paris, France, November 27.

Woolf, S. H., and L. Y. Aron. 2013. "The US health disadvantage relative to other high-income countries: Findings from a National Research Council/Institute of Medicine Report." *JAMA* 309(8): 771–772. https://doi.org/10.1001/jama.2013.91.

World Health Organization. 2000. *Mental Health and Work: Impact, Issues and Good Practices*. Geneva, Switzerland: World Health Organization.

Zagorsky, J. L., and P. K. Smith. 2016. "Does asthma impair wealth accumulation or does wealth protect against asthma?" *Soc Sci Q* 97(5): 1070–1081. https://doi.org/10.1111/ssqu.12293.

Zaw, K., J. Bhattacharya, A. Price, D. Hamilton, and W. Darity, Jr. 2017. *Women, Race & Wealth*. Oakland, CA: Insight Center.

Zell, E., J. E. Strickhouser, and Z. Krizan. 2018. "Subjective social status and health: A meta-analysis of community and society ladders." *Health Psychol* 37(10): 979–987. https://doi.org/10.1037/hea0000667.

CHAPTER 3

Education Shapes Health and Health Disparities in Many Ways

3.1. INTRODUCTION

Few people would disagree with the statement that without a good education, prospects for a good job with decent earnings are slim. Few people, however, think of education as a crucial path to health. Yet a large body of evidence strongly—and, with very rare exceptions, consistently—links education with health, even when, as in some studies, other related factors such as income are taken into account (Cutler and Lleras-Muney 2010; Ross and Mirowsky 1999; Mirowsky and Ross 2003; Gakidou et al. 2010; Kaplan, Spittel, and Zeno 2014; Hummer and Hernandez 2013; Sasson 2016; Luy et al. 2019). In this chapter and generally in this book, "education" refers to what is more technically called educational attainment, the number of years or level (high school, college, etc.) of overall schooling a person has; this is distinguished from health education—that is, targeted instruction on health topics such as diet, exercise, or managing a chronic disease. Although the quality, not just the quantity, of education also is important for health, educational quality is more difficult to measure and consensus is lacking about how to measure it; consequently, information is rarely available on educational quality in studies containing health information.

It has repeatedly been shown that people with more education are likely to live longer (Figure 3.1) and experience better health outcomes and are more likely to practice health-promoting behaviors such as exercising regularly, maintaining a healthy weight, and refraining from smoking and excess alcohol (Hamad et al. 2018; Cutler and Lleras-Muney 2010; Brunello et al. 2016; de Walque 2010). The positive relationship between education and health has been observed not only overall in the United States but also among all racial/ethnic groups in the United States (Figure 3.2) and in every country in which it has been studied (Gallus et al. 2020; Gwatkin et al. 2007; Gakidou et al. 2021). As shown in Figure 3.3, educational attainment among adults is linked with the health of not only adults but also their children (Lawrence, Rogers, and Hummer 2020; Currie and Moretti 2003). This relationship can be seen beginning early in life: Infants of more-educated mothers are less likely to die before their first birthdays (Gage et al. 2013), and children of more-educated parents experience better health (see Figure 3.3). Moreover,

The Social Determinants of Health and Health Disparities. Paula Braveman, Oxford University Press. © Oxford University Press 2023.
DOI: 10.1093/oso/9780190624118.003.0003

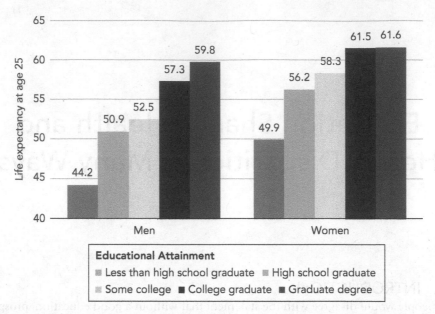

FIGURE 3.1 Life expectancy at age 25 years by educational attainment. This chart describes the number of years that adults with different levels of education can expect to live beyond age 25 years. For example, a 25-year-old man with only a high school diploma can expect to live 50.9 more years and reach an age of 75.9 years, whereas a 25-year-old man with a graduate-level degree can expect to live 61.6 more year and reach the age of 84.8 years—almost a 9-year difference. *Source*: Rostron, Boies, and Arias (2010).

the associations are multigenerational: Links have been observed between the educational attainment of grandparents and the likelihood of low birth weight and neonatal complications in infants (McFarland et al. 2017).

Repeated, pervasive, and strong associations between education and health are well-documented in the United States and globally. It is reasonable, however, to question whether these associations reflect causation. It is challenging to study this question in part because education and income, although distinct, are highly related to each other, and at least in theory, income rather than education could be the cause of observed links between education and health. It also is challenging to establish a causal role of education in health because it would not be feasible or ethical (given the well-known economic and other social benefits of education) to randomize people to different levels of education and then observe their health over a period of time thereafter. Appropriate research methods, including longitudinal studies, have, however, shed light on the issue; several scholars have examined this question in depth (Kawachi, Adler, and Dow 2010; Grossman and Kaestner 1997; Feinstein et al. 2006). They have concluded that although there is evidence of some "reverse causation"—that is, of ill children having their schooling curtailed by illness—this is likely to account for only a small part of the observed associations between education and health. A more important role is seen for unmeasured factors that shape both education and health, such as family economic resources; however, even after considering potential confounders, which do play a role, scholars have concluded that education has substantial causal effects on health,

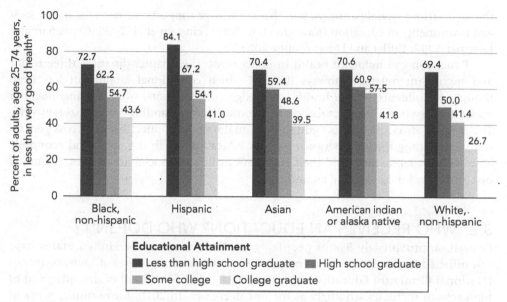

FIGURE 3.2 In every racial/ethnic group, higher educational attainment of adults aged 25–74 years is associated with better health (lower likelihood of being in less-than-very-good health). Based on self-report and measured as poor, fair, good, very good, or excellent. *Age-adjusted. *Source*: Behavioral Risk Factor Surveillance System survey data, 2005–2007.

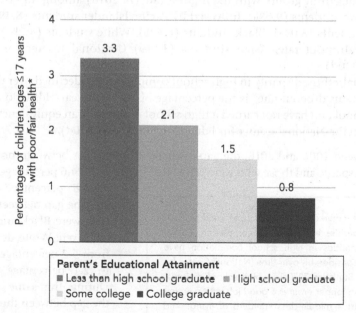

FIGURE 3.3 Children's health by parent's educational attainment. *Based on parental assessment. *Source*: National Survey of Children's Health, 2017–2018.

through various causal pathways, and this knowledge supports the need for major societal investments in education (Kawachi et al. 2010; Feinstein et al. 2006; Grossman and Kaestner 1997; Cutler and Lleras-Muney 2006).

Education can influence health in many ways. This chapter discusses three major and highly interrelated pathways through which educational attainment has been thought to influence health: health knowledge and behaviors; work and income; and social and psychological resources such as control, social standing, and social networks. The chapter also explores how educational attainment can affect health across generations, examining the links between parents' education—with the social and economic advantages it represents—and their children's health and social advantages, including opportunities for educational attainment.

3.2. WHO RECEIVES AN EDUCATION? WHO DOESN'T?

Overall, approximately 9% of people aged 25–64 years in the United States have not finished high school, a rate comparable to that of many other affluent countries (National Center for Education Statistics 2020b). The likelihood of dropping out of high school increases strikingly as income decreases. In 2016, for example, 9.7% of 16- to 24-year-olds from families in the lowest income quartile were not enrolled in high school (and lacked a high school equivalency credential such as a GED) compared to 2.6% of those from families in the highest income quartile (National Center for Education Statistics 2019). High school dropout rates also vary markedly by racial/ethnic group, with the highest rate (in 2018) among American Indian/Alaska Native students (9.5%), followed by Pacific Islander students (8.1%), Latino/Hispanic students (8.0%), Black students (6.4%), White students (4.2%), and, with the lowest dropout rate, Asian students (1.9%) (National Center for Education Statistics 2020d).

The racial/ethnic disparity in high school completion has declined over time (Figure 3.4). The "status dropout rate" is the percentage of 16- to 24-year-olds who are not currently in school and have not earned a high school diploma or an equivalency certificate. According to the National Center for Education Statistics (2020d),

> Between 2006 and 2018, the gap in status dropout rates between those who were Hispanic and those who were White decreased from 14.6 percentage points to 3.8 percentage points and the gap between those who were Black and those who were White decreased from 5.2 percentage points to 2.1 percentage points. During the same period, the gap between those who were Hispanic and those who were Black decreased from 9.5 percentage points to 1.7 percentage points.

There are marked socioeconomic and racial/ethnic disparities in high school completion. Racial/ethnic disparities in high school completion have narrowed considerably over time (National Center for Education Statistics 2020c). A high school diploma, however, no longer ensures a good job with pay that can support a middle-class standard of living. And large racial/ethnic disparities in income have been observed among people with similar levels of education (National Center for Education Statistics 2020a).

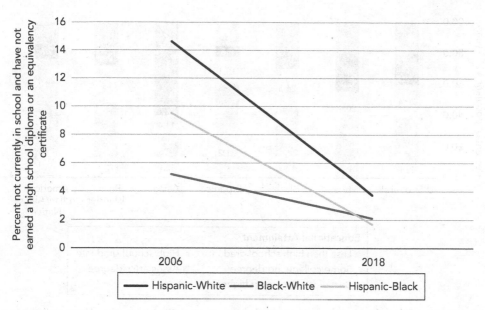

FIGURE 3.4 The racial/ethnic gap in drop-out rates has decreased over time, along with drop-out rates themselves. *Source*: National Center for Education Statistics.

The reduction in racial/ethnic disparities in high school completion is encouraging, particularly given the record achievement in 2017 of a 90.6% rate of high school (or equivalency) completion in the overall population aged 25 years or older. This is a first in U.S. history, and it contrasts with a 24% overall rate of high school completion in 1940 (Schmidt 2018). At the same time, however, that the racial/ethnic disparity in high school dropout rates has diminished, a high school diploma has come to mean increasingly less in an economy heavily dependent on technology.

Post-secondary education—and, generally receiving at least a bachelor's degree—has become a prerequisite for an increasing number of jobs (Rolen 2019). Reflecting systemic and structural racism, the likelihood of having a bachelor's (or higher) degree varies markedly by racial/ethnic group (Figure 3.5). In 2017, the lowest rates of having a bachelor's degree or higher were observed among American Indians/Alaska Natives (15.0%) and Latinos/Hispanics (16.0%), followed by Pacific Islanders (18.9%), Blacks (21.6%), and Whites (35.8%), with the highest rate among Asians (54.1%) (National Center for Education Statistics 2020e).

College has become unaffordable for low- and middle-income families. Figure 3.6 displays the average cost of a year of college (for the 2017–2018 academic year) according to family income. The burden appears excessive for all income groups and prohibitive (over 67.7% and 42.9% of total family income, respectively) for the two lowest income groups. Between 2008 and 2018, in response to budget constraints, 19 states cut funding for public colleges and universities; in six of these states, the cut exceeded 30% (Mitchell, Leachman, and Saenz 2019).

Systemic racism has limited the educational opportunities of African Americans in many ways for hundreds of years. Under slavery, educating slaves was prohibited. After

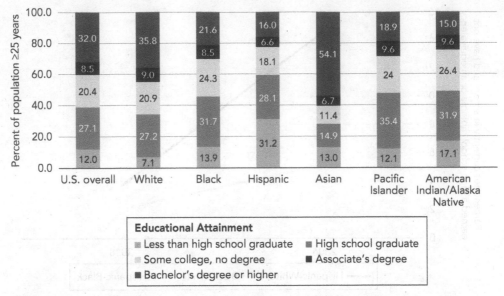

FIGURE 3.5 Educational attainment among U.S. adults aged 25+ years varies substantially by race/ethnicity. *Source*: National Center for Education Statistics (2020e, Table 104.40).

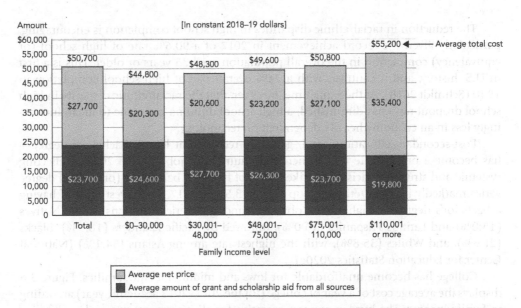

FIGURE 3.6 In 2017–2018, the net cost (after considering all financial aid received) of a year of college was more than two-thirds of the family income for the lowest income group. Average total cost, grant and scholarship aid, and net price for first-time, full-time degree/certificate-seeking undergraduate students awarded Title IV aid at private nonprofit 4-year institutions, by family income level: Academic year 2017–2018. Calculated using the highest income in each income group. *Source*: U.S. Department of Education, National Center for Education Statistics, Integrated Postsecondary Education Data Systems, Winter 2018–2019, Student Financial Aid component.

the end of the Civil War, the nearly 100 years of Jim Crow laws enforced strict segregation in all domains; separate schools for African Americans were overwhelmingly unequal, underfunded, and underresourced. Although civil rights laws in the 1960s achieved some integration of schools, the persistence of racial residential segregation and White resistance to school busing have made it difficult to achieve more educational integration. In the United States, school funding is based heavily on local property taxes, putting low-wealth communities at significant educational disadvantage. Obstacles to accumulating wealth for people of color (see Chapter 5) have continued to limit the tax base particularly for schools in segregated areas, limiting local schools' resources and thus putting them at a particularly severe educational disadvantage. Lack of wealth also limits the ability of families to send their children to college. Dependence on local property taxes limits the resources of schools in low-wealth communities of all racial/ethnic groups, but particularly for people of color because their opportunities to accumulate wealth have been so severely constrained.

3.3. HOW DOES EDUCATION INFLUENCE HEALTH?

Education can influence health in many and often complex ways. Figure 3.7 displays in greatly simplified form three general and highly interrelated causal pathways from educational attainment to health effects that are supported by considerable scientific literature. It is important to note that for the sake of readability, the figure does not indicate all possible intermediate steps along the displayed pathways in Figure 3.7, nor the many plausible interactions among the displayed factors or among displayed factors and factors that are not displayed. This figure also does not capture how educational advantage or disadvantage is transmitted across generations; Figure 3.8, which is discussed later in this section, aims to illustrate that.

Education Can Lead to Improved Health by Increasing Health Knowledge and Healthy Behaviors

Figures 3.7a, 3.7b, and 3.7c show three general pathways through which education can influence health. The causal pathway that most people are likely to think of first to explain the strong links between education and health is one that involves how education increases knowledge and skills that are relevant to health-related behaviors (Figure 3.7a). Education can increase people's knowledge, comprehension, problem-solving, and coping skills, enabling them to make better-informed choices among the health-related options available for themselves and their families, including those related to self-care and to obtaining and managing medical care. Greater educational attainment has been associated, for example, with health-promoting behaviors including healthy eating, engaging in regular physical activity, and refraining from smoking (Zimmerman, Woolf, and Haley 2014). Changes in health-related behaviors in response to new evidence, health advice, and public health campaigns (e.g., about the risks of smoking) tend to occur earlier among more-educated people (de Walque 2010). For example, Figure 3.9 displays marked differences over time in smoking rates in the United States according to educational attainment. Not all unhealthy behaviors are associated with lower educational attainment, however; binge drinking has been observed to be more frequent among people with higher education levels (Centers for Disease Control and Prevention 2013).

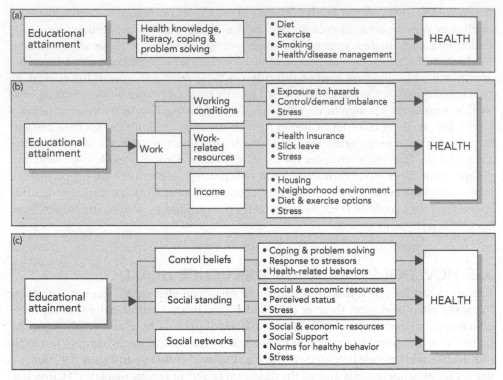

FIGURE 3.7 Education can influence health through multiple causal pathways. (a) Education is linked with improved health through its effects on knowledge and behaviors. (b) More education leads to better employment opportunities and higher income, which are linked with better health. (c) Education is linked with social and psychological resources that affect health.

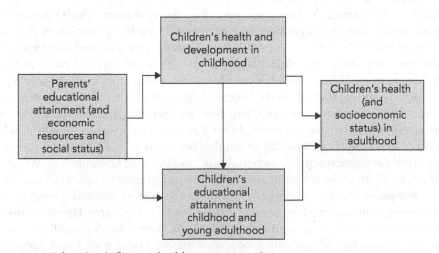

FIGURE 3.8 Education influences health across generations.

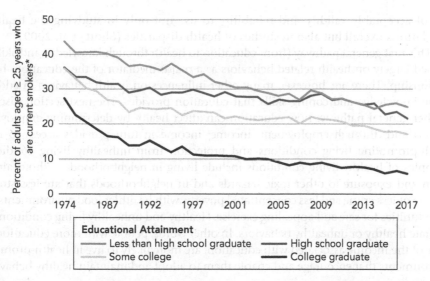

FIGURE 3.9   Rates of cigarette smoking are strongly associated with educational attainment among adults aged 25+ years. *Age adjusted. Source: b, National Center for Health Statistics (2018, Table 018).

The links between education and health through health knowledge and behaviors are likely to be explained at least in part by literacy, the ability to read and write at a basic level (Lundetrae and Gabrielsen 2016; Dewalt et al. 2004; Yamashita and Kunkel 2015). Low literacy is common in the United States. Surveys conducted in 2012 and 2014 found that 13% of U.S. residents aged 16–34 years had low English literacy levels; not surprisingly, low literacy had a higher prevalence among people with lower educational attainment (Rampey et al. 2016). A large study of Nordic countries observed an association between low literacy and ill health even after controlling for educational attainment (Lundetrae and Gabrielsen 2016), suggesting that literacy could be a major mediator of the effect of education on health.

Distinguishing overall literacy from *health* literacy (i.e., the degree to which individuals have the capacity to obtain, process, and understand basic health information and services needed to make appropriate health decisions and adhere to disease management protocols), health literacy also increases with educational attainment (Mantwill, Monestel-Umana, and Schulz 2015). The proportion of Americans with "below basic" health literacy, for example, ranged in 2003 (the most recent year of data) from 3% of college graduates to 15% of high school graduates and 49% of adults who had not completed high school (National Center for Education Statistics 2006). Levels of health literacy have been associated with self-reported health (overall). Compared with adults who have adequate health literacy, for example, adults with inadequate health literacy are more likely to rate their health as poor (Berkman et al. 2011). These associations, of course, do not answer questions about the direction of causation. Evidence of the correlation between self-reported health and clinical assessments, furthermore, is mixed. It appears to vary with characteristics of respondents and mode of survey administration. Some sources, however, have concluded that it generally correlates well with objective clinical assessments (Idler and Benyamini 1997), and it is of acceptable validity and reliability to use not only in studying the health of populations overall but also in studies of health disparities (Short et al. 2009).

This first general pathway (from education to health through knowledge and skills) is focused largely on health-related behaviors as a major mediator of the education–health relationship. There are, however, many other influences on health behaviors in addition to the knowledge and coping skills that education provides. The next section discusses another general pathway: how education can affect health by determining employment options and, through employment, income; income in turn provides access to many health-promoting living conditions and protection from unhealthy living conditions. Examples of healthy living conditions include living in neighborhoods without air pollution and exposure to other toxic hazards and in neighborhoods that are less stressful because of less crime and less concentrated poverty, with healthier food environments, and opportunities for safe and appealing exercise. Healthy and unhealthy living conditions can facilitate healthy or unhealthy behaviors. In other words, people with more education, because of the income associated with education, are more likely to live in health-promoting environments that encourage and enable them to adopt and maintain healthy behaviors.

Greater Educational Attainment Leads to Better Employment Opportunities and Higher Income, Which Are Linked with Better Health

Another important causal pathway (Figure 3.7b) through which education can influence health is by providing the knowledge, skills, and credentials necessary for employment, which in turn can shape health in many ways. More education generally means a greater likelihood of being employed at all and of having a job with healthier working conditions, better employment-based benefits, and higher income (Zimmerman et al. 2014). Reflecting racism, however, for a given level of education, people of color earn less than their White peers (National Center for Education Statistics 2020a; Braveman et al. 2005; Chiswick 2020; Assari and Bazargan 2019b).

- *Education, job security, financial instability, and health.* Americans with lower educational attainment are more likely to be affected by fluctuations in the economy. Although unemployment rates reached historic lows in 2019, they varied markedly by educational attainment: Unemployment rates were 5.4% for adults who had not graduated from high school, 3.7% for high school graduates, 3.3% for those who had attended but not completed college, 2.7% for those with an Associate's degree, and 2.2% for those with a bachelor's degree (U.S. Bureau of Labor Statistics 2020). These differences have major health implications; compared with their employed counterparts, people who are unemployed experience poorer health and higher mortality rates (Clemens, Popham, and Boyle 2015; McLeod et al. 2012; Vågerö and Garcy 2016). Stress (discussed below) is likely to play a role. The COVID-19 pandemic has made unemployment rates, job insecurity, and financial insecurity skyrocket globally, with the most severe effects falling on those with less skilled and lower paid jobs that require less education; people of color are disproportionately represented among those most affected (Galea and Abdalla 2020).
- *Education, working conditions, and health.* Workers with less formal education and training are more likely to hold lower paying jobs with more exposure to occupational hazards, including environmental and chemical exposures (e.g., pesticides

and asbestos) and poor working conditions (e.g., shift work with few breaks, potentially dangerous tools, and speed-ups) that put them at higher risk of injury and death (Zimmerman et al. 2014). Less-educated workers are also likely to experience more psychosocial stress at work (Lunau et al. 2015) due to jobs that make high demands on them yet offer few opportunities for control and skill utilization. Relevant psychosocial aspects of work include the perceived balance between a worker's efforts and rewards, perceived justice and discrimination in the workplace, and social support among co-workers—have been shown to have both short-term and longer term impacts on health, particularly through pathways related to psychosocial stress (Pan et al. 2019; McCluney et al. 2018). (See Chapter 9.)

- *Education, work-related benefits, and health.* Less-educated workers in lower wage jobs also are less likely to have health-related benefits, including paid sick and personal leave, workplace wellness programs, child and elder care resources, and retirement benefits, in addition to employer-sponsored health insurance. Although most Americans receive their health insurance through their jobs, many workers do not have access to this benefit. Employers with lower wage workers offer health insurance less frequently, and, even if employment-sponsored benefits are available, low-wage workers may be unable to afford the premiums, copayments, or deductibles (Claxton et al. 2019).

- *Education, employment, income, and health.* For the vast majority of people, employment is their sole or main source of income—a work-related resource that affects health through multiple well-documented direct and indirect pathways (see Chapter 2). Overall, with limited exceptions, greater educational attainment generally corresponds with higher paying employment: Median yearly earnings in the United States in 2018 were $40,500 for a full-time year-round worker with only a high school degree, $46,300 for a worker with some college, and $65,400 for a worker with a bachelor's degree (Ma, Pender, and Welch 2019). These differences are particularly dramatic when compounded over a person's lifetime: Consider, for example, lifetime earnings in 2009 dollars and based on a 50-year full-time work life. For men who have graduated from high school but not attended college, lifetime earnings have been estimated at $1.54 million, compared with $2.43 million for those with bachelor's degrees and $3.05 million for those with graduate degrees (Tamborini, Kim, and Sakamoto 2015). Among women, those who have graduated from high school but not attended college can expect to earn a total of approximately $811,000 over their lifetime (in 2009 dollars), compared to $1.44 and $1.87 million for those with bachelor's and graduate degrees, respectively (Tamborini, Kim, and Sakamoto 2015).

The relationship between education and income has been shown to vary by race or ethnic group (National Center for Education Statistics 2020a; Braveman et al. 2005; Chiswick 2020; Assari and Bazargan 2019b). Blacks and Latinos experience a lower rate of return on their investment in education than do their White counterparts. In 2007, for example, the average annual earnings of a White man with a graduate degree (beyond bachelor's degree) were estimated at $80,000, whereas the earnings of Black and Latino men with the same level of educational attainment were approximately $61,000 and $65,000, respectively (National Center for Education Statistics 2020a). This pattern may be explained both by discrimination in the labor market in access to high-paying jobs and by indirect effects of residential segregation, which effectively marginalizes people of color in multiple ways even in the absence of labor-market discrimination (Assari and Bazargan 2019b).

Higher paying jobs also tend to offer greater economic security and increased ability to accumulate wealth; this makes it more possible for individuals to obtain health care when needed, to provide themselves and their families with more nutritious foods, and to live in safer and healthier homes and neighborhoods with supermarkets, parks, and places to exercise—all of which can promote good health by making it easier to adopt and maintain healthy behaviors (Zimmerman et al. 2014).

- *Education, employment, income, stress, and health.* Income may also affect health through pathways involving stress. Chronically stressful experiences have been linked repeatedly with many adverse health outcomes across the life course, through physiological mechanisms including neuroendocrine, immune, and vascular responses to stressors (see Chapter 4). Stress can trigger the release of hormones and other substances in the body, which, over time, can damage immune defenses and vital organs (McEwen 2017). Chronic stress, even when it is relatively undramatic, appears more likely to damage health than a single, dramatic acute but time-limited stressor (McEwen and Seeman 1999). The physiologic chain of events initiated by stressful experiences can, when chronic, accelerate aging and lead to serious chronic illnesses, including cardiovascular disease (Lagraauw, Kuiper, and Bot 2015). People with lower levels of education may experience greater stress due to having fewer financial resources to cope with everyday challenges, such as child care, transportation to work, and illness. Coping with the constant challenges of daily living—balancing the demands of work and family, for example—can be particularly stressful for people whose financial and social opportunities and resources have been limited by low educational attainment. Jobs that require lower levels of education also may be more stressful in that they are likely to be of lower status and authority and thus involve less control or autonomy. The combination of low control over work with high external demands, referred to as "job strain," has been linked with health and with socioeconomic disparities in health (Karasek et al. 1981). Black and Latino workers of high educational attainment do not always experience less occupational stress than their less-educated counterparts (Assari and Bazargan 2019b); the phenomenon referred to as "the hidden costs of upward mobility" for people of color is discussed in Chapter 5.

Education Can Affect Health by Conferring Social and Psychological Resources

Yet another general pathway from education to health is through psychosocial factors in addition to those mentioned above. This is illustrated in Figure 3.7d. Education is strongly linked with social and psychological resources, including sense of control, social standing, and social support. These resources can improve health by reducing stress or helping one to manage it, by influencing health-related behaviors, and by providing practical and emotional support.

- *Control beliefs.* Education may influence health by shaping people's sense of personal control—their perceptions of the extent to which they, rather than external factors, can influence their life circumstances. Several studies have concluded that more education confers a greater sense of personal control (or the related notions of mastery, self-efficacy, and internal locus of control) (Specht, Egloff, and Schmukle 2013; Mirowsky and Ross 2007; Festin et al. 2017; Lehto et al. 2013), which would not be surprising, given the well-documented influence of education on prospects for jobs and income (Lehto et al. 2013). Festin et al. (2017), however, did not find an association between educational attainment and mastery or social support in a study of 45- to 69-year-olds in Sweden, after adjusting for other socioeconomic indicators; and a large Finnish study (Lehto et al. 2013) did not find an association between education and control. Similarly, Cutler and Lleras-Muney (2010) did not find that sense of control explained the links between education and health-related behaviors. The relationships may vary in different contexts and populations. Higher levels of education generally have been associated with the development of skills, habits, and attitudes—such as problem-solving, purposefulness, self-directedness, perseverance, and confidence—that contribute to people's expectations that their own actions and behaviors shape what happens to them. Lower levels of education, however, may lead to experiences that produce fatalism, a sense of powerlessness, or the belief that one's own efforts are less important than the influence of chance or powerful others when it comes to health or life outcomes (Matthews and Gallo 2011; Lachman and Weaver 1998; Zimmerman et al. 2014). Positive beliefs about personal control have been linked with health outcomes including higher levels of self-rated health (Bailis et al. 2001) and decreased risk of all-cause mortality (Infurna, Ram, and Gerstorf 2013; Turiano et al. 2014; Lachman and Weaver 1998); they also have been associated with health-related behaviors including smoking, alcohol consumption, physical activity, and diet (Thomas et al. 2020; Mirowsky and Ross 1998; Sheeran et al. 2016; Leganger and Kraft 2003). These relationships, however, appear to vary according to individuals' other characteristics. Turiano (2014) observed, for example, that the link between sense of control and mortality only held among individuals with low levels of education. Two studies, furthermore, found that low self-efficacy and sense of control were associated with short-term mortality among Whites but not among Blacks (Assari 2017a, 2017b). Sense of control may also influence health through employment-related pathways—for example, by affecting a person's job seeking and/or performance (Dicke et al. 2018; Carter et al. 2018; McGee and McGee 2016). It is important to note that an individual with a greater sense of control may also be more likely to achieve higher educational attainment, making it difficult to separate out the effects of sense of control and education on health.

- *Social standing.* Many scholars believe that social standing—relative position in a social hierarchy reflecting status, prestige, and influence—is another important factor linking education with health. Along with income and occupation, educational attainment is an important determinant of where individuals rank within social hierarchies. Greater educational attainment typically is associated with higher social standing, which in turn has been linked with better health status (Kawachi et al. 2010). An individual's perception of where they rank in a social hierarchy—referred to as *subjective social status*—has been shown to powerfully predict health status even after adjusting for conventional measures of socioeconomic status (Hoebel and Lampert 2020; Tang et al. 2016; Zell, Strickhouser, and Krizan 2018; Kawachi et al. 2010). Although the pathways linking it to health are not well understood, subjective social status may be a more comprehensive reflection of social and economic resources than the traditional measures (Singh-Manoux, Marmot, and Adler 2005).

- *Social support.* Higher educational attainment, income, and occupational status all have been associated with higher levels of social support (Aartsen, Veenstra, and Hansen 2017). Higher levels of social support—emotional and/or practical—have repeatedly been linked with better physical and mental health outcomes (Guilaran et al. 2018; Uchino et al. 2018). Social contact has been associated with lower mortality rates, although recent findings show a lack of significance in some subgroups (Shor and Roelfs 2015). Disruptions in family stability (viewed as breakdowns in social support) have been linked with worse health among adults and with higher rates of externalizing behaviors, delinquency, and risky health behaviors among children (Fomby and Osborne 2017; Ryan, Claessens, and Markowitz 2015). Emotional support is hypothesized to affect health by buffering the health-damaging effects of stress; this may be achieved by reducing negative emotional and behavioral responses to stressful situations (García-Herrero et al. 2013; Thoits 2010, 2011). Social support has also been linked with reductions in cardiovascular risk, depression risk, and health-related behaviors, especially among older adults (Malcolm, Frost, and Cowie 2019; Gariépy, Honkaniemi, and Quesnel-Vallée 2016; Serlachius et al. 2016). Perceived social support has been linked to lower risks of mortality and depression in some populations (Holt-Lunstad, Smith, and Layton 2010). Material support also may have health consequences; for example, financial help, help with transportation or child care, or connections to opportunities for employment or other resources may reduce stress or its health-damaging effects or increase resources.
- *Social networks.* Education also may be linked to health through its influence on social networks, which can be a source of both emotional support (having someone to turn to for comfort or advice) and practical support (having someone to turn to for practical or material help, or someone who can connect one to educational or employment opportunities, for example). Larger and more privileged social networks can provide access to employment, housing, and other opportunities and resources that influence health (Yi, Huang, and Fan 2016; Brucker 2015; Hanley et al. 2018). Higher educational attainment increases a person's likelihood of having close friends who would have the resources to provide help if needed and also of experiencing greater family stability, including a stable and supportive marriage (Mirowsky and Ross 2003). Formal educational settings may also encourage the development of long-term friendships and interpersonal skills; people with more education and related social advantages may also have more time and resources to maintain relationships and support friends emotionally and financially (Aartsen et al. 2017). Behavioral norms within social groups can influence health-related behaviors such as smoking (Giordano and Lindström 2011), physical exercise (Aliyas 2020), alcohol consumption (Ng Fat, Scholes, and Jivraj 2017), and healthy eating (Chen et al. 2019). Conversely, social networks may be sources of adverse effects when, for example, they expose a person to pressure to use harmful substances or to excessive demands

for financial help; the latter may occur when a person who grew up in poverty achieves some measure of financial success and is frequently faced with requests for financial support from struggling family and friends.

Transgenerational Effects: Parents' Education Influences Children's Prospects for Lifelong Health

Parents' educational attainment and their other socioeconomic resources (income, accumulated wealth, and social status) have repeatedly been linked to children's health and development and to children's educational attainment—both of which influence children's health as adults.

Figure 3.8 (shown earlier in this chapter) illustrates how child health may vary according to parents' educational attainment; it is only one example of the many strong associations between parents' education and children's health that have been observed across diverse health outcomes. It schematically depicts a number of plausible general explanations, based on the literature. For example, Figure 3.8 indicates that parents' education (along with their economic resources and social status) is linked indirectly to children's health in adulthood through pathways involving both (a) children's health and cognitive, emotional, and physical development in childhood; and (b) children's educational attainment in childhood and young adulthood. The figure also notes the influence of children's health and development on their educational attainment. Note that in the first box on the left in Figure 3.8, education appears along with economic resources and social status. This is intended as a reminder that although each of these aspects of socioeconomic status is a distinct entity, they are often so intertwined that it may be difficult for a study to fully disentangle the independent effects of education alone. This issue should be considered in designing and evaluating policies.

Parents' educational attainment can shape children's prospects for healthy lives through links with children's development and health, which in turn affect their educational attainment in childhood and young adulthood and directly and indirectly affect their health later in life. Many studies have observed associations between parental education and children's developmental, educational, and health outcomes (Dickson, Gregg, and Robinson 2016; Kaushal 2014). In addition, parental education is related to child nutrition (Vollmer et al. 2017) and physical activity (Glozah and Pevalin 2015).

Differences in parental education level have been linked with differences in children's brain structure and cognitive (Holochwost et al. 2018) and neurocognitive (Noble et al. 2015) development (see Chapter 2). Parents with lower educational attainment often face greater obstacles—notably lack of money and time and sometimes lack of knowledge, skills, or other resources—to optimal fostering of their children's development, providing healthy home and neighborhood environments, and modeling healthy behaviors for their children (Kaushal 2014). Conversely, higher parental educational attainment has been associated with higher levels of parental investment (time and money) in children's health (Kaushal 2014; Prickett and Augustine 2016), better educational outcomes over the life course (Ludeke et al. 2021; Erola, Jalonen, and Lehti 2016), and better cognitive and behavioral outcomes (Harding 2015).

Recent analyses of U.S. data have revealed that parental education may benefit White families more than Black families in terms of effects on both health and upward socioeconomic mobility (Assari 2018a, 2018b). This is consistent with what some have called the theory of "diminished returns" from higher socioeconomic status for people of color (Assari and Bazargan 2019a). This theory holds that because of a range of effects of racism, people of color often experience lower "returns"—that is, benefits, in the form of social status, health, and/or well-being—from achieving higher socioeconomic status (as represented by income and education) than their White counterparts. This phenomenon also has been observed—described as the "hidden costs of upward mobility"—for a number of health outcomes, including preterm birth, which is a strong predictor of infant mortality, childhood disability, and adult chronic disease (Braveman et al. 2017; Hudson et al. 2020; Assari 2018c).

Not all studies have concurred about the effects of parental education on children's health. Some have concluded that unobserved factors—such as unmeasured characteristics of parents or children—are likely to explain many aspects of the observed associations between parental education and child health. Dickson et al. (2016) state,

> It is a consistent finding across numerous countries that individuals with higher levels of schooling have children who also attain higher levels of schooling. There are two main sources of this intergenerational correlation and distinguishing between them is of considerable importance. The first explanation of the intergenerational link is a selection story—characteristics that lead parents to select into higher levels of education may also impact their abilities in child-raising or be related to other genetic and environmental factors shared with their children that will lead the children to also achieve higher levels of education. The second explanation is a causal story—as a result of attaining more education, the parents with high levels of schooling provide a better childhood experience and educational environment and consequently their children do better in school. (p. 184)

In addition, a study of low- and middle-income countries observed a weakening of the association between education and health over time, but that may be explained by other factors that were changing over the study period (Karlsson, De Neve, and Subramanian 2018), such as social programs benefiting people of lower educational levels.

Although some authors remain reluctant to attribute causality to the relationship between parental education and children's health, many scholars, including Dickson et al. (2016), have concluded that the overall body of evidence does support a causal relationship, with an understanding that the relationship will vary over time and across different contexts and populations. As noted previously, they have concluded, furthermore, that the important and persistent causal effects of parents' education on children's health and well-being justify societal investments in education (Kaushal 2014; Dickson et al. 2016; Kawachi et al. 2010; Andriano and Monden 2019; De Neve and Subramanian 2017; Mensch et al. 2019).

3.4. POLICIES TO IMPROVE EDUCATION AND REDUCE THE EDUCATIONAL DISPARITIES RESULTING IN HEALTH DISPARITIES

Current knowledge discussed in this chapter indicates that one of the most effective strategies for improving health and reducing health disparities in the United States may be to take steps to close the gaps in educational attainment across different racial/ethnic, family income, and parental education groups. By providing the knowledge and skills necessary to fully participate in the workforce, education can play a key role in promoting social mobility and breaking the cycle of intergenerational social disadvantage and the associated health disparities (Rouse and Barrow 2006; Haveman and Smeeding 2006). Investments to promote and increase educational attainment could have both human and economic benefits; for example, an analysis showed that if adult Americans who have not completed college experienced the lower death rates and better health of college graduates, the resulting improvements in health status and life expectancy would translate into potential gains estimated at more than $1 trillion annually (Braveman and Egerter 2008). Implementing policies to increase educational attainment may not succeed, however, without simultaneous efforts to reduce poverty and systemic racism.

Policy issues regarding preschool are explored in Chapter 6. There are ongoing debates about many kindergarten through grade 12 (K–12) policies, including optimal and acceptable ratios of teachers to students (Woods 2015), the credentials that teachers should have (Lewis and Young 2013), and the salary levels that teachers should earn (Reilly 2018) to achieve the best educational outcomes. These issues are key determinants of the costs of education. There also are ongoing debates about the best approaches and resources needed for teaching students who have disabilities or are at risk for other reasons, such as poverty(Kauffman and Badar 2013; Schwartz, Schmitt, and Lose 2012); for teaching literacy (Schwartz et al. 2012; Street 2013), reading (Street 2013), math, and science(English 2016); and for providing education to develop good citizenship (Roosevelt 2008), including critical thinking (Walker 2003) and an understanding and appreciation of democracy.

The range of important education policy issues and the ongoing debates about them is so wide and deep that it is well beyond the scope of this chapter to cover them. Rather, the following text notes and briefly discusses a few selected issues in education policy that have major implications for health and for health equity: how K–12 schools are funded, charter schools, school discipline issues, and paying for higher education (college).

Equitable funding. Currently, as mentioned previously in relation to racial/ethnic disparities in education, a considerable portion of the funding for U.S. K–12 public schools comes from local property taxes. The effect of this is extremely inequitable, in that schools in affluent neighborhoods are far better funded than those in poor neighborhoods. An equitable approach would provide the same funding per student throughout the United States, allocating additional funds based on the number of students with special needs, such as disability and poverty, that are obstacles to learning.

Charter schools. Charter schools receive public funds but are operated by private companies, sometimes including for-profit companies. Proponents of charter schools argue that they improve the quality of schools because they are free of the constraints faced by public schools, particularly in relation to how they treat teachers. Opponents argue that they undermine public education; they sometimes obtain good outcomes not because they are more effective but, rather, because they siphon off the low-risk students whose outcomes would be good in any school environment.

School discipline. It has been well documented that Black students receive harsher punishment than White students for similar behavioral infractions (Wallace et al. 2008; Gopalan and Nelson 2019). Harsh discipline is often meted out for behaviors that should be addressed through counseling and support, not punishment (Biolcati, Palareti, and Mameli 2018). Suspension and expulsion and involvement of the police are used disproportionately with Black students, increasing the likelihood of students dropping out and creating what has been referred to as the "school-to-prison pipeline" because it can lead to incarceration (Raible and Irizarry 2010; Mizel et al. 2016).

Paying for college. The increasing expense of a college education has impacted both middle-income and lower income families (Kim and Ko 2015). This has led to calls for free college tuition at state-funded schools (Rocque 2018).

3.5. KEY POINTS

- One's educational attainment (level of completed schooling) is strongly determined by the education, income, and wealth of one's parents. Systemic (structural) racism deprives people of color of educational opportunities.
- A graded relationship (with incremental improvement in health accompanying greater educational attainment) has repeatedly been observed between education and health for many health outcomes. This relationship is seen overall and within all racial/ethnic groups.
- The relationship between health and educational credentials (completed educational levels or degrees, such as high school graduation or GED, college graduation, and post-graduate degree) appears stronger than the relationship with completed years of schooling. This suggests the importance of the economic and social recognition of educational credentials, distinguished from simply the number of years spent in a classroom.
- Reflecting a long history of disparities in social advantage, there are large disparities in educational attainment according to racial/ethnic group. These quantitative disparities are likely to understate the racial/ethnic differences in schooling because they do not reflect disparities in the *quality* of education. By limiting schools' resources, racial residential segregation has limited the quality of schools in areas in which there are many people of color.
- Although some scholars continue to question whether the association between education and health is causal, many others have concluded that the body of evidence that has accumulated by now, including evidence from longitudinal studies, provides an adequate basis for a causal inference.
- Education plays a major role in determining the income a person will earn, because it strongly determines the kind of work one can obtain. It can be difficult at times to separate out the effects of education from those of income, because they are strongly associated with each other.

3.6. QUESTIONS FOR DISCUSSION

1. Discuss at least three general causal pathways through which education is thought to influence health, based on the literature. How plausible do you think these pathways are as explanations for the associations between education and health? Are there additional or alternative explanations that you find to be as (or more) plausible?

2. What are the obstacles to educational opportunity that are faced by low-income/low-wealth communities in general? What are the particular obstacles faced by many people of color? What role does racial segregation play in educational disparities?

ACKNOWLEDGMENTS

Susan Egerter, PhD, made major contributions to this chapter, which builds on the 2011 issue brief *Education Matters for Health*, by Susan Egerter, Paula Braveman, Tabashir Sadegh-Nobari, Rebecca Grossman-Kahn, and Mercedes Dekker, which was produced as part of the Robert Wood Johnson Foundation's Commission to Build a Healthier America and subsequently as part of the Foundation's Vulnerable Populations portfolio. Tram Nguyen, MPH, also contributed to the research for this chapter.

REFERENCES

Aartsen, M., M. Veenstra, and T. Hansen. 2017. "Social pathways to health: On the mediating role of the social network in the relation between socio-economic position and health." *SSM – Popul Health* 3: 419–426. https://doi.org/10.1016/j.ssmph.2017.05.006.

Aliyas, Z. 2020. "Social capital and physical activity level in an urban adult population." *Am J Health Educ* 51(1): 40–49. https://doi.org/10.1080/19325037.2019.1691092.

Andriano, L., and C. W. S. Monden. 2019. "The causal effect of maternal education on child mortality: Evidence from a quasi-experiment in Malawi and Uganda." *Demography* 56(5): 1765–1790. https://doi.org/10.1007/s13524-019-00812-3.

Assari, S. 2017a. "General self-efficacy and mortality in the USA: Racial differences." *J Racial Ethn Health Disparities* 4(4): 746–757. https://doi.org/10.1007/s40615-016-0278-0.

Assari, S. 2017b. "Race, sense of control over life, and short-term risk of mortality among older adults in the United States." *Arch Med Sci* 13(5): 1233–1240. https://doi.org/10.5114/aoms.2016.59740.

Assari, S. 2018a. "Parental education attainment and educational upward mobility: Role of race and gender." *Behav Sci* 8(11): 107. https://doi.org/10.3390/bs8110107.

Assari, S. 2018b. "Parental education better helps White than Black families escape poverty: National Survey of Children's Health." *Economies* 6(2): 30.

Assari, S. 2018c. "Parental educational attainment and mental well-being of college students: Diminished returns of Blacks." *Brain Sci* 8(11): 193.

Assari, S., and M. Bazargan. 2019a. "Minorities' diminished returns of educational attainment on hospitalization risk: National Health Interview Survey (NHIS)." *Hosp Pract Res* 4(3): 86–91. https://doi.org/10.15171/HPR.2019.17.

Assari, S., and M. Bazargan. 2019b. "Unequal associations between educational attainment and occupational stress across racial and ethnic groups." *Int J Environ Res Public Health* 16(19): 3539.

Bailis, D. S., A. Segall, M. I. Mahon, J. G. Chipperfield, and E. M. Dunn. 2001. "Perceived control in relation to socioeconomic and behavioral resources for health." *Soc Sci Med* 52(11): 1661–1676. https://doi.org/10.1016/S0277-9536(00)00280-X.

Berkman, N. D., S. L. Sheridan, K. E. Donahue, D. J. Halpern, and K. Crotty. 2011. "Low health literacy and health outcomes: An updated systematic review." *Ann Intern Med* 155(2): 97–107. https://doi.org/10.7326/0003-4819-155-2-201107190-00005.

Biolcati, R., L. Palareti, and C. Mameli. 2018. "What adolescents seeking help teach us about a school-based counseling service." *Child Adolesc Soc Work J* 35(1): 45–56. https://doi.org/10.1007/s10560-017-0503-7.

Braveman, P. A., C. Cubbin, S. Egerter, S. Chideya, K. S. Marchi, M. Metzler, and S. Posner. 2005. "Socioeconomic status in health research: One size does not fit all." *JAMA* 294(22): 2879–2888. https://doi.org/10.1001/jama.294.22.2879.

Braveman, P. A., and S. Egerter. 2008. *Overcoming Obstacles to Health: Report from the Robert Wood Johnson Foundation to the Commission to Build a Healthier America*. Washington, DC: Robert Wood Johnson Foundation Commission to Build a Healthier America.

Braveman, P., K. Heck, S. Egerter, T. P. Dominguez, C. Rinki, K. S. Marchi, and M. Curtis. 2017. "Worry about racial discrimination: A missing piece of the puzzle of Black–White disparities in preterm birth?" *PLoS One* 12(10): e0186151. https://doi.org/10.1371/journal.pone.0186151.

Brucker, D. L. 2015. "Social capital, employment and labor force participation among persons with disabilities." *J Vocat Rehabil* 43: 17–31. https://doi.org/10.3233/JVR-150751.

Brunello, G., M. Fort, N. Schneeweis, and R. Winter-Ebmer. 2016. "The causal effect of education on health: What is the role of health behaviors?" *Health Econ* 25(3): 314–336. https://doi.org/10.1002/hec.3141.

Carter, W. R., P. L. Nesbit, R. J. Badham, S. K. Parker, and L.-K. Sung. 2018. "The effects of employee engagement and self-efficacy on job performance: A longitudinal field study." *Int J Hum Resour Manage* 29(17): 2483–2502. https://doi.org/10.1080/09585192.2016.1244096.

Centers for Disease Control and Prevention. 2013. "CDC health disparities and inequalities report—United States, 2013." *Morb Mortal Wkly Rep* 62(3): 1–187.

Chen, W.-L., C.-G. Zhang, Z.-Y. Cui, J.-Y. Wang, J. Zhao, J.-W. Wang, X. Wang, and J.-M. Yu. 2019. "The impact of social capital on physical activity and nutrition in China: The mediating effect of health literacy." *BMC Public Health* 19(1): 1713. https://doi.org/10.1186/s12889-019-8037-x.

Chiswick, B. R. 2020. "Differences in education and earnings across racial and ethnic groups: Tastes, discrimination and investments in child quality." In *Jews at Work: Their Economic Progress in the American Labor Market*, edited by B. R. Chiswick, 227–250. Cham, Switzerland: Springer.

Claxton, G., M. Rae, A. Damico, G. Young, D. McDermott, and H. Whitmore. 2019. *Employer Health Benefits 2019 Annual Survey*. Washington, DC: Kaiser Family Foundation.

Clemens, T., F. Popham, and P. Boyle. 2015. "What is the effect of unemployment on all-cause mortality? A cohort study using propensity score matching." *Eur J Public Health* 25(1): 115–121. https://doi.org/10.1093/eurpub/cku136.

Currie, J., and E. Moretti. 2003. "Mother's education and the intergenerational transmission of human capital: Evidence from college openings." *Q J Econ* 118(4): 1495–1532. https://doi.org/10.1162/003355303322552856.

Cutler, D. M., and A. Lleras-Muney. 2006. "Education and health: Evaluating theories and evidence." National Bureau of Economic Research. Accessed November 13, 2020. https://www.nber.org/papers/w12352.

Cutler, D. M., and A. Lleras-Muney. 2010. "Understanding differences in health behaviors by education." *J Health Econ* 29(1): 1–28. https://doi.org/10.1016/j.jhealeco.2009.10.003.

De Neve, J.-W., and S. V. Subramanian. 2017. "Causal effect of parental schooling on early childhood undernutrition: Quasi-experimental evidence from Zimbabwe." *Am J Epidemiol* 187(1): 82–93. https://doi.org/10.1093/aje/kwx195.

de Walque, D. 2010. "Education, information, and smoking decisions: Evidence from smoking histories in the United States, 1940–2000." *J Hum Resour* 45(3): 682–717.

Dewalt, D. A., N. D. Berkman, S. Sheridan, K. N. Lohr, and M. P. Pignone. 2004. "Literacy and health outcomes: A systematic review of the literature." *J Gen Intern Med* 19(12): 1228–1239. https://doi.org/10.1111/j.1525-1497.2004.40153.x.

Dicke, T., F. Stebner, C. Linninger, M. Kunter, and D. Leutner. 2018. "A longitudinal study of teachers' occupational well-being: Applying the job demands-resources model." *J Occup Health Psychol* 23(2): 262.

Dickson, M., P. Gregg, and H. Robinson. 2016. "Early, late or never? When does parental education impact child outcomes?" *Econ J* 126(596): F184–F231. https://doi.org/10.1111/ecoj.12356.

English, L. D. 2016. "STEM education K–12: Perspectives on integration." *Int J STEM Educ* 3(1): 3. https://doi.org/10.1186/s40 594-016-0036-1.

Erola, J., S. Jalonen, and H. Lehti. 2016. "Parental education, class and income over early life course and children's achievement." *Res Soc Stratif Mobil* 44: 33–43. https://doi. org/10.1016/j.rssm.2016.01.003.

Feinstein, L., R. Sabates, A. M. Tashweka, A. Sorhaindo, and C. Hammond. 2006. "What are the effects of education on health?" In *Measuring the effects of education on health and civic engagement: Proceedings of the Copenhagen symposium*, 171–354. Paris, France: Organisation for Economic Co-operation and Development.

Festin, K., K. Thomas, J. Ekberg, and M. Kristenson. 2017. "Choice of measure matters: A study of the relationship between socioeconomic status and psychosocial resources in a middle-aged normal population." *PLoS One* 12(8): e0178929. https://doi. org/10.1371/journal.pone.0178929.

Fomby, P., and C. Osborne. 2017. "Family instability, multipartner fertility, and behavior in middle childhood." *J Marriage Fam* 79(1): 75–93. https://doi.org/10.1111/jomf.12349.

Gage, T. B., F. Fang, E. O'Neill, and G. Dirienzo. 2013. "Maternal education, birth weight, and infant mortality in the United States." *Demography* 50(2): 615–635. https://doi.org/ 10.1007/s13524-012-0148-2.

Gakidou, E., K. Cowling, R. Lozano, and C. J. Murray. 2010. "Increased educational attainment and its effect on child mortality in 175 countries between 1970 and 2009: A systematic analysis." *Lancet* 376(9745): 959–974. https:// doi.org/10.1016/s0140-6736(10)61257-3.

Galea, S., and S. M. Abdalla. 2020. "COVID-19 pandemic, unemployment, and civil unrest: Underlying deep racial and socioeconomic divides." *JAMA* 324(3): 227–228. https://doi.org/10.1001/jama.2020.11132.

Gallus, S., A. Lugo, X. Liu, P. Behrakis, R. Boffi, C. Bosetti, G. Carreras, et al. 2021. "Who smokes in Europe? Data from 12 European countries in the TackSHS survey (2017–2018)." *J Epidemiol* 31(2): 145–151. https:// doi.org/10.2188/jea.JE20190344.

García-Herrero, S., M. A. Mariscal, J. M. Gutiérrez, and D. O. Ritzel. 2013. "Using Bayesian networks to analyze occupational stress caused by work demands: Preventing stress through social support." *Accid Anal Prev* 57: 114–123. https://doi.org/10.1016/ j.aap.2013.04.009.

Gariépy, G., H. Honkaniemi, and A. Quesnel-Vallée. 2016. "Social support and protection from depression: Systematic review of current findings in Western countries." *Br J Psychiatry* 209(4): 284–293. https://doi.org/10.1192/ bjp.bp.115.169094.

Giordano, G. N., and M. Lindström. 2011. "The impact of social capital on changes in smoking behaviour: A longitudinal cohort study." *Eur J Public Health* 21(3): 347–354. https://doi.org/10.1093/eurpub/ckq048.

Glozah, F. N., and D. J. Pevalin. 2015. "Perceived social support and parental education as determinants of adolescents' physical activity and eating behaviour: A cross-sectional survey." *Int J Adolesc Med Health* 27(3): 253–259. https://doi.org/10.1515/ ijamh-2014-0019.

Gopalan, M., and A. A. Nelson. 2019. "Understanding the racial discipline gap in schools." *AERA Open* 5(2): 2332858419844613. https://doi.org/10.1177/2332858419844613.

Grossman, M., and R. Kaestner. 1997. "Effects of education on health." In *The Social Benefits of Education*, edited by J. R. Behrman and N. Stacey, 69–123. Ann Arbor, MI: University of Michigan Press.

Guilaran, J., I. de Terte, K. Kaniasty, and C. Stephens. 2018. "Psychological outcomes in disaster responders: A systematic review and meta-analysis on the effect of social support." *Int J Disaster Risk Sci* 9(3): 344–358. https:// doi.org/10.1007/s13753-018-0184-7.

Gwatkin, D. R., S. Rutstein, K. Johnson, E. Suliman, A. Wagstaff, and A. Amouzou. 2007. *Socio-economic Difference in Health, Nutrition and Population Within Developing Countries*. Washington, DC: World Bank.

Hamad, R., H. Elser, D. C. Tran, D. H. Rehkopf, and S. N. Goodman. 2018. "How and why studies disagree about the effects of education on health: A systematic review and meta-analysis of studies of compulsory schooling laws." *Soc Sci Med* 212: 168–178. https://doi. org/10.1016/j.socscimed.2018.07.016.

Hanley, J., A. A. Mhamied, J. Cleveland, O. Hajjar, G. Hassan, N. Ivies, R. Khyar, and

M. Hynie. 2018. "The social networks, social support and social capital of Syrian refugees privately sponsored to settle in Montreal: Indications for employment and housing during their early experiences of integration." *Can Ethnic Stud* 50(2): 123–148.

Harding, J. F. 2015. "Increases in maternal education and low-income children's cognitive and behavioral outcomes." *Dev Psychol* 51(5): 583–599. doi:10.1037/a0038920.

Haveman, R., and T. Smeeding. 2006. "The role of higher education in social mobility." *Future Child* 16(2): 125–150. https://doi.org/10.1353/foc.2006.0015.

Hoebel, J., and T. Lampert. 2020. "Subjective social status and health: Multidisciplinary explanations and methodological challenges." *J Health Psychol* 25(2): 173–185. https://doi.org/10.1177/1359105318800804.

Holochwost, S. J., V. V. Volpe, N. Gueron-Sela, C. B. Propper, and W. R. Mills-Koonce. 2018. "Sociodemographic risk, parenting, and inhibitory control in early childhood: The role of respiratory sinus arrhythmia." *J Child Psychol Psychiatry* 59(9): 973–981. https://doi.org/10.1111/jcpp.12889.

Holt-Lunstad, J., T. B. Smith, and J. B. Layton. 2010. "Social relationships and mortality risk: A meta-analytic review." *PLoS Med* 7(7): e1000316. https://doi.org/10.1371/journal.pmed.1000316.

Hudson, D., T. Sacks, K. Irani, and A. Asher. 2020. "The price of the ticket: Health costs of upward mobility among African Americans." *Int J Environ Res Public Health* 17(4): 1179.

Hummer, R. A., and E. M. Hernandez. 2013. "The effect of educational attainment on adult mortality in the United States." *Popul Bull* 68(1): 1–16.

Idler, E. L., and Y. Benyamini. 1997. "Self-rated health and mortality: A review of twenty-seven community studies." *J Health Soc Behav* 38(1): 21–37.

Infurna, F. J., N. Ram, and D. Gerstorf. 2013. "Level and change in perceived control predict 19-year mortality: Findings from the Americans' Changing Lives Study." *Dev Psychol* 49(10): 1833–1847. https://doi.org/10.1037/a0031041.

Kaplan, R. M., M. L. Spittel, and T. L. Zeno. 2014. "Educational attainment and life expectancy." *Policy Insights Behav Brain Sci* 1(1): 189–194. https://doi.org/10.1177/2372732214549754.

Karasek, R., D. Baker, F. Marxer, A. Ahlbom, and T. Theorell. 1981. "Job decision latitude, job demands, and cardiovascular disease: A prospective study of Swedish men." *Am J Public Health* 71(7): 694–705. https://doi.org/10.2105/ajph.71.7.694.

Karlsson, O., J.-W. De Neve, and S. V. Subramanian. 2018. "Weakening association of parental education: Analysis of child health outcomes in 43 low- and middle-income countries." *Int J Epidemiol* 48(1): 83–97. https://doi.org/10.1093/ije/dyy158.

Kauffman, J. M., and J. Badar. 2013. "How we might make special education for students with emotional or behavioral disorders less stigmatizing." *Behav Disord* 39(1): 16–27.

Kaushal, N. 2014. "Intergenerational payoffs of education." *Future Child* 24(1): 61–78. https://doi.org/10.1353/foc.2014.0005.

Kawachi, I., N. E. Adler, and W. H. Dow. 2010. "Money, schooling, and health: Mechanisms and causal evidence." *Ann N Y Acad Sci* 1186: 56–68. https://doi.org/10.1111/j.1749-6632.2009.05340.x.

Kim, M. M., and J. Ko. 2015. "The impacts of state control policies on college tuition increase." *Educ Policy* 29(5): 815–838. https://doi.org/10.1177/0895904813518100.

Lachman, M. E., and S. L. Weaver. 1998. "The sense of control as a moderator of social class differences in health and well-being." *J Pers Soc Psychol* 74(3): 763.

Lagraauw, H. M., J. Kuiper, and I. Bot. 2015. "Acute and chronic psychological stress as risk factors for cardiovascular disease: Insights gained from epidemiological, clinical and experimental studies." *Brain Behav Immun* 50: 18–30. https://doi.org/10.1016/j.bbi.2015.08.007.

Lawrence, E. M., R. G. Rogers, and R. A. Hummer. 2020. "Maternal educational attainment and child health in the United States." *Am J Health Promot* 34(3): 303–306. https://doi.org/10.1177/0890117119890799.

Leganger, A., and P. Kraft. 2003. "Control constructs: Do they mediate the relation between educational attainment and health behaviour?" *J Health Psychol* 8(3): 361–372. https://doi.org/10.1177/13591053030083006.

Lehto, E., H. Konttinen, P. Jousilahti, and A. Haukkala. 2013. "The role of psychosocial factors in socioeconomic differences in physical activity: A population-based study." *Scand J Public Health* 41(6): 553–559. https://doi.org/10.1177/1403494813481642.

Lewis, W. D., and T. V. Young. 2013. "The politics of accountability: Teacher education policy." *Educ Policy* 27(2): 190–216. https://doi.org/10.1177/0895904812472725.

Ludeke, S. G., M. Gensowski, S. Y. Junge, R. M. Kirkpatrick, O. P. John, and S. C. Andersen. 2021. "Does parental education influence child educational outcomes? A developmental analysis in a full-population sample and adoptee design." *J Pers Soc Psychol* 120(4): 1074–1090. https://doi.org/10.1037/pspp0000314.

Lunau, T., J. Siegrist, N. Dragano, and M. Wahrendorf. 2015. "The association between education and work stress: Does the policy context matter?" *PLoS One* 10(3): e0121573. https://doi.org/10.1371/journal.pone.0121573.

Lundetrae, K., and E. Gabrielsen. 2016. "Relationship between literacy skills and self-reported health in the Nordic countries." *Scand J Public Health* 44(8): 758–764. https://doi.org/10.1177/1403494816668082.

Luy, M., M. Zannella, C. Wegner-Siegmundt, Y. Minagawa, W. Lutz, and G. Caselli. 2019. "The impact of increasing education levels on rising life expectancy: A decomposition analysis for Italy, Denmark, and the USA." *Genus* 75(1): 11. https://doi.org/10.1186/s41118-019-0055-0.

Ma, J., M. Pender, and M. Welch. 2019. "Education pays 2019: The benefits of higher education for individuals and society." CollegeBoard. https://distance-educator.com/https-research-collegeboard-org-pdf-education-pays-2019-full-report-pdf.

Malcolm, M., H. Frost, and J. Cowie. 2019. "Loneliness and social isolation causal association with health-related lifestyle risk in older adults: A systematic review and meta-analysis protocol." *System Rev* 8 (1): 48. https://doi.org/10.1186/s13643-019-0968-x.

Mantwill, S., S. Monestel-Umana, and P. J. Schulz. 2015. "The relationship between health literacy and health disparities: A systematic review." *PLoS One* 10(12): e0145455. https://doi.org/10.1371/journal.pone.0145455.

Matthews, K. A., and L. C. Gallo. 2011. "Psychological perspectives on pathways linking socioeconomic status and physical health." *Annu Rev Psychol* 62(1): 501–530. https://doi.org/10.1146/annurev.psych.031809.130711.

McCluney, C. L., L. L. Schmitz, M. T. Hicken, and A. Sonnega. 2018. "Structural racism in the workplace: Does perception matter for health inequalities?" *Soc Sci Med* 199: 106–114. https://doi.org/10.1016/j.socscimed.2017.05.039.

McEwen, B. S. 2017. "Neurobiological and systemic effects of chronic stress." *Chronic Stress* 1: 2470547017692328.

McEwen, B. S., and T. Seeman. 1999. "Protective and damaging effects of mediators of stress: Elaborating and testing the concepts of allostasis and allostatic load." *Ann N Y Acad Sci* 896: 30–47. https://doi.org/10.1111/j.1749-6632.1999.tb08103.x.

McFarland, M. J., S. S. McLanahan, B. J. Goosby, and N. E. Reichman. 2017. "Grandparents' education and infant health: Pathways across generations." *J Marriage Fam* 79(3): 784–800. https://doi.org/10.1111/jomf.12383.

McGee, A., and P. McGee. 2016. "Search, effort, and locus of control." *J Econ Behav Organ* 126:89–101. https://doi.org/10.1016/j.jebo.2016.03.001.

McLeod, C. B., J. N. Lavis, Y. C. MacNab, and C. Hertzman. 2012. "Unemployment and mortality: A comparative study of Germany and the United States." *Am J Public Health* 102(8): 1542–1550. https://doi.org/10.2105/ajph.2011.300475.

Mensch, B. S., E. K. Chuang, A. J. Melnikas, and S. R. Psaki. 2019. "Evidence for causal links between education and maternal and child health: Systematic review." *Trop Med Int Health* 24(5): 504–522. https://doi.org/10.1111/tmi.13218.

Mirowsky, J., and C. E. Ross. 1998. "Education, personal control, lifestyle and health: A human capital hypothesis." *Res Aging* 20(4): 415–449. https://doi.org/10.1177/0164027598204003.

Mirowsky, J., and C. E. Ross. 2003. *Education, Social Status, and Health*. Hawthorne, NY: Aldine de Gruyter.

Mirowsky, J., and Ross, C. E. 2007. "Life course trajectories of perceived control and their relationship to education." *Am J Sociol* 112(5): 1339–1382. https://doi.org/10.1086/511800.

Mitchell, M., M. Leachman, and M. Saenz. 2019. "State higher education funding cuts have pushed costs to students, worsened inequality." Center on Budget and Policy Priorities. Accessed November 9, 2020. https://www.cbpp.org/research/state-budget-and-tax/state-higher-education-funding-cuts-have-pushed-costs-to-students.

Mizel, M. L., J. N. V. Miles, E. R. Pedersen, J. S. Tucker, B. A. Ewing, and E. J. D'Amico. 2016. "To educate or to incarcerate: Factors in disproportionality in school discipline." *Child Youth Serv Rev.* 70: 102–111. https://doi.org/10.1016/j.childyouth.2016.09.009.

National Center for Education Statistics. 2006. *The Health Literacy of America's Adults: Results from the 2003 National Assessment of Adult Literacy.* Washington, DC: U.S. Department of Education.

National Center for Education Statistics. 2019. "Percentage of high school dropouts among persons 16 to 24 years old (status dropout rate), by income level, and percentage distribution of status dropouts, by labor force status and years of school completed: Selected years, 1970 through 2016." Accessed April 2019. https://nces.ed.gov/programs/digest/d17/tables/dt17_219.75.asp.

National Center for Education Statistics. 2020a. "Figure 29. Median annual earnings of full-time, full-year wage and salary workers ages 25 and older, by sex, race/ethnicity, and educational attainment: 2007." Accessed November 10, 2020. https://nces.ed.gov/pubs2010/2010015/figures/figure_29.asp.

National Center for Education Statistics. 2020b. "Percentage of the population 25 to 64 years old who completed high school, by age group and country: Selected years, 2000 through 2017." Accessed May 11, 2020. https://nces.ed.gov/programs/digest/d18/tables/dt18_603.10.asp.

National Center for Education Statistics. 2020c. "Rates of high school completion and bachelor's degree attainment among persons age 25 and over, by race/ethnicity and sex: Selected years, 1910 through 2018." Accessed May 11, 2020. https://nces.ed.gov/programs/digest/d18/tables_1.asp.

National Center for Education Statistics. 2020d. "Status dropout rates." Accessed May 11, 2020. https://nces.ed.gov/programs/coe/indicator_coj.asp.

National Center for Education Statistics. 2020e. "Table 104.40. Percentage of persons 18 to 24 years old and age 25 and over, by educational attainment, race/ethnicity, and selected racial/ethnic subgroups: 2010 and 2017." Accessed November 17, 2020. https://nces.ed.gov/programs/digest/d18/tables/dt18_104.40.asp?current=yes.

National Center for Health Statistics. 2018. *Health, United States, 2018.* Hyattsville, MD: National Center for Health Statistics.

Ng Fat, L., S. Scholes, and S. Jivraj. 2017. "The relationship between drinking pattern, social capital, and area-deprivation: Findings from the Health Survey for England." *J Stud Alcohol Drugs* 78(1): 20–29. https://doi.org/10.15288/jsad.2017.78.20.

Noble, K. G., S. M. Houston, N. H. Brito, H. Bartsch, E. Kan, J. M. Kuperman, N. Akshoomoff, et al. 2015. "Family income, parental education and brain structure in children and adolescents." *Nat Neurosci* 18(5): 773–778. https://doi.org/10.1038/nn.3983.

Pan, K. Y., W. Xu, F. Mangialasche, R. Wang, S. Dekhtyar, A. Calderon-Larranaga, L. Fratiglioni, and H. X. Wang. 2019. "Psychosocial working conditions, trajectories of disability, and the mediating role of cognitive decline and chronic diseases: A population-based cohort study." *PLoS Med* 16(9): e1002899. https://doi.org/10.1371/journal.pmed.1002899.

Prickett, K. C., and J. M. Augustine. 2016. "Maternal education and investments in children's health." *J Marriage Family* 78(1): 7–25. https://doi.org/10.1111/jomf.12253.

Raible, J., and J. G. Irizarry. 2010. "Redirecting the teacher's gaze: Teacher education, youth surveillance and the school-to-prison pipeline." *Teaching Teacher Educ* 26(5): 1196–1203. https://doi.org/10.1016/j.tate.2010.02.006.

Rampey, B. D., R. Finnegan, M. Goodman, L. Mohadjer, T. Krenzke, J. Hogan, and S. Provasnik. 2016. *Skills of U.S. Unemployed, Young, and Older Adults in Sharper Focus: Results from the Program for the International Assessment of Adult Competencies (PIAAC) 2012/2014: First Look.* Washington, DC: U.S. Department of Education, National Center for Education Statistics.

Reilly, K. 2018, September 13. "'I work 3 jobs and donate blood plasma to pay the bills.' This is what it's like to be a teacher in America." *TIME*.

Rocque, M. 2018. "The prison school: Educational inequality and school discipline in the age of mass incarceration." *J Criminal Justice Educ* 29(3): 476–479. https://doi.org/10.1080/10511253.2017.1310476.

Rolen, E. 2019. *Occupational Employment Projections Through the Perspective of Education and Training*. Washington, DC: U.S. Bureau of Labor Statistics.

Roosevelt, E. 2008. "Good citizenship: The purpose of education." *Yearbook Natl Soc Stud Educ* 107(2): 312–320. https://doi.org/10.1111/j.1744-7984.2008.00228.x.

Ross, C. E., and J. Mirowsky. 1999. "Refining the association between education and health: The effects of quantity, credential, and selectivity." *Demography* 36(4): 445–460. https://doi.org/10.2307/2648083.

Rostron, B. L., J. L. Boies, and E. Arias. 2010. Education reporting and classification on death certificates in the United States. *Vital Health Stat 2* (151): 1–21.

Rouse, C. E., and L. Barrow. 2006. "U.S. elementary and secondary schools: Equalizing opportunity or replicating the status quo?" *Future Child* 16(2): 99–123. https://doi.org/10.1353/foc.2006.0018.

Ryan, R. M., A. Claessens, and A. J. Markowitz. 2015. "Associations between family structure change and child behavior problems: The moderating effect of family income." *Child Dev* 86(1): 112–127. https://doi.org/10.1111/cdev.12283.

Sasson, I. 2016. "Trends in life expectancy and lifespan variation by educational attainment: United States, 1990–2010." *Demography* 53(2): 269–293. https://doi.org/10.1007/s13524-015-0453-7.

Schmidt, E. 2018. *For the First Time, 90 Percent Completed High School or More*. Washington, DC: U.S. Census Bureau.

Schwartz, R. M., M. C. Schmitt, and M. K. Lose. 2012. "Effects of teacher–student ratio in response to intervention approaches." *Elementary School J* 112(4): 547–567. https://doi.org/10.1086/664490.

Serlachius, A., M. Elovainio, M. Juonala, S. Shea, M. Sabin, T. Lehtimäki, O. Raitakari, L. Keltikangas-Järvinen, and L. Pulkki-Råback. 2016. "High perceived social support protects against the intergenerational transmission of obesity: The Cardiovascular Risk in Young Finns Study." *Prev Med* 90: 79–85. https://doi.org/10.1016/j.ypmed.2016.07.004.

Sheeran, P., A. Maki, E. Montanaro, A. Avishai-Yitshak, A. Bryan, W. M. P. Klein, E. Miles, and A. J. Rothman. 2016. "The impact of changing attitudes, norms, and self-efficacy on health-related intentions and behavior: A meta-analysis." *Health Psychol* 35(11): 1178.

Shor, E., and D. J. Roelfs. 2015. "Social contact frequency and all-cause mortality: A meta-analysis and meta-regression." *Soc Sci Med* 128: 76–86. https://doi.org/10.1016/j.socscimed.2015.01.010.

Short, M. E., R. Z. Goetzel, X. Pei, M. J. Tabrizi, R. J. Ozminkowski, T. B. Gibson, D. M. Dejoy, and M. G. Wilson. 2009. "How accurate are self-reports? Analysis of self-reported health care utilization and absence when compared with administrative data." *J Occup Environ Med* 51(7): 786–796. https://doi.org/10.1097/JOM.0b013e3181a86671.

Singh-Manoux, A., M. G. Marmot, and N. E. Adler. 2005. "Does subjective social status predict health and change in health status better than objective status?" *Psychosom Med* 67(6): 855–861. https://doi.org/10.1097/01.psy.0000188434.52941.a0.

Specht, J., B. Egloff, and S. Schmukle. 2013. "Everything under control? The effects of age, gender, and education on trajectories of perceived control in a nationally representative German sample." *Dev Psychol* 49: 353–364. https://doi.org/10.1037/a0028243.

Street, B. 2013. "Literacy in theory and practice: Challenges and debates over 50 years." *Theory Practice* 52 (Sup1): 52–62. https://doi.org/10.1080/00405841.2013.795442.

Tamborini, C. R., C. H. Kim, and A. Sakamoto. 2015. "Education and lifetime earnings in the United States." *Demography* 52(4): 1383–1407. https://doi.org/10.1007/s13524-015-0407-0.

Tang, K. L., R. Rashid, J. Godley, and W. A. Ghali. 2016. "Association between subjective social status and cardiovascular disease and cardiovascular risk factors: A systematic review and meta-analysis." *BMJ Open* 6(3): e010137. https://doi.org/10.1136/bmjopen-2015-010137.

Thoits, P. A. 2010. "Stress and health: Major findings and policy implications." *J Health Soc Behav* 51(Suppl): S41–S53. https://doi.org/10.1177/0022146510383499.

Thoits, P. A. 2011. "Mechanisms linking social ties and support to physical and mental health." *J Health Soc Behav* 52(2): 145–161. https://doi.org/10.1177/0022146510395592.

Thomas, K., E. Nilsson, K. Festin, P. Henriksson, M. Lowén, M. Löf, and M. Kristenson. 2020. "Associations of psychosocial factors with multiple health behaviors: A population-based study of middle-aged men and women." *Int J Environ Res Public Health* 17(4): 1239. https://doi.org/10.3390/ijerph17041239.

Turiano, N. A., B. P. Chapman, S. Agrigoroaei, F. J. Infurna, and M. Lachman. 2014. "Perceived control reduces mortality risk at low, not high, education levels." *Health Psychol* 33(8): 883–890. https://doi.org/10.1037/hea0000022.

Uchino, B. N., R. Trettevik, R. G. Kent de Grey, S. Cronan, J. Hogan, and B. R. W. Baucom. 2018. "Social support, social integration, and inflammatory cytokines: A meta-analysis." *Health Psychol* 37(5): 462–471. https://doi.org/10.1037/hea0000594.

U.S. Bureau of Labor Statistics. 2020. "Unemployment rates and earnings by educational attainment." Accessed May 15, 2020. https://www.bls.gov/emp/tables/unemployment-earnings-education.htm.

Vågerö, D., and A. M. Garcy. 2016. "Does unemployment cause long-term mortality? Selection and causation after the 1992–96 deep Swedish recession." *Eur J Public Health* 26(5): 778–783. https://doi.org/10.1093/eurpub/ckw053.

Vollmer, S., C. Bommer, A. Krishna, K. Harttgen, and S. V. Subramanian. 2017. "The association of parental education with childhood undernutrition in low- and middle-income countries: Comparing the role of paternal and maternal education." *Int J Epidemiol* 46(1): 312–323. https://doi.org/10.1093/ije/dyw133.

Walker, S. E. 2003. "Active learning strategies to promote critical thinking." *J Athletic Training* 38(3): 263–267.

Wallace, J. M., S. Goodkind, C. M. Wallace, and J. G. Bachman. 2008. "Racial, ethnic, and gender differences in school discipline among U.S. high school students: 1991–2005." *Negro Educ Rev* 59(1-2): 47–62.

Woods, D. 2015. "The class size debate: What the evidence means for education policy." Goldman School of Public Policy. Accessed November 13, 2020. https://bppj.berkeley.edu/2015/09/23/the-class-size-debate-what-the-evidence-means-for-education-policy.

Yamashita, T., and S. R. Kunkel. 2015. "An international comparison of the association among literacy, education, and health across the United States, Canada, Switzerland, Italy, Norway, and Bermuda: Implications for health disparities." *J Health Commun* 20(4): 406–415. https://doi.org/10.1080/10810730.2014.977469.

Yi, D., Y. Huang, and G.-Z. Fan. 2016. "Social capital and housing affordability: Evidence from China." *Emerg Markets Finance Trade* 52(8): 1728–1743. https://doi.org/10.1080/1540496X.2016.1181856.

Zell, E., J. E. Strickhouser, and Z. Krizan. 2018. "Subjective social status and health: A meta-analysis of community and society ladders." *Health Psychol* 37(10): 979–987. https://doi.org/10.1037/hea0000667.

Zimmerman, E. B., S. H. Woolf, and A. Haley. 2015. "Understanding the relationship between education and health: a review of the evidence and an examination of community perspectives. Population health: behavioral and social science insights." Rockville, MD: Agency for Health-care Research and Quality, 347–384.

CHAPTER 4

Stress Mediates the Health Effects of Many Social Determinants

4.1. INTRODUCTION

Almost all of us have, at some point, experienced the feeling of being overwhelmed or struggling to maintain balance and perform adequately in the face of heavy demands, responsibilities, or uncertainties. When we feel like this, we say we are "stressed" or "stressed out." Sometimes, the stress we experience is acute (i.e., temporary or short term)—for example, when we have to meet a tight deadline at work or are involved in an automobile accident. At other times, stress may arise from a chronic (i.e., ongoing or longer term) hardship, such as caring for a seriously ill family member; having a supervisor or colleagues at work who we believe treat us unfairly; or constantly worrying about being able to adequately feed, clothe, educate, or otherwise care for our children in the face of inadequate financial resources.

As discussed in other chapters, research during the past few decades has revealed dramatic differences in important child and adult health outcomes based on social factors such as income and wealth, education, and racism. These differences in health often begin early in life—sometimes even before birth—and accumulate over lifetimes and across generations. A growing body of evidence indicates that the effects of stress play a powerful role; many social determinants of health affect our bodies by producing and/or buffering the effects of stress (Box 4.1). This chapter provides an overview of current knowledge about the links between stress and health; it examines how social advantage or disadvantage can influence one's experiences of stress and the consequences for health and health disparities. Understanding these relationships can help inform and guide policies and programs in all of the sectors that influence health.

4.2. STRESS HAS BEEN LINKED REPEATEDLY WITH MANY HEALTH OUTCOMES

Exposure to stress and stressful conditions has been implicated repeatedly in a wide array of health outcomes across the life course. For example, a growing body of evidence suggests that stressful experiences both during and before conception can increase

The Social Determinants of Health and Health Disparities. Paula Braveman, Oxford University Press. © Oxford University Press 2023.
DOI: 10.1093/oso/9780190624118.003.0004

BOX 4.1   **Stress Versus Stressors Versus the Stress Response**

Stress (or *feeling "stressed"* or *"stressed out"*) refers to the uncomfortable experiences people have when they face challenging or threatening events or conditions that they feel strain their resources for coping.

The terms *stressor, hardships,* or *stressful conditions* refer to the challenging events or conditions that produce the experience of stress. Stressors include not only dramatic, short-term challenges or threats but also the kinds of on-going, everyday hassles that can strain a person's ability to cope. Douros et al. (2017) defined a stressor as any factor "able to threaten the homeostasis of an organism."

Stress response refers to the behavioral and physiologic processes provoked by a stressor.

---

a woman's risk of delivering a baby preterm (before 37 completed weeks of gestation) (Witt et al. 2014; Almeida et al. 2018). Cumulative effects of stress over the entire life course, including in childhood, may increase the risk of preterm birth (McDonald et al. 2014; Lu et al. 2003; Smith, Gotman, and Yonkers 2016). This elevated risk can have long-lasting effects for the affected infant and the family: Preterm birth is a powerful risk factor not only for infant mortality and cognitive, behavioral, and physical developmental disability in childhood but also for serious chronic disease—including heart disease, hypertension, and diabetes—later in life (Institute of Medicine Committee on Understanding Premature Birth and Assuring Healthy Outcomes 2007; Crump et al. 2019; Parkinson et al. 2013).

Research examining a range of individual and family stressors such as food insecurity, family disruption or conflict, parents' psychological distress, and financial strain indicates that children and adolescents exposed to high levels of stress due to any of these factors have increased risks of being overweight and/or obese even after considering other factors, such as family income, parents' body mass index, or racial/ethnic group (Gundersen et al. 2011). A growing body of evidence links stressful experiences in childhood and adolescence with increased risk of serious adult health problems, including heart disease and diabetes (Suglia et al. 2018). Among adults, multiple studies have linked exposure to work-related and other stressors with cardiovascular illness such as coronary heart disease and heart attacks, as well as with cardiovascular disease risk factors (Marmot et al. 1997; Nyberg et al. 2013; Steptoe and Kivimäki 2013; Rosengren et al. 2004; Kivimäki et al. 2015).

Acute, short-lived experiences of stress due to isolated dramatic events certainly can have adverse health impacts; for example, a study of the 2011 Tōhoku earthquake and tsunami in Japan found a nearly twofold increase in heart attacks during the 4 weeks following the disaster compared to the 4 weeks that preceded it (Tanaka et al. 2015). Hospitalizations for acute cardiovascular disease events in a large Southern California health care system were 1.62 times higher in the 2 days after the 2016 U.S. presidential election, which researchers attributed to election-related stress (Mefford et al. 2020). Although severe acute stressors can have adverse health consequences, current research indicates that overall, prolonged (vs. short-term) activation of the stress response due to chronic stressors is more likely to lead to poor health (Cohen, Murphy, and Prather 2019).

"Good Stress," "Bad Stress," and Resilience

Stress can adversely affect health when a perceived challenge exceeds a person's ability to cope. This seems to occur especially when the imbalance between stressful conditions and available coping resources is severe or chronic. *Resilience* is another term for coping resources, which McEwen et al. (2015) defined as the ability to achieve "a positive outcome in the face of adversity"(McEwen, Gray, and Nasca 2015; see also Schetter and Dolbier 2011, p. 1).

Experiencing challenges does not always have harmful effects, however. For example, meeting and overcoming a challenge may have paradoxically positive health effects, presumably by leading to growth, adaptation, and learning; this is referred to in the literature as "good stress" or "positive stress" (Dhabhar 2014, 2019). McEwen (2017) described "tolerable stress" as "situations where bad things happen, but the individual with healthy brain architecture . . . is able to cope with the support of family, friends, and other individuals" (p. 2). Both "good" and "tolerable" stress, in the presence of social support and other internal and external resources needed to meet a challenge, can promote a person's resilience and capacity for coping with future hardships (McEwen 2017).

"Good" (or "tolerable") stress is contrasted with "toxic" (or "bad") stress (McEwen 2017; Dhabhar 2014). Chronic stress is more likely to be toxic than acute stress. The health-damaging effects of toxic stress are more likely to occur when people experience ongoing or chronic exposure to multiple stressors in aspects of everyday life over which they have limited control—for example, if they must try to fulfill both family and job commitments without having adequate income, flexible work schedules, or paid family leave (McNamara, Bohle, and Quinlan 2011) or if they repeatedly encounter discrimination (e.g., based on their race, religion, gender, sexual orientation, or disability status) at work and lack other employment options. This type of chronic stress can lead to a cascade of adverse cognitive, physiological, and behavioral changes over time that in turn increase one's vulnerability to poor mental or physical health, particularly chronic disease (McEwen 2017).

The term *toxic stress* first appeared in the writings of child development expert Jack Shonkoff at Harvard University. He defined it as "strong, frequent, and/or prolonged activation of the body's stress response systems in the absence of the buffering protection of adult support " (Shonkoff, Boyce, and McEwen 2009, p. 2256). In common usage, however, this vivid term has been used more broadly to refer to stress in a child or adult that is at a level of severity and duration exceeding the body's capacity to react physiologically without producing collateral damage to health.

McEwen (2017) states,

> "Toxic stress" refers to the situation in which bad things happen to an individual who has limited support and who may also have brain architecture that reflects effects of adverse early life events that have impaired the development of good impulse control and judgment and adequate self-esteem. Here, the degree and/or duration of "distress" may be greater. With toxic stress, the inability to cope is likely to have adverse effects on behavior and physiology, and this will result in a higher degree of allostatic overload [defined in Box 4.2] (p. 2).

| BOX 4.2 | Allostatic Load |

Allostatic load (or *allostatic overload*) is the physiological reflection of the consequences of toxic stress. It is the cumulative wear and tear on the body's systems caused by endocrine and neural responses to prolonged or excessive stress. Allostatic load/overload is measured using multiple biological markers of autonomic, endocrine, metabolic, immune, cardiovascular, and respiratory mediators of the stress response (e.g., salivary cortisol, insulin-like growth factor-1, C-reactive protein, fibrinogen, immunoglobulin E, high-density lipoprotein, low-density lipoprotein, triglycerides, hemoglobin A1c, systolic blood pressure, heart rate, and peak [respiratory] expiratory flow), as well as anthropometric measures (i.e., body mass index and waist-to-hip ratio) (Juster, McEwen, and Lupien 2010). In addition to direct physiologic effects, allostatic load/overload has also been linked indirectly with health through its connection with health-damaging behaviors, including poor sleeping and eating patterns (Jackson, Knight, and Rafferty 2010).

Chronic exposure to stressful conditions can be particularly damaging to health, especially when it begins early in life (see Chapter 6). Chronic stress, particularly early in life, can result in long-term damage to multiple body organs and systems; it also can interfere with one's ability to respond to stress cognitively and physiologically, permanently impairing the body's ability to appropriately "switch off" the stress response under circumstances in which it is not needed later in life (McEwen 2001; Karatsoreos and McEwen 2013; Miller, Chen, and Zhou 2007).

Stressful experiences—including both ongoing everyday hassles and more dramatic acute events such as job loss with inadequate resources to cope—tend to compound one another, creating higher levels of stress over a person's lifetime (Pearlin 2010). For example, a person with lower educational attainment typically has more limited employment opportunities. Limited job options may raise the likelihood of needing to accept stressful work that is insecure, lower paying, potentially hazardous, and lacking in benefits such as medical insurance and paid family and sick leave. All of these could make it more difficult to balance family and work obligations. Chronic exposure—particularly in childhood—to the kinds of stressful conditions related to social disadvantage (e.g., poverty and racism or other forms of discrimination) may disrupt regulation of the body's physiologic (neuroendocrine and immune) response to stress, leading to impaired functioning with potentially lifelong adverse impacts on health.

4.3. HOW DOES STRESS GET INTO THE BODY TO CAUSE DISEASE? THE BIOLOGY OF STRESS

Stress Can Influence Health Indirectly by Influencing Behaviors That Influence Health

Stress can influence health indirectly through causal pathways involving behaviors. For example, exposure to stressful conditions has been associated with onset of smoking in adolescence (Wills, Sandy, and Yaeger 2002) and alcohol abuse and/or dependence in early adulthood (Boden, Fergusson, and Horwood 2014). Although findings on the relationship between stress and diet or physical activity have been less consistent, a number of studies have linked stressful experiences with overeating, unhealthy food choices, and less frequent exercise (Sominsky and Spencer 2014; Razzoli et al. 2017; Stults-Kolehmainen and Sinha 2014; Mouchacca, Abbott, and Ball 2013).

Advances in Neuroscience Have Informed Our Understanding of How Stress More Directly Gets into the Body to Damage Health

During the past three decades, there has been a dramatic growth in knowledge about the biological processes through which stressful experiences may more directly (than by shaping behaviors) lead to disease and premature (before age 75 years) death. The brain is the link between stress and health. The experience of stress begins when the brain registers the occurrence of a stressor—that is, a stressful event or condition (McEwen et al. 2015). Several areas within the brain have been identified as mediators of the body's responses to stress; they play key roles both in assessing whether events or circumstances are threatening and in regulating the body's responses through complex interactions between two main physiological systems: the neuroendocrine system, which includes the brain and the hormonal systems directly activated by the brain, and the immune system (McEwen et al. 2015; Dhabhar 2014). Two components of the neuroendocrine system play major roles in the stress response: the hypothalamic–pituitary–adrenal (HPA) axis and the sympathetic nervous system.

As shown in Figure 4.1, the body's stress response begins in the brain, with the detection of a challenge or threat. Within seconds of registering the existence of a stressor, one part of the brain, the hypothalamus, releases corticotropin-releasing hormone, which triggers another part of the brain, the anterior pituitary gland, to release another hormone, adrenocorticotropic hormone (ACTH). ACTH then acts on the cortex (outer portion) of the adrenal glands, stimulating them to secrete a type of steroid hormone called glucocorticoids, including cortisol. Adequate levels of cortisol are needed for healthy functioning of a number of bodily systems. When secreted at excessive levels or for prolonged periods in response to stress, however, cortisol can have major adverse effects on multiple organs and systems; these effects can alter physiologic regulation mechanisms and lead to premature aging of the immune system; adverse changes in the brain; and metabolic disturbances known to contribute to cardiovascular disease risk (McEwen 2005; Sorrells and Sapolsky 2007).

In addition to the HPA axis, the sympathetic nervous system is the other major component of the neuroendocrine system involved in the stress response. Perceiving an external threat activates what is called the "sympathetic" branch of the autonomic nervous system, stimulating the release of substances (hormones) called catecholamines—including epinephrine (also called adrenaline) and norepinephrine (also called noradrenaline)—from the adrenal medulla (inner portion of the adrenal glands). The catecholamines act to increase heart rate and blood pressure; mobilize energy stores from the liver; and direct blood flow to the heart, brain, and skeletal muscles (and away from the skin, digestive tract, and kidneys) (Piazza et al. 2010). This set of physiologic responses can greatly enhance performance, especially when one confronts a physical threat. This is the so-called fight-or-flight response, which is thought to have had evolutionary value long ago: It could make the difference between life or death when our prehistoric ancestors not infrequently faced immediate, potentially catastrophic physical threats, such as hungry lions, tigers, or bears. These threats required our ancestors to react

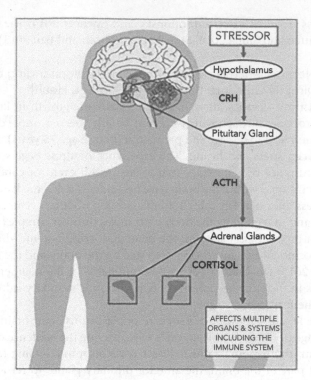

FIGURE 4.1   A simplified illustration of the hypothalamic–pituitary–adrenal axis and its involvement in the stress response. ACTH, adrenocorticotropic hormone; CRH, corticotropin-releasing hormone.

with relatively short but intense spurts of superior mental and physical performance. The fight-or-flight response to stressors encountered in modern society, however, may not have evolutionary value now, when the most serious challenges and threats we commonly face in our daily lives are generally likely to be less dramatic, more persistent, and, regrettably, often not solved by running away.

Immune system processes also are involved in the stress response. The primary role of the immune system is to defend the body against infection; it does so through several mechanisms, including inflammation, with effects that in certain circumstances are beneficial and in others may be harmful to health (Sorrells and Sapolsky 2007; Dhabhar 2014). Ongoing exposure to stressful conditions can produce significant and long-lasting changes in immune processes, referred to as immune dysregulation (Cohen, Janicki-Deverts, and Miller 2007; Fagundes, Glaser, and Kiecolt-Glaser 2013; Elenkov 2004; Elenkov and Chrousos 2002; Bauer, Jeckel, and Luz 2009); these changes have been linked with multiple adverse health effects (Cohen et al. 2007; Elenkov 2004; Elenkov and Chrousos 2002). The immune system appears to be most susceptible to the adverse effects of stress both early and late in life. Animal research suggests that stress during the prenatal period can lead to elevated risk of childhood asthma in the offspring (Douros et al. 2017), and paternal stress has been observed to affect offspring's HPA axis regulation, which could contribute to neuropsychiatric disease risk (Rodgers et al. 2013).

Stress early in life—particularly when experienced on a chronic basis—may compromise the immune system's ability to respond adequately to stress in adulthood (Fagundes et al. 2013). Chronic stress also may exacerbate changes in the immune response associated with aging (Gouin, Hantsoo, and Kiecolt-Glaser 2008; Kiecolt-Glaser et al. 2003). Geronimus, of the University of Michigan, hypothesized that African Americans experience a process of "weathering"—that is, physiologically premature aging—as a result of having to cope with chronic stress due to experiences of racism (Geronimus et al. 2019).

Both biology and context matter. Two individuals faced with the same external stressor may react very differently. Although genetic predisposition and other biological factors can play a role (McEwen 2008; Taylor 2010; Brody et al. 2013), evidence indicates that some people are more vulnerable than others to the health-harming effects of stress as a result of the nature, severity, frequency, and/or duration of the stressors they encounter and the resources they have available to respond. For example, a 2010 study found that among children in families with generally low levels of stress, children who were more biologically sensitive (i.e., who physiologically reacted more) to stressful conditions coped more effectively—were more resilient—than their less stress-reactive peers. However, among families facing greater financial and social stressors, the more stress-reactive children fared worse (Obradović et al. 2010).

Not surprisingly, the resources available for coping matter. Social support from family, friends, and co-workers may reduce the health-damaging effects of stress by helping people cope more effectively with stressful situations (Uchino et al. 2018). For example, among physicians, support from colleagues has been shown to buffer against the effects of increased workload on sleep quality and other indicators of well-being (Aalto et al. 2018). Access to greater financial resources also can greatly help a person cope with stress. People with a wide range of income and wealth levels lost their jobs or businesses due to the COVID-19 pandemic in 2020, for example. Those with financial resources—such as high incomes, accumulated wealth, and/or family economic resources—to fall back on, however, did not have to worry about their children going hungry or becoming homeless. Those with lower incomes and limited or no savings, and those whose extended families had little or no resources to spare, likely experienced a very different level and duration of stress associated with job loss.

The complexity of the elements involved in the response to stress is indicated by Figure 4.2, a diagram created by neuroscientists Bruce McEwen and Teresa Seeman (McEwen and Seeman 1999). Stressors include factors in the social or physical environments in which we live, work, study, and play; major life events; and experiences of trauma or abuse. When the brain registers a stressor (a perceived threat), this triggers physiologic responses with health consequences that can be favorable (adaptation) or potentially harmful (allostatic load, wear and tear on vital organs/systems). The stress response also produces behavioral responses (e.g., the well-known fight-or-flight response) and personal behaviors (e.g., smoking, alcohol consumption, exercise, and diet) that have health consequences. There are individual differences in the stress response, based on genetic factors ("nature") and experiences ("nurture").

Stress can trigger epigenetic effects with health consequences. Epigenetic effects (gene–environment interactions) are thought likely to play a role in the health effects of stress (Cao-Lei et al. 2020; McEwen et al. 2015). Epigenetic effects do not alter a person's

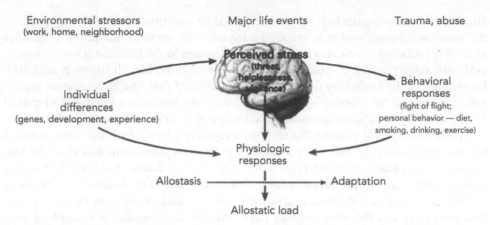

FIGURE 4.2   Multiple factors influence the stress response. *Source*: McEwen and Seeman (1999).

DNA. They can be thought of as "on/off" switches that control whether one's DNA is expressed or is suppressed. An individual may have a genetic predisposition for disease X, for example. Disease X, however, may only be expressed if that person is exposed to chronic stress. The significance of this is tremendous. It turns on its head the "nature versus nurture" question (whether genetic makeup or experiences are more influential in shaping a person): "Nurture" may be able to overcome "nature." It is thought that traumatic experiences, furthermore, may have epigenetic effects that can be inherited from one generation to another (Thayer and Kuzawa 2011; Yehuda and Lehrner 2018); this suggests the possibility of enduring contemporary health effects of severe historical trauma, such as slavery.

4.4. EXPERIENCING SOCIAL DISADVANTAGE, SUCH AS POVERTY OR RACISM, IS STRESSFUL

Having Inadequate Economic Resources to Meet Basic Needs, Such as Food, Shelter, Child Care, Elder Care, Transportation, and Medical Care, Is Stressful

Striking differences in health and life expectancy have been seen repeatedly in the United States and other countries based on differences in educational attainment, occupational ranking, income, and accumulated wealth. The differences are not only between groups at the very top and bottom of the socioeconomic ladder; they often follow a stepwise gradient pattern in which health improves incrementally with increasing levels of social and economic advantage (Hajat et al. 2010; Braveman et al. 2010; Lahelma et al. 2005; Avendano et al. 2006; Sasson 2016; Chetty et al. 2016). (See Chapter 2 for discussion of the implications of the socioeconomic gradient observed in so many health outcomes.)

How could stress contribute to the links between socioeconomic advantage and health? Does it make intuitive sense that people at the bottom of the socioeconomic ladder experience greater levels of stress than those at the top? One could argue, for example, that executives and professionals, who typically have considerable pressure to perform well at challenging tasks, encounter high levels of stress on a daily basis; by contrast, workers in

> Economic disadvantage means having to face stressful living and working conditions with inadequate resources, every day and over time.

lower status positions do not face the same levels of decision-making or high-level performance pressures. As discussed above, however, neuroscientists have learned that certain kinds of stress appear to be more damaging to the body than others. People in high-status jobs typically have more control over their work and how they accomplish it than workers in low-status jobs. They have more financial resources to cope with, for example, child care transportation, or other logistical challenges. The challenges typically faced by high-status workers therefore may not result in the wear and tear on bodily systems provoked by the chronic—and sometimes toxic—stress more often experienced by people in low-status jobs (Kivimäki et al. 2015). (See Chapter 9 for discussion of stress and control at work.) Seeman et al. (2010) examined the relationship between different measures of allostatic load and socioeconomic status and found that the predominant pattern was an increase in allostatic load with decreasing levels of income and education.

People with greater economic or socioeconomic advantage—for example, those who have higher levels of education, income, and/or accumulated wealth—may in fact be more likely to experience stress in ways that, perhaps surprisingly, have beneficial effects on their health. "Good stress," discussed previously, can occur when prior experiences (particularly in childhood) of successfully meeting challenges reinforce one's confidence in being able to manage current challenges (McEwen 2019; Aschbacher et al. 2013). In contrast, those with less education and lower incomes typically face more frequent and numerous stressors in many aspects of their lives while at the same time having less control over addressing those stressors; they often have more limited social and material resources for coping with "bad stress."

Even before the massive job losses due to the COVID-19 pandemic, social disadvantage and the stress that accompanies it were not rare in the United States, which lacks the safety nets of many other high-income countries. A sizable proportion of the U.S. population—10.5% overall and 14.4% of U.S. children younger than age 18 years in 2019—lived in poverty before the COVID-19 pandemic.(U.S. Census Bureau 2020). (Official poverty guidelines for 2020 classify households as poor if they earn less than $21,720 for a family of three or $26,172 for a family of four.) Several months into the pandemic, estimates of poverty had risen to approximately 15% overall and approximately 20% among children (Center on Poverty and Social Policy 2020). Pre-pandemic, more than one-fourth of the U.S. population (26.3%) was considered "low-income"—that is, having incomes up to twice the federal poverty guidelines (Semega et al. 2020); this doubtlessly increased dramatically during the pandemic.

Low-income and poor people face daunting stressors, including food insecurity (Holben 2010), housing insecurity (Kushel et al. 2006), and job insecurity (Semega, Fontenot, and Kollar 2016). The COVID-19 pandemic has been extremely stressful for many people, but particularly those who had low incomes and little or no wealth before the pandemic began.

Chronic Stress due to Financial Hardship in Childhood Is Common and Likely to Be Damaging to Health

Chronic stress due to financial hardship is likely to be particularly damaging to health when experienced during early childhood (see Chapter 6).

A pre-pandemic survey of women in California (where more than one in eight U.S. births occur) who had given birth within the prior 2–9 months found even higher rates of poverty and low income around the time of childbirth compared with rates in the population overall. Furthermore, many of the women had experienced financial hardships during their childhoods; these stressors included hunger in their families because of inability to afford enough food (9.5%), their families having to move because of inability to pay the rent/mortgage (13.8%), and their families frequently having difficulty paying for basic needs such as food or housing (21.2%) (Braveman et al. 2018). As shown in Figure 4.3, the level of serious hardships (reflecting both severity and number of hardships) that women bearing children in California had experienced during their childhoods was correlated with their current income around the time of childbirth.

Children in low-income families are often exposed to more physical stressors (e.g., substandard housing, noise, and crowding) and psychosocial stressors (e.g., family turmoil, separation from caregivers, and community violence) than those in middle-income families (Evans and Kim 2013; Duncan et al. 2019). Financial difficulties put families with limited means under great stress, contributing to family disruption (Evans and Kim 2013; Duncan et al. 2019). Lower levels of both family income and educational attainment have been associated with greater financial, marital, and parental stress among U.S. adults older than age 25 years (Lantz et al. 2005). Several studies have found that lower levels of family income, accumulated wealth, or educational attainment correspond with higher rates of adverse or traumatic life events or chronic stress (Lê-Scherban et al. 2018; Sherman and Mehta 2020; Turner and Avison 2003; Hatch and Dohrenwend 2007; Matthews, Gallo, and Taylor 2010).

A series of groundbreaking studies of severe childhood psychosocial stressors, referred to as adverse childhood experiences (ACEs), revealed an unexpectedly high rate of ACEs among a large, representative sample of California children of virtually all socioeconomic levels. These studies examined severe psychosocial stressors such as child abuse, domestic violence, and family disruption, and they showed that these exceedingly stressful experiences were associated with a wide range of illness in adulthood (Felitti et al. 2019). They did not, unfortunately, also examine severe socioeconomic stressors such as food insecurity, housing insecurity, or homelessness suffered in childhood—neither their prevalence, their associations with adverse health outcomes, nor the role that socioeconomic stressors may have played in producing the severe psychosocial stressors.

Racism Is an Important Stressor

Dramatic racial and ethnic disparities in health have repeatedly been observed in the United States, even after taking into account socioeconomic differences between groups;

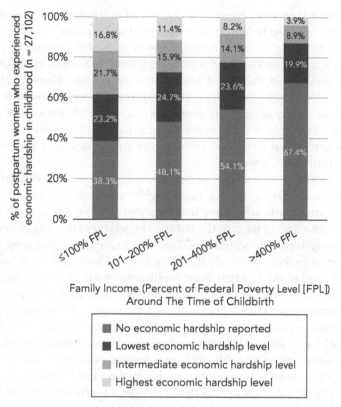

FIGURE 4.3 Economic hardship in childhood, according to women's income around the time of childbirth. Lower income of a childbearing woman often reflects economic hardship during her offspring's childhood. The percentage of postpartum (2–9 months after giving birth) women in California who experienced economic hardships during childhood (i.e., hunger/food insecurity, rent/mortgage problems, and/or difficulty paying for basic needs such as food or housing), as well as the number of and the chronicity of those hardships, increased with decreasing levels of family income. *Source*: Braveman et al. (2018).

for many health outcomes, African Americans as a group fare worse than Whites at every socioeconomic level (Williams et al. 2010). A number of scholars have concluded that stress, due to the direct and indirect consequences of racism, is likely to be a major contributor to racial disparities in health (Williams 2018; Krieger 2014). Plausible neurobiological mechanisms have been described (Berger and Sarnyai 2015). People of color encounter racial discrimination in various forms and settings. Overt interpersonal discrimination, e.g., insults, threats, physical attacks, are only a part of it, and now in many settings it may be less important than structural or systemic sources of stress, which are often hidden. Deeply embedded practices of institutions—for example, in employment, housing, credit, and banking, determining who receives a favorable loan to buy a home or launch or expand a business—have been shown to be discriminatory (Pager and Shepherd 2008). Racial residential discrimination exposes people of color to a range of stressors (Rothstein 2017). Discrimination is built so deeply into many institutions and structures that it operates even in the absence of individuals consciously wanting to discriminate. Studies have linked chronic racism-related vigilance, a measure of chronic stress, to sleep difficulty, which is associated with ill health (Hicken et al. 2013) and preterm birth, a salient predictor of infant mortality (Braveman et al., 2017). People of color may believe that they must outperform their White peers to disprove racial stereotypes; this can be stressful (Felix et al. 2019). These damaging physiologic effects of racism-related stress may accumulate over time from multiple sources. In addition, because racism tracks people of color into economic disadvantage—and makes it difficult to escape—racism-related stress also includes the stress associated with racism-related economic hardship (see Chapter 5).

Some studies have found that, perhaps paradoxically, racial disparities in some health outcomes are larger among more highly educated or affluent people than among their counterparts who have fewer socioeconomic resources. This has been hypothesized to be due, in part, to the stressful experiences that many people of color who are currently highly educated or affluent had to endure over time to overcome discrimination in order to reach their current level of socioeconomic success. It also has been attributed to the fact that more highly educated/affluent people of color are more likely to be in the minority in their workplaces and, therefore, potentially more exposed to discrimination, including less overt forms of it (Braveman et al. 2017; Bell et al. 2018; Hudson et al. 2012). A growing body of research suggests that stress related to living in a society with a legacy of persistent racial discrimination is a major factor in explaining poorer health outcomes among people of color (Williams and Mohammed 2013). Even for someone who has not personally faced major incidents of overt bias, the constant awareness that they—or a loved one—might be perceived or treated unfairly based on race may be a potent source of chronic stress (Nuru-Jeter et al. 2009; Williams, Lawrence, and Davis 2019). Also, even after considering other risk factors, perceptions of racial/ethnic discrimination have been linked with poorer mental and physical health outcomes (Lewis, Cogburn, and Williams 2015), including adverse birth outcomes (Alhusen et al. 2016) and cardiovascular disease (Lockwood et al. 2018; Hermosura, Haynes, and Kaholokula 2018), indicating that stress-related pathways are likely to be involved. One study examining physiologic markers of stress found that at every age and in both poor and non-poor households, Black people had higher levels of allostatic load—evidence of bodily wear and tear associated with chronic stress (defined previously)—than White people (Geronimus et al. 2006).

4.5. ACTIONS TO IMPROVE HEALTH AND REDUCE HEALTH DISPARITIES BY ADDRESSING STRESS

What can be done to address the damage that "bad stress" inflicts on health, particularly among those experiencing the most stress? The health care sector has, not surprisingly, focused on trying to buffer the harmful effects of stress on health rather than addressing its causes. In the clinical setting, ways to help people cope with stress have included counseling, medications for anxiety, home visiting or group interventions for social support, and increasing stress-management skills (e.g., to help people avoid turning to health-damaging behaviors in response to stress). Approaches taken by some health care systems or third-party payers have attempted to remove financial, cultural, and geographic barriers to counseling, social support, and stress management interventions. Such efforts include making relevant services more acceptable and accessible to affected populations, for example, by employing staff ethnically and linguistically concordant with the target population, locating services in the communities where the target population lives, and reducing or eliminating the cost of such services. Such efforts may help narrow stress-related health disparities. Efforts to build resilience to the health-harming effects of stress may make a worthwhile contribution. Their effects, however, may be limited. The success rates of such stress reduction/management efforts have been modest at best (American Psychological Association 2017). In addition, these approaches would not address the upstream sources of ongoing stress, which would continue to produce their downstream damage.

Current knowledge indicates that both public- and private-sector programs and policies—including, but not limited to, those within the health sector—could have profound effects on health, health disparities, and health care costs across the entire life span by reducing stressful conditions, particularly in childhood. Some innovative health care sector interventions reach beyond the walls of health care institutions to focus more broadly on changing the conditions in people's lives that are the causes of chronic stress (e.g., see Social Interventions Research & Evaluation Network; https://sirenetwork.ucsf.edu). Some programs have focused on integrating social and medical services in medical care settings, with the goal of reducing the number and severity of stressors experienced by low-income families. For example, the Medical–Legal Partnership (Lawton and Sandel 2014) provides onsite access to legal assistance at more than 300 hospitals and health centers nationally. Legal action may be needed to improve living conditions—for example, when landlords refuse to remove health hazards such as mold from housing—or to force the cleanup of toxic waste sites, contaminated drinking water, or air pollution that put nearby residents' health at risk.

A range of relevant strategies outside the health care sector have focused on reducing stressful conditions (as opposed to merely buffering the damaging effects of stressful conditions on health). Many examples of these strategies are discussed in other chapters in this book—focusing, for example, on improving living conditions in early childhood; reducing the prevalence and depth of poverty, especially childhood poverty; building wealth (so that people have resources to fall back on in times of unexpected need, such as during the COVID-19 pandemic); and improving education, work, neighborhood conditions, and housing. For example, programs focused on early childhood education (e.g., Head Start and Early Head Start) and increasing educational and employment opportunities can translate into greater social and economic resources to cope with life's challenges, thereby actually reducing stress. Making high-quality child care and pre-kindergarten universally accessible could have a substantial impact on the stress levels experienced by both low- and middle-income families, as could high-quality affordable housing. Improving access to affordable medical care (e.g., by expanding eligibility for publicly subsidized coverage or providing financial access to everyone through Medicare) could reduce a major source of stress and economic insecurity for many American families—the inability to afford health care.

Existing safety-net programs could be expanded, with wider eligibility and more generous assistance; examples include unemployment benefits, tax credits for low-income working families (e.g., the Earned Income Tax Credit), cash assistance/"welfare" benefits (e.g., Temporary Assistance for Needy Families), subsidized housing and child care, and transportation benefits for low-income working families. These could greatly reduce the ongoing daily stress experienced by low-income and many middle-class families. In both the public and private sectors, family-friendly workplace programs and policies—including flexible scheduling, family leave, breastfeeding support, and onsite or subsidized child care—also could reduce stress among employees as they seek to balance their work and family responsibilities. Initiatives to reduce and ultimately eliminate racism in all forms (see Chapter 5) are a crucial component of any strategy to reduce health-damaging stress. As the upstream (fundamental) source of all forms of racial discrimination and, as such, the source of considerable stress, addressing systemic or structural racism should receive particular attention in efforts to reduce health disparities by reducing stress.

The growing scientific—including biomedical—knowledge about the links between stress and health has tremendous practical significance. Understanding these links—and appreciating the magnitude of the toll that avoidable stress takes on health—can help raise awareness among the public and policymakers about the importance of policies and programs that can help make life less stressful, particularly for those who experience the most stress and are most vulnerable to its health-damaging effects because of poverty and/or racial discrimination. Although much remains to be learned, current knowledge makes it clear that addressing both the causes and the effects of stress—particularly chronic stress, and particularly among children—must be part of a long-range strategy to advance health and eliminate health disparities.

4.6. KEY POINTS

- Stress (the experience of feeling "stressed" or "stressed out") should be distinguished from a stressor (an event or condition that causes stress) and from the stress response—that is, the body's physiologic response to stress.
- Advances in neuroscience have indicated that stress is likely to be an important link between many social factors and health.
- Chronic exposure to stressful everyday hardships appears to be more damaging to health than acute stressors, even when the latter are more dramatic.
- Having inadequate economic resources to cope with basic everyday needs—such as food, shelter, child care, elder care, or medical care—is likely to be stressful, as is experiencing discrimination (unfair treatment based on attributes such as race/ethnic group, skin color, religion, gender, disability, or LGBTQ status).
- The health-damaging effects of stress appear more likely to occur when people experience ongoing or chronic exposure to multiple stressors in aspects of everyday life over which they have limited control.
- Social support appears to help buffer the health-damaging effects of stress.

4.7. QUESTIONS FOR DISCUSSION

1. How plausible is it to you that stress is an important way in which both low income and discrimination can damage health? Why or why not?
2. What major bodily systems are thought to be involved in the effects of stress on health?
3. How can a person's context (e.g., social and financial resources) be important in determining both the stressors they experience and the effects of a given stressor on their health?
4. What should be done to address the toll that stress appears to take on health? Name at least two strategies—including at least one upstream approach—that seem worthwhile and explain why.

ACKNOWLEDGMENTS

This chapter builds on the 2011 issue brief How Social Factors Shape Health: The Role of Stress, by Susan Egerter, Paula Braveman, and Colleen Barclay, which was produced as part of the work of the Robert Wood Johnson Foundation's Vulnerable Populations portfolio. Julia Acker, Nicole Holm, and Tram Nguyen contributed to the research for this chapter.

REFERENCES

Aalto, A.-M., T. Heponiemi, K. Josefsson, M. Arffman, and M. Elovainio. 2018. "Social relationships in physicians' work moderate relationship between workload and wellbeing—9-year follow-up study." *Eur J Public Health* 28(5): 798–804. https://doi.org/10.1093/eurpub/ckx232.

Alhusen, J. L., K. M. Bower, E. Epstein, and P. Sharps. 2016. "Racial discrimination and adverse birth outcomes: An integrative review." *J Midwifery Women's Health* 61(6): 707–720. https://doi.org/10.1111/jmwh.12490.

Almeida, J., L. Bécares, K. Erbetta, V. R. Bettegowda, and I. B. Ahluwalia. 2018. "Racial/ethnic inequities in low birth weight and preterm birth: The role of multiple forms of stress." *Matern Child Health J* 22(8): 1154–1163. https://doi.org/10.1007/s10995-018-2500-7.

American Psychological Association. 2017. *Stress and Health Disparities: Contexts, Mechanisms, and Interventions Among Racial/Ethnic Minority and Low-Socioeconomic Status Populations.* Washington, DC: American Psychological Association.

Aschbacher, K., A. O'Donovan, O. M. Wolkowitz, F. S. Dhabhar, Y. Su, and E. Epel. 2013. "Good stress, bad stress and oxidative stress: Insights from anticipatory cortisol reactivity." *Psychoneuroendocrinology* 38(9): 1698–1708. https://doi.org/10.1016/j.psyneuen.2013.02.004.

Avendano, M., I. Kawachi, F. Van Lenthe, H. C. Boshuizen, J. P. Mackenbach, G. A. M. Van den Bos, M. E. Fay, and L. F. Berkman. 2006. "Socioeconomic status and stroke incidence in the US elderly." *Stroke* 37(6): 1368–1373. https://doi.org/10.1161/01.STR.0000221702.75002.66.

Bauer, M. E., C. M. Jeckel, and C. Luz. 2009. "The role of stress factors during aging of the immune system." *Ann N Y Acad Sci* 1153: 139–152. https://doi.org/10.1111/j.1749-6632.2008.03966.x.

Behrman, R. E., A. S. Butler, and Institute of Medicine (US) Committee on Understanding Premature Birth and Assuring Healthy Outcomes (Eds.). 2007. *Preterm Birth: Causes, Consequences, and Prevention.* Washington, DC: National Academies Press.

Bell, M. P., J. Leopold, D. Berry, and A. V. Hall. 2018. "Diversity, discrimination, and persistent inequality: Hope for the future through the solidarity economy movement." *J Soc Issues* 74(2): 224–243. https://doi.org/10.1111/josi.12266.

Berger, M., and Z. Sarnyai. 2015. "'More than skin deep': Stress neurobiology and mental health consequences of racial discrimination." *Stress* 18(1): 1–10. https://doi.org/10.3109/10253890.2014.989204.

Boden, J. M., D. M. Fergusson, and L. J. Horwood. 2014. "Associations between exposure to stressful life events and alcohol use disorder in a longitudinal birth cohort studied to age 30." *Drug Alcohol Depend* 142: 154–160. https://doi.org/10.1016/j.drugalcdep.2014.06.010.

Braveman, P., C. Cubbin, S. Egerter, D. R. Williams, and E. Pamuk. 2010. "Socioeconomic disparities in health in the United States: What the patterns tell us." *Am J Public Health* 100(Suppl 1): S186–S196. https://doi.org/10.2105/AJPH.2009.166082.

Braveman, P., K. Heck, S. Egerter, T. P. Dominguez, C. Rinki, K. S. Marchi, and M. Curtis. 2017. "Worry about racial discrimination: A missing piece of the puzzle of Black–White disparities in preterm birth?" *PLoS One* 12(10): e0186151.

Braveman, P., K. Heck, S. Egerter, C. Rinki, K. Marchi, and M. Curtis. 2018. "Economic hardship in childhood: A neglected issue in ACE studies?" *Matern Child Health J* 22(3): 308–317. https://doi.org/10.1007/s10995-017-2368-y.

Brody, G. H., T. Yu, Y. F. Chen, S. M. Kogan, G. W. Evans, S. R. Beach, M. Windle, et al. 2013. "Cumulative socioeconomic status risk, allostatic load, and adjustment: A prospective latent profile analysis with contextual and genetic protective factors." *Dev Psychol* 49(5): 913–927. https://doi.org/10.1037/a0028847.

Cao-Lei, L., S. R. de Rooij, S. King, S. G. Matthews, G. A. S. Metz, T. J. Roseboom, and M. Szyf. 2020. "Prenatal stress and epigenetics." *Neurosci Biobehav Rev* 117: 198–210. https://doi.org/10.1016/j.neubiorev.2017.05.016.

Center on Poverty and Social Policy. 2020. "Monthly poverty data." https://www.povertycenter.columbia.edu/forecasting-monthly-poverty-data.

Chetty, R., M. Stepner, S. Abraham, S. Lin, B. Scuderi, N. Turner, A. Bergeron, and D. Cutler. 2016. "The association between income and life expectancy in the United States, 2001–2014." *JAMA* 315(16): 1750–1766. https://doi.org/10.1001/jama.2016.4226.

Cohen, S., D. Janicki-Deverts, and G. E. Miller. 2007. "Psychological stress and disease." *JAMA* 298(14): 1685–1687. https://doi.org/10.1001/jama.298.14.1685.

Cohen, S., M. L. M. Murphy, and A. A. Prather. 2019. "Ten surprising facts about stressful life events and disease risk." *Annu Rev Psychol* 70(1): 577–597. https://doi.org/10.1146/annurev-psych-010418-102857.

Crump, C., E. A. Howell, A. Stroustrup, M. A. McLaughlin, J. Sundquist, and K. Sundquist. 2019. "Association of preterm birth with risk of ischemic heart disease in adulthood." *JAMA Pediatr* 173(8): 736–743. https://doi.org/10.1001/jamapediatrics.2019.1327.

Dhabhar, F. S. 2014. "Effects of stress on immune function: The good, the bad, and the beautiful." *Immunol Res* 58(2–3): 193–210. https://doi.org/10.1007/s12026-014-8517-0.

Dhabhar, F. S. 2019. "The power of positive stress—A complementary commentary." *Stress* 22(5): 526–529. https://doi.org/10.1080/10253890.2019.1634049.

Douros, K., M. Moustaki, S. Tsabouri, A. Papadopoulou, M. Papadopoulos, and K. N. Priftis. 2017. "Prenatal maternal stress and the risk of asthma in children." *Front Pediatr* 5(202). https://doi.org/10.3389/fped.2017.00202.

Duncan, G., K. Magnuson, R. Murnane, and E. Votruba-Drzal. 2019. "Income inequality and the well-being of American families." *Family Relat* 68(3): 313–325. https://doi.org/10.1111/fare.12364.

Elenkov, I. J. 2004. "Glucocorticoids and the Th1/Th2 balance." *Ann N Y Acad Sci* 1024(1): 138–146. https://doi.org/10.1196/annals.1321.010.

Elenkov, I. J., and G. P. Chrousos. 2002. "Stress hormones, proinflammatory and antiinflammatory cytokines, and autoimmunity." *Ann N Y Acad Sci* 966: 290–303. https://doi.org/10.1111/j.1749-6632.2002.tb04229.x.

Evans, G. W., and P. Kim. 2013. "Childhood poverty, chronic stress, self-regulation, and coping." *Child Dev Perspect* 7(1): 43–48. https://doi.org/10.1111/cdep.12013.

Fagundes, C. P., R. Glaser, and J. K. Kiecolt-Glaser. 2013. "Stressful early life experiences and immune dysregulation across the lifespan." *Brain Behav Immun* 27: 8–12. https://doi.org/10.1016/j.bbi.2012.06.014.

Felitti, V. J., R. F. Anda, D. Nordenberg, D. F. Williamson, A. M. Spitz, V. Edwards, M. P. Koss, and J. S. Marks. 2019. "Reprint of: Relationship of childhood abuse and household dysfunction to many of the leading causes of death in adults: The Adverse Childhood Experiences (ACE) study." *Am J Prev Med* 56(6): 774–786. https://doi.org/10.1016/j.amepre.2019.04.001.

Felix, A. S., R. Shisler, T. S. Nolan, B. J. Warren, J. Rhoades, K. S. Barnett, and K. P. Williams. 2019. "High-effort coping and cardiovascular disease among women: A systematic review of the John Henryism hypothesis." *J Urban Health* 96(1): 12–22. https://doi.org/10.1007/s11524-018-00333-1.

Geronimus, A. T., J. Bound, T. A. Waidmann, J. M. Rodriguez, and B. Timpe. 2019. "Weathering, drugs, and Whack-a-Mole: Fundamental and proximate causes of widening educational inequity in U.S. life expectancy by sex and race, 1990–2015." *J Health Soc Behav* 60(2): 222–239. https://doi.org/10.1177/0022146519849932.

Geronimus, A. T., M. Hicken, D. Keene, and J. Bound. 2006. ""Weathering" and age patterns of allostatic load scores among Blacks and Whites in the United States." *Am J Public Health* 96(5): 826–833. https://doi.org/10.2105/AJPH.2004.060749.

Gouin, J. P., L. Hantsoo, and J. K. Kiecolt-Glaser. 2008. "Immune dysregulation and chronic stress among older adults: A review." *Neuroimmunomodulation* 15(4–6): 251–259. https://doi.org/10.1159/000156468.

Gundersen, C., D. Mahatmya, S. Garasky, and B. Lohman. 2011. "Linking psychosocial stressors and childhood obesity." *Obes Rev* 12(5): e54–e63. https://doi.org/10.1111/j.1467-789X.2010.00813.x.

Hajat, A., J. S. Kaufman, K. M. Rose, A. Siddiqi, and J. C. Thomas. 2010. "Long-term effects of wealth on mortality and self-rated health status." *Am J Epidemiol* 173(2): 192–200. https://doi.org/10.1093/aje/kwq348.

Hatch, S. L., and B. P. Dohrenwend. 2007. "Distribution of traumatic and other stressful life events by race/ethnicity, gender, SES and age: A review of the research." *Am J Community Psychol* 40(3–4): 313–332. https://doi.org/10.1007/s10464-007-9134-z.

Hermosura, A. H., S. N. Haynes, and J. K. Kaholokula. 2018. "A preliminary study of the relationship between perceived racism and cardiovascular reactivity and recovery in Native Hawaiians." *J Racial Ethnic Health Disparities* 5(5): 1142–1154. https://doi.org/10.1007/s40615-018-0463-4.

Hicken, M. T., H. Lee, J. Ailshire, S. A. Burgard, and D. R. Williams. 2013. ""Every shut eye, ain't sleep': The role of racism-related vigilance in racial/ethnic disparities in sleep difficulty." *Race Soc Probl* 5(2): 100–112. https://doi.org/10.1007/s12552-013-9095-9.

Holben, D. 2010. "Position of the American Dietetic Association: Food insecurity in the United States." *J Am Dietetic Assoc* 110(9): 1368–1377. https://doi.org/10.1016/j.jada.2010.07.015.

Hudson, D. L., K. M. Bullard, H. W. Neighbors, A. T. Geronimus, J. Yang, and J. S. Jackson. 2012. "Are benefits conferred with greater socioeconomic position undermined by racial discrimination among African American men?" *J Men's Health* 9(2): 127–136. https://doi.org/10.1016/j.jomh.2012.03.006.

Jackson, J. S., K. M. Knight, and J. A. Rafferty. 2010. "Race and unhealthy behaviors: Chronic stress, the HPA axis, and physical and mental health disparities over the life course." *Am J Public Health* 100(5): 933–939. https://doi.org/10.2105/ajph.2008.143446.

Juster, R.-P., B. S. McEwen, and S. J. Lupien. 2010. "Allostatic load biomarkers of chronic stress and impact on health and cognition." *Neurosci Biobehav Rev* 35(1): 2–16. https://doi.org/10.1016/j.neubiorev.2009.10.002.

Karatsoreos, I. N., and B. S. McEwen. 2013. "Annual research review: The neurobiology and physiology of resilience and adaptation across the life course." *J Child Psychol Psychiatry* 54(4): 337–347. https://doi.org/10.1111/jcpp.12054.

Kiecolt-Glaser, J. K., K. J. Preacher, R. C. MacCallum, C. Atkinson, W. B. Malarkey, and R. Glaser. 2003. "Chronic stress and age-related increases in the proinflammatory cytokine IL-6." *Proc Natl Acad Sci USA* 100(15): 9090. https://doi.org/10.1073/pnas.1531903100.

Kivimäki, M., M. Jokela, S. T. Nyberg, A. Singh-Manoux, E. I. Fransson, L. Alfredsson, J. B. Bjorner, et al. 2015. "Long working hours and risk of coronary heart disease and stroke: A systematic review and meta-analysis of published and unpublished data for 603,838 individuals." *Lancet* 386(10005): 1739–1746. https://doi.org/10.1016/S0140-6736(15)60295-1.

Krieger, N. 2014. "Discrimination and health inequities." *Int J Health Services* 44(4): 643–710.

Kushel, M. B., R. Gupta, L. Gee, and J. S. Haas. 2006. "Housing instability and food insecurity as barriers to health care among low-income Americans." *J Gen Intern Med* 21(1): 71–77. https://doi.org/10.1111/j.1525-1497.2005.00278.x.

Lahelma, E., P. Martikainen, O. Rahkonen, E. Roos, and P. Saastamoinen. 2005. "Occupational class inequalities across key domains of health: Results from the Helsinki Health Study." *Eur J Public Health* 15(5): 504–510. https://doi.org/10.1093/eurpub/cki022.

Lantz, P. M., J. S. House, R. P. Mero, and D. R. Williams. 2005. "Stress, life events, and socioeconomic disparities in health: Results from the Americans' Changing Lives Study." *J Health Soc Behav* 46(3): 274–288. https://doi.org/10.1177/002214650504600305.

Lawton, E. M., and M. Sandel. 2014. "Investing in legal prevention: Connecting access to civil justice and healthcare through medical–legal partnership." *J Leg Med* 35(1): 29–39. https://doi.org/10.1080/01947648.2014.884430.

Lê-Scherban, F., A. B. Brenner, M. T. Hicken, B. L. Needham, T. Seeman, R. P. Sloan, X. Wang, and A. V. Diez Roux. 2018. "Child and adult socioeconomic status and the cortisol response to acute stress: Evidence from the Multi-Ethnic Study of Atherosclerosis." *Psychosom Med* 80(2): 184–192. https://doi.org/10.1097/PSY.0000000000000543.

Lewis, T. T., C. D. Cogburn, and D. R. Williams. 2015. "Self-reported experiences of discrimination and health: Scientific advances, ongoing controversies, and emerging issues." *Annu Rev Clin Psychol* 11(11): 407–440.

Lockwood, K. G., A. L. Marsland, K. A. Matthews, and P. J. Gianaros. 2018. "Perceived discrimination and cardiovascular health disparities: A multisystem review and health neuroscience perspective." *Ann N Y Acad Sci* 1428(1): 170–207. https://doi.org/10.1111/nyas.13939.

Lu, M. C., V. Tache, G. R. Alexander, M. Kotelchuck, and N. Halfon. 2003. "Preventing low birth weight: Is prenatal care the answer?" *J Maternal–Fetal Neonatal Med* 13(6): 362–380. https://doi.org/10.1080/jmf.13.6.362.380.

Marmot, M. G., H. Bosma, H. Hemingway, E. Brunner, and S. Stansfeld. 1997. "Contribution of job control and other risk factors to social variations in coronary heart disease incidence." *Lancet* 350(9073): 235–239. https://doi.org/10.1016/s0140-6736(97)04244-x.

Matthews, K. A., L. C. Gallo, and S. E. Taylor. 2010. "Are psychosocial factors mediators of socioeconomic status and health connections?" *Ann N Y Acad Sci* 1186(1): 146–173. https://doi.org/10.1111/j.1749-6632.2009.05332.x.

McDonald, S. W., D. Kingston, H. Bayrampour, S. M. Dolan, and S. C. Tough. 2014. "Cumulative psychosocial stress, coping resources, and preterm birth." *Arch Women's Mental Health* 17(6): 559–568. https://doi.org/10.1007/s00737-014-0436-5.

McEwen, B. S. 2001. "Plasticity of the hippocampus: Adaptation to chronic stress and allostatic load." *Ann N Y Acad Sci* 933(1): 265–277. https://doi.org/10.1111/j.1749-6632.2001.tb05830.x.

McEwen, B. S. 2005. "Stressed or stressed out: What is the difference?" *J Psychiatry Neurosci* 30(5): 315–318.

McEwen, B. S. 2008. "Central effects of stress hormones in health and disease: Understanding the protective and damaging effects of stress and stress mediators." *Eur J Pharmacol* 583(2): 174–185. https://doi.org/10.1016/j.ejphar.2007.11.071.

McEwen, B. S. 2017, February. "Neurobiological and systemic effects of chronic stress." *Chronic Stress.* https://doi.org/10.1177/2470547017692328.

McEwen, B. S. 2019. "The good side of 'stress.'" *Stress* 22(5): 524–525. https://doi.org/10.1080/10253890.2019.1631794.

McEwen, B. S., J. D. Gray, and C. Nasca. 2015. "Recognizing resilience: Learning from the effects of stress on the brain." *Neurobiol Stress* 1: 1–11. s.

McEwen, B. S., and T. Seeman. 1999. "Protective and damaging effects of mediators of stress: Elaborating and testing the concepts of allostasis and allostatic load." *Ann N Y Acad Sci* 896: 30–47. https://doi.org/10.1111/j.1749-6632.1999.tb08103.x.

McNamara, M., P. Bohle, and M. Quinlan. 2011. "Precarious employment, working hours, work-life conflict and health in hotel work." *Appl Ergon* 42(2): 225–232. https://doi.org/10.1016/j.apergo.2010.06.013.

Mefford, M. T., M. A. Mittleman, B. H. Li, L. X. Qian, K. Reynolds, H. Zhou, T. N. Harrison, et al. 2020. "Sociopolitical stress and acute cardiovascular disease hospitalizations around the 2016 presidential election." *Proc Natl Acad Sci USA* 117(43): 27054–27058. https://doi.org/10.1073/pnas.2012096117.

Miller, G. E., E. Chen, and E. S. Zhou. 2007. "If it goes up, must it come down? Chronic stress and the hypothalamic–pituitary–adrenocortical axis in humans." *Psychol Bull* 133(1): 25–45. http://dx.doi.org/10.1037/0033-2909.133.1.25.

Mouchacca, J., G. R. Abbott, and K. Ball. 2013. "Associations between psychological stress, eating, physical activity, sedentary behaviours and body weight among women: A longitudinal study." *BMC Public Health* 13(1): 828. https://doi.org/10.1186/1471-2458-13-828.

Nuru-Jeter, A., T. P. Dominguez, W. P. Hammond, J. Leu, M. Skaff, S. Egerter, C. P. Jones, and P. Braveman. 2009. "'It's the skin you're in': African-American women talk about their experiences of racism: An exploratory study to develop measures of racism for birth outcome studies." *Matern Child Health J* 13(1): 29–39. https://doi.org/10.1007/s10995-008-0357-x.

Nyberg, S. T., E. I. Fransson, K. Heikkilä, L. Alfredsson, A. Casini, E. Clays, D. De Bacquer, et al.; for the IPD-Work Consortium. 2013. "Job strain and cardiovascular disease risk factors: Meta-analysis of individual-participant data from 47,000 men and women." *PLoS One* 8(6): e67323. https://doi.org/10.1371/journal.pone.0067323.

Obradović, J., N. R. Bush, J. Stamperdahl, N. E. Adler, and W. T. Boyce. 2010. "Biological sensitivity to context: The interactive effects of stress reactivity and family adversity on socioemotional behavior and school readiness." *Child Dev* 81(1): 270–289. https://doi.org/10.1111/j.1467-8624.2009.01394.x.

Pager, D., and H. Shepherd. 2008. "The sociology of discrimination: Racial discrimination in employment, housing, credit, and consumer markets." *Annu Rev Sociol* 34(1): 181–209. https://doi.org/10.1146/annurev.soc.33.040406.131740.

Parkinson, J. R. C., M. J. Hyde, C. Gale, S. Santhakumaran, and N. Modi. 2013. "Preterm birth and the metabolic syndrome in adult life: A systematic review and meta-analysis." *Pediatrics* 131(4): e1240–e1263. https://doi.org/10.1542/peds.2012-2177.

Pearlin, L. I. 2010. "The life course and the stress process: Some conceptual comparisons." *J Gerontol B Psychol Sci Soc Sci* 65b(2): 207–215. https://doi.org/10.1093/geronb/gbp106.

Piazza, J. R., D. M. Almeida, N. O. Dmitrieva, and L. C. Klein. 2010. "Frontiers in the use of biomarkers of health in research on stress and aging." *J Gerontol Ser B* 65B(5): 513–525. https://doi.org/10.1093/geronb/gbq049.

Razzoli, M., C. Pearson, S. Crow, and A. Bartolomucci. 2017. "Stress, overeating, and obesity: Insights from human studies and preclinical models." *Neurosci Biobehav Rev* 76: 154–162. https://doi.org/10.1016/j.neubiorev.2017.01.026.

Rodgers, A. B., C. P. Morgan, S. L. Bronson, S. Revello, and T. L. Bale. 2013. "Paternal stress exposure alters sperm microRNA content and reprograms offspring HPA stress axis regulation." *J Neurosci* 33(21): 9003. https://doi.org/10.1523/JNEUROSCI.0914-13.2013.

Rosengren, A., S. Hawken, S. Ôunpuu, K. Sliwa, M. Zubaid, W. A. Almahmeed, K. N. Blackett, C. Sitthi-amorn, H. Sato, and S. Yusuf. 2004. "Association of psychosocial risk factors with risk of acute myocardial infarction in 11,119 cases and 13,648 controls from 52 countries (the INTERHEART study): Case–control study." *Lancet* 364(9438): 953–962. https://doi.org/10.1016/S0140-6736(04)17019-0.

Rothstein, R. 2017. The *Color of Law: A Forgotten History of How Our Government Segregated America*. Liveright.

Sasson, I. 2016. "Trends in life expectancy and lifespan variation by educational attainment: United States, 1990–2010." *Demography* 53(2): 269–293. https://doi.org/10.1007/s13524-015-0453-7.

Schetter, C. D., and C. Dolbier. 2011. "Resilience in the context of chronic stress and health in adults." *Soc Personal Psychol Compass* 5(9): 634–652. https://doi.org/10.1111/j.1751-9004.2011.00379.x.

Seeman, T., E. Epel, T. Gruenewald, A. Karlamangla, and B. S. McEwen. 2010. "Socio-economic differentials in peripheral biology: Cumulative allostatic load." *Ann N Y Acad Sci* 1186: 223–239. https://doi.org/10.1111/j.1749-6632.2009.05341.x.

Semega, J., K. R. Fontenot, and M. A. Kollar. 2016. *Income and Poverty in the United States: 2016*. U.S. Census Bureau.

Semega, J., M. Kollar, E. A. Shrider, and J. Creamer. 2020. *Income and Poverty in the United States: 2019* (Table B-3). U.S. Census Bureau.

Sherman, G. D., and P. H. Mehta. 2020. "Stress, cortisol, and social hierarchy." *Curr Opin Psychol* 33: 227–232. https://doi.org/10.1016/j.copsyc.2019.09.013.

Shonkoff, J. P., W. T. Boyce, and B. S. McEwen. 2009. "Neuroscience, molecular biology, and the childhood roots of health disparities: Building a new framework for health promotion and disease prevention." *JAMA* 301(21): 2252–2259. https://doi.org/10.1001/jama.2009.754.

Smith, M. V., N. Gotman, and K. A. Yonkers. 2016. "Early childhood adversity and pregnancy outcomes." *Matern Child Health J* 20(4): 790–798. https://doi.org/10.1007/s10995-015-1909-5.

Sominsky, L., and S. J. Spencer. 2014. "Eating behavior and stress: A pathway to obesity." *Front Psychol* 5(434). https://doi.org/10.3389/fpsyg.2014.00434.

Sorrells, S. F., and R. M. Sapolsky. 2007. "An inflammatory review of glucocorticoid actions in the CNS." *Brain Behav Immun* 21(3): 259–272. https://doi.org/10.1016/j.bbi.2006.11.006.

Steptoe, A., and M. Kivimäki. 2013. "Stress and cardiovascular disease: An update on current knowledge." *Annu Rev Public Health* 34(1): 337–354. https://doi.org/10.1146/annurev-publhealth-031912-114452.

Stults-Kolehmainen, M. A., and R. Sinha. 2014. "The effects of stress on physical activity and exercise." *Sports Med* 44(1): 81–121. https://doi.org/10.1007/s40279-013-0090-5.

Suglia, S. F., K. C. Koenen, R. Boynton-Jarrett, P. S. Chan, C. J. Clark, A. Danese, M. S. Faith, et al. 2018. "Childhood and adolescent adversity and cardiometabolic outcomes: A scientific statement from the American Heart Association." *Circulation* 137(5): e15–e28. https://doi.org/10.1161/cir.0000000000000536.

Tanaka, F., S. Makita, T. Ito, T. Onoda, K. Sakata, and M. Nakamura. 2015. "Relationship between the seismic scale of the 2011 northeast Japan earthquake and the incidence of acute myocardial infarction: A population-based study." *Am Heart J* 169(6): 861–869. https://doi.org/10.1016/j.ahj.2015.02.007.

Taylor, S. E. 2010. "Mechanisms linking early life stress to adult health outcomes." *Proc Natl Acad Sci USA* 107(19): 8507–8512. https://doi.org/10.1073/pnas.1003890107.

Thayer, Z. M., and C. W. Kuzawa. 2011. "Biological memories of past environments: Epigenetic pathways to health disparities." *Epigenetics* 6(7): 798–803. https://doi.org/10.4161/epi.6.7.16222.

Turner, R. J., and W. R. Avison. 2003. "Status variations in stress exposure: Implications for the interpretation of research on race, socioeconomic status, and gender." *J Health Soc Behav* 44(4): 488–505. https://doi.org/10.2307/1519795.

Uchino, B. N., K. Bowen, R. K. de Grey, J. Mikel, and E. B. Fisher. 2018. "Social support and physical health: Models, mechanisms, and opportunities." In *Principles and Concepts of Behavioral Medicine: A Global Handbook*, edited by E. B. Fisher, L. D. Cameron, A. J. Christensen, U. Ehlert, Y. Guo, B. Oldenburg, and F. J. Snoek, 341–372. New York, NY: Springer.

U.S. Census Bureau. 2020. *Income, Poverty and Health Insurance Coverage in the United States: 2019*. U.S. Census Bureau.

Williams, D. R. 2018. "Stress and the mental health of populations of color: Advancing our understanding of race-related stressors." *J Health Soc Behav* 59(4): 466–485. https://doi.org/10.1177/0022146518814251.

Williams, D. R., J. A. Lawrence, and B. A. Davis. 2019. "Racism and health: Evidence and needed research." *Annu Rev Public Health* 40(1): 105–125. https://doi.org/10.1146/annurev-publhealth-040218-043750.

Williams, D. R., and S. A. Mohammed. 2013. "Racism and health I: Pathways and scientific evidence." *Am Behav Sci* 57(8): 1152–1173. https://doi.org/10.1177/0002764213487340.

Williams, D. R., S. A. Mohammed, J. Leavell, and C. Collins. 2010. "Race, socioeconomic status, and health: Complexities, ongoing challenges, and research opportunities." *Ann N Y Acad Sci* 1186: 69–101. https://doi.org/10.1111/j.1749-6632.2009.05339.x.

Wills, T. A., J. M. Sandy, and A. M. Yaeger. 2002. "Stress and smoking in adolescence: A test of directional hypotheses." *Health Psychol* 21(2): 122–130.

Witt, W. P., E. R. Cheng, L. E. Wisk, K. Litzelman, D. Chatterjee, K. Mandell, and F. Wakeel. 2014. "Preterm birth in the United States: The impact of stressful life events prior to conception and maternal age." *Am J Public Health* 104(Suppl 1): S73–S80. https://doi.org/10.2105/ajph.2013.301688.

Yehuda, R., and A. Lehrner. 2018. "Intergenerational transmission of trauma effects: Putative role of epigenetic mechanisms." *World Psychiatry* 17(3): 243–257.

CHAPTER 5

Racism Damages Health Through Many Causal Pathways

5.1. INTRODUCTION

This chapter examines the ways in which racism is linked with health and health disparities. *Discrimination*—unfair treatment based on belonging to (or being perceived as belonging to) a particular social group—is a product of racism. Discriminatory treatment can be directed toward people based on a wide array of characteristics, including, but not limited to, a person's racial/ethnic group, immigration status, national origin, religion, gender, gender identity, disability, or sexual orientation. This chapter focuses largely on race-based unfair treatment—racism and racial discrimination—and concludes with a brief discussion of other types of discrimination and their likely health effects.

5.2. HEALTH VARIES DRAMATICALLY AMONG PEOPLE IN DIFFERENT RACIAL/ETHNIC GROUPS

An extensive body of literature has accumulated showing large and pervasive disparities in health adversely affecting African Americans/Black people (Williams, Priest, and Anderson 2016; Wheeler and Bryant 2017), American Indians/Alaska Natives (Adakai et al. 2018), Hispanics/Latinos (Velasco-Mondragon et al. 2016), some Asian/Pacific Islander subgroups (Le et al. 2017; Huang et al. 2012), and immigrants (Williams et al. 2016; Wheeler and Bryant 2017; Huang et al. 2012; Abuelezam, El-Sayed, and Galea 2018). These differences are seen for a wide range of health indicators and across the life span. The largest and most consistent racial/ethnic

In this chapter and this book, the six major racial/ethnic groups routinely identified in health data are referred to as Black or African American, American Indian/Alaska Native, Asian American, Latino or Hispanic, Native Hawaiian and other Pacific Islanders, and White or European American. For brevity, often only Black, American Indian, Asian, Latino, or White are used. Where data are available, Native Hawaiians/other Pacific Islanders are distinguished from other Asian people.

The Social Determinants of Health and Health Disparities. Paula Braveman, Oxford University Press. © Oxford University Press 2023.
DOI: 10.1093/oso/9780190624118.003.0005

BOX 5.1   **Racial/Ethnic Disparities in Health: Examples from the United States**

- American Indians and Alaska Natives have the lowest average life expectancies at birth and highest rates of diabetes and hypertension among all racial/ethnic groups in the United States (Arias, Xu, and Jim 2014; Adakai et al. 2018).
- A baby born to a Black mother is more than twice as likely to die before reaching their first birthday as a baby born to a White mother (Ely and Driscoll 2019).
- Black women are more than twice as likely as White women to die from causes connected with childbirth (Rossen et al. 2020).
- The average life expectancy at birth of a non-Latino Black male is 4.6 years shorter than that of his White counterpart (Arias and Xu 2019).
- Although Latinos/Hispanics have a longer average life expectancy at birth and fare better on many health indicators (a "paradox" discussed later in this chapter), they experience disproportionately higher

rates of diabetes and liver diseases relative to some or all other racial or ethnic groups (Lazo, Bilal, and Perez-Escamilla 2015; Velasco-Mondragon et al. 2016). Rates also vary according to countries or areas of origin.

- Asian Americans considered as a whole group generally experience favorable health outcomes. Aggregated health data, however, mask disproportionate rates of poor health outcomes experienced by some Asian subgroups (Yi et al. 2016; Holland and Palaniappan 2012). For example, in a study of records from a large California health plan, middle-aged or older Filipino, South Asian, and Native Hawaiian/Pacific Islanders had higher rates of diabetes, hypertension, and coronary artery disease compared with Whites and Latinos. Rates for these groups were similar to or greater than rates for Black people (Gordon et al. 2019).

health disparities generally have been observed when comparing Black people and (when data are available) American Indians with White people, although Latinos and some Asian subgroups also have significantly worse health than Whites on some measures. Despite some evidence that disparities in infant mortality and life expectancy by racial/ethnic group have narrowed over time, sizable racial/ethnic disparities persist in these and many other health measures, including maternal mortality (Petersen et al. 2019). Box 5.1 lists examples.

This chapter focuses on racism as a fundamental social determinant of racial disparities in health, discussing the roles of a range of factors. Racism should be understood as an upstream factor that can cause racial disparities in health by triggering cascades of multiple downstream causes (causes that occur closer to the biological mechanisms that result in health outcomes). Downstream causes may include, but are not limited to, differences in environmental exposures (physical and social), stressful experiences (including racial discrimination and/or economic hardship), behaviors, health care, and gene expression.

5.3. RACE VERSUS RACISM
The Concept of Race
To understand the causes of racial disparities in health, it is important to consider the meaning of race. Is there just one race—the human race? Or are there intrinsically different groups of humans who are biologically distinct from each other? Despite extensive scientific evidence to the contrary (discussed below), there has been a long-standing,

widely held, and deeply rooted belief that "race"—as reflected by skin color, hair texture, facial features, and other superficial secondary physical characteristics—reflects fundamental biological differences. This unfounded belief is that the differences are encoded in a person's genetic makeup, making people of different races fundamentally, biologically different. In colonial America, that belief co-evolved with the emerging trans-Atlantic slave trade in the 1600s and 1700s as a justification for the enslavement of African people (Smedley 2007; Krieger 1987; Bailey et al. 2017). Globally, the separation of groups into "superior" and "inferior" races not only has been foundational to slavery but also has justified genocide (Shirer 1991). These notions also have been used to justify many discriminatory laws, policies, and practices that deny equal rights and opportunities based on race—including the "Jim Crow" laws in formerly Confederate states that prevailed for almost 100 years after legal slavery officially ended, severely restricting the rights of African Americans (Bailey et al. 2017; Wormser 2014). Pro-slavery doctors used pseudo-science to explain Black–White differences in anatomy and disease as innate and evidence of Black inferiority. Pro-slavery politicians amplified this science to resist calls for abolition (Krieger 1987; Washington 2006). Reflecting the belief in an underlying biological basis for race, official birth and death records and other health data in the United States have long been reported separately by race, age, and sex. Because age and sex do indeed reflect fundamental biological differences, this reporting practice implicitly tends to reinforce the erroneous notion of race as a biological construct.

If race were biologically based, one might expect to find consistency in classification and consensus about some standard set of mutually exclusive racial groups. The concept of race has been very fluid, however, and operationalized in different ways at different times, which is a further indication of the primarily social nature of the construct. For example, the Nazi movement in 20th-century Germany regarded Jewish people as a race; the rationale for the mass extermination of Jews was that they were an inferior race (Shirer 1991). In the United States during the late 19th/early 20th centuries, many economically struggling White people felt threatened by an influx of immigrants willing to work for lower wages; immigrants from countries such as Ireland, Italy, and Poland were widely regarded as being from races distinct from and inferior to "Whites" (Roediger 2006; Ignatiev 2009). More established European immigrants began to express political power through various institutions (e.g., labor unions) and processes (e.g., race riots) to establish their ethnic groups' superiority to others. Over time, the ethnic identities of the more recently arrived European immigrants were subsumed into "Whiteness," and members of these groups benefited from the legal, political, and social advantages enjoyed by White people in the United States (Roediger 2006; Ignatiev 2009).

To examine the health advantage of Whiteness, Jones et al. (2008) studied how self-reported health varied depending on whether it was examined in relation to survey respondents' "socially assigned race," meaning the race that people generally assumed them to be, or respondents' self-identified race. There were considerable differences in health according to self-identified versus socially assigned race. They found that among respondents who self-identified as Black, Hispanic, or multiracial, the prevalence of excellent or good self-reported health was significantly higher among those who were perceived by others to be White. The same pattern was seen for American Indians but was not statistically significant. A 2020 review of 18 studies of associations between a range of health indicators and socially assigned race reported that most studies have found an association between socially assigned race and health (White et al. 2020). This research reinforces that it is the social experience of living in bodies perceived to be of different races—which society treats differently—as opposed to fundamental biological differences between people of different racial backgrounds, that generally drives differential health outcomes.

Reflecting changing social, economic, and political forces over time, races have been officially categorized in the United States in various ways. The earliest U.S. Census surveys distinguished only Whites, all other free persons, and slaves. Later Census racial categories included White (European ancestry), Black (African ancestry), or Mulatto (mixed), and, in the 1890 census, "Quadroon" (one-quarter Black) and "Octoroon" (one-eighth Black). Census racial categories have changed and expanded to reflect emancipation, immigration, social movements, and political pressure (Pratt, Hixson, and Jones 2015; Karklis and Badger 2015). Currently, the established "racial" categories for reporting federal statistics in the United States are African American/Black, American Indian/Alaska Native, Asian, Native Hawaiian or Other Pacific Islander, and White. Each of these groupings corresponds to ancestry in a continent or other large geographic region (Executive Office of the President 1997).

Since the 1980s, the U.S. Census and vital statistics have collected data on a separate field in addition to "race," to specify whether a person is of "Hispanic origin." This information is officially referred to as a measure of Hispanic *ethnicity* and not of race. This implies that whereas African Americans, Asian Americans, European Americans (Whites), and Indigenous Americans each constitute a separate race, Latinos or Hispanics do not; they are an "ethnic group." This practice implicitly tends to reinforce a notion of race as biological, in contrast to ethnicity, which is social. In practice, however, public health and medical research frequently classifies people into five or six mutually exclusive categories referred to as "racial/ethnic" groups, based on the continent or other large geographic region of ancestry. This is done by creating a category for Latinos/Hispanics regardless of "race" and restricting each of the other groups to non-Latinos/Hispanics (non-Hispanic American Indian, non-Hispanic Black, etc.).

The term "race" often carries the connotation of physical characteristics such as skin color, facial features, and hair texture, whereas "ethnicity" evokes cultural characteristics such as language, beliefs, manner of dress, and dietary practices. Based on recognition that these two categories are not distinct, the term "race/ethnicity" is often used instead of either term alone. In reaction to the "race"-based genocide of 6 million people that occurred during World War II, in much of Europe today the term ethnicity is widely used to encompass characteristics that in the United States would span both race and ethnicity. This approach—using "ethnic group" or "ethnicity" instead of "race" or "racial group"—is more consistent with current science than prevailing approaches in the United States (Braveman and Dominguez 2021). There is no scientific basis for considering African Americans, Asian Americans, European Americans, or American Indians/Alaska Natives to be races rather than ethnic groups while at the same time viewing Latin Americans as an ethnic group but not a race. Each of these racial/ethnic designations reflects ancestral origin in a particular continent or other large region of the world. Given human migrations over tens of thousands of years, each of these groupings also reflects extensive genetic admixture across and within continents/regions. Studies of human genetics have shown that there is more genetic variation among people with the same geographic ancestry than there is between groups of people with different geographic ancestry (Rosenberg et al. 2002). The scientific consensus about racial categories today is that they are primarily social rather than biological constructs (Yudell et al. 2016; Cooper, Kaufman, and Ward 2003; Duster 2005; Witherspoon et al. 2007; Graves and Goodman 2021).

Craig Venter, head of Celera, the private genetics company that partnered with the National Institutes of Health on the Human Genome Project (HGP), stated the following in a White House briefing on the HGP in June 2000:

> The method used by Celera has determined the genetic code of five individuals. We have sequenced the genome of three females and two males, who have identified themselves as Hispanic, Asian, Caucasian, or African American. We did this sampling not in an exclusionary way, but out of respect for the diversity that is America, and to help illustrate that the concept of race has no genetic or scientific basis. In the five Celera genomes, there is no way to tell one ethnicity from another.

This does not imply that there cannot be any genetic differences among people in groups with different geographic ancestry—that is, different racial/ethnic groups. Rather, it means that these minor differences—which typically affect risk of a particular disease, such as Tay–Sachs disease among Jews of Northern European origin—do not define biologically distinct groups. It means that in the vast majority of cases, social differences are most important in shaping health and health disparities. It is also important to understand, furthermore, that even when there are minor, nonfundamental genetic differences between groups of people with different geographic ancestry, those minor differences may not be expressed (i.e., the genes may not have their potential effects on the body) unless people are exposed to certain environmental influences, which are shaped by social policies. (These are referred to as epigenetic effects, which are discussed later) In other words, social differences often control whether or not genetic differences are expressed or suppressed, which further underscores the social nature of racial categories.

Although not useful as a biological category, race is a crucially important social category for monitoring, understanding, and intervening on differences in health (Williams 2001). As used in this book and widely, the terms race, ethnicity, race/ethnicity, or racial/ethnic group all refer to groups of people identified by the large geographic region (often a continent) of their ancestral origin. For example, "Black" denotes African or African American ancestry, "White" denotes European or European American ancestry, and Latino/Hispanic denotes Latin American ancestry. ("Latino" is arguably a more appropriate term than "Hispanic," given that many Latin Americans—for example, those from Brazil, Latin America's largest country—are not Spanish-speaking, and people from Spain—who one would expect to be included as "Hispanics"—are Europeans.) Although many authors and institutions continue to use a separate field for "Hispanic ethnicity" and do not include Hispanic/Latino as a racial category, in this book and in much of the health literature, the major racial/ethnic groups are considered to be African American or Black, American Indian/Alaska Native, Asian American, non-Latino/Hispanic European American, Latino/Hispanic, Native Hawaiian/Other Pacific Islander, and non-Latino/

Hispanic White. These groups are generally treated as mutually exclusive, although an increasing number of people identify with multiple racial/ethnic categories.

This book uses the term "people of color," which technically refers to all racial/ethnic groups whose skin is darker than that of Whites—that is, all groups other than Whites. In practice, however, "person/people of color" is often used to refer only to African Americans, American Indians/Alaska Natives, and Latinos. As fluid racial categories change over time, the term may come to include or exclude additional groups of people. For example, Arab Americans, who have been counted as White in official reports, at times have been viewed and treated prejudicially as an ethnic group—for example, after the September 11, 2001 (9/11), terrorist attacks (Vidal-Ortiz 2008). Shah et al. (2008) observed an increase in threats and experiences of physical violence against women wearing a hijab in New York City following 9/11. The term people of color suggests that people who are not White share elements of their social experiences in the United States or other nations where Europeans are the dominant racial/ethnic group (Vidal-Ortiz 2008). Sometimes, however, there have been objections to the term in that it may obscure the unique identity, history, or contemporary experiences of people of some racial/ethnic groups in the United States—for example, the uniquely brutal histories of chattel slavery for Black Americans and the systematic genocide of American Indians, which were not experienced by other people of color.

It is sometimes unclear whether Asian Americans, who have experienced considerable discrimination, are included under "people of color." History, however, indicates that they should be. Approximately 120,000 residents of West Coast states who were Japanese immigrants or their citizen children were disenfranchised and forcibly interned (imprisoned) in concentration camps during World War II; this was mandated by Executive Order 9066, signed by President Franklin Delano Roosevelt (Park 2008). Increases in anti-Asian violence were observed after President Trump blamed China for the coronavirus pandemic in early 2020 (Nguyen et al. 2020). Based on anti-Chinese sentiment fomented by politicians, the Chinese Exclusion Act of 1882 prohibited all immigration of laborers from China for 10 years and barred all Chinese workers from citizenship. Many Chinese immigrants already living in the United States at the time of the Chinese Exclusion Act suffered discrimination (Zhang 2019; Boswell 1986; E. Lee 2002). In 1935, Filipinos in Seattle were among the targets of a bill prohibiting marriage between White persons and "Negroes, Orientals, Malays, and persons of Eastern European extraction" (Strandjord 2009). Numerous instances of apparent hate-crime attacks, some fatal, against Asian people have occurred since former President Trump repeatedly and publicly referred to the virus responsible for the COVID-19 pandemic as the "Chinese virus" (Gover, Harper, and Langton 2020).

Racism

Most people use the terms "racism" and "racial discrimination" interchangeably. Both terms are widely understood to refer to physical, verbal, or other incidents of unfair treatment motivated by a conscious intention to discriminate based on a person's race or ethnic group. Such incidents are sometimes referred to as *interpersonal racism* or race-based *interpersonal discrimination*. Unfairly rejecting a qualified person of color for hiring or promotion based on race would be an example of interpersonal racial discrimination, as would the use of a racial slur or inflicting racially motivated physical harm.

> Racism includes not only interpersonal acts of race-based unfair treatment but also internalized racism, which can undermine self-esteem, and systemic or structural racism. Systemic or structural racism is embedded in systems, laws, policies, and institutions, along with long-standing practices and entrenched beliefs. The passage of the Civil Rights Act of 1964, the Voting Rights Act of 1965, and the Fair Housing Act of 1968 made discrimination based on race illegal in multiple domains. However, largely because of systemic or structural racism, the road between enactment and enforcement of these laws has been long and many obstacles remain.

Racism extends beyond unfair interpersonal treatment based on race, however. It can also manifest as *internalized racism*—when members of a group that experiences discrimination actually accept and incorporate into their own thinking the negative attitudes, beliefs, and stereotypes and accordingly feel inferior. The resulting loss of self-esteem can affect health by increasing the risk of unhealthy behaviors (Williams and Mohammed 2013; Kwate and Meyer 2011) and may also have more direct psychological effects (Euteneuer 2014). Someone who has internalized racist beliefs may treat members of their own group in a prejudicial way (Uzogara and Jackson 2016). Williams and Mohammed (2009) wrote,

> The term, racism, refers to an organized system that categorizes population groups into "races," and uses this ranking to preferentially allocate societal goods and resources to groups regarded as superior (Bonilla-Silva 1996). Fundamental to racism is cultural racism that undergirds an ideology of inferiority that ranks some racial groups as inherently or culturally superior to others and supports the social norms and institutions that implement this ideology (Jones 1997). Racism often leads to the development of negative attitudes and beliefs toward racial outgroups (prejudice), and differential treatment of members of these groups by both individuals and social institutions (discrimination). Importantly, because racism is deeply embedded in the culture and institutions of society, discrimination can persist in institutional structures and policies even in the context of marked declines in individual-level racial prejudice and discrimination. . . . Considerable evidence indicates that racial discrimination persists in multiple contexts of American society including housing, labor markets, criminal justice and education (Blank et al. 2004; Fix and Struyk 1993, p. 21).

Systemic (or Structural) Racism

In addition to interpersonal and internalized racism, racism may also be *structural* or *systemic*. Systemic or structural racism refers to race-based inequities that are deeply embedded within systems, laws, policies, institutions, practices, ways of thinking, and values as a result of historical and ongoing injustice and their legacy. Although racial discrimination is no longer legal, socioeconomic and health inequities along racial lines persist because of deeply rooted, unfair systems that continue to operate, at times unconsciously or unintentionally, to sustain a legacy of overtly discriminatory practices, policies, and laws. Systemic or structural racism systematically puts African Americans/Blacks, Hispanics/Latinos, and American Indians/Alaska Natives at an economic and health disadvantage within society. Whether or not the structure or system in its current

form is intentionally discriminatory, it can generally be traced to deliberate acts of racial discrimination
in the past, such as laws mandating
residential segregation by race.
Once in place, structural or systemic

> Systemic racism refers to systems, laws, and policies
> (written and unwritten) that have the effect of discrim-
> inating, regardless of intent.

racism is often self-perpetuating, with damaging effects on health even after the original
explicitly discriminatory law or policy is no longer in place. Racial residential segregation
illustrates this well.

Systemic and structural racism are sometimes used interchangeably, but they have
somewhat different emphases. Systemic racism emphasizes the involvement of entire
systems—such as the criminal justice system, the political system, the economic system,
etc.—including the structures (laws, policies, and practices) that form the framework of
the systems. Structural racism emphasizes the structures themselves. Because systemic
racism includes structural racism, this book often uses "systemic racism" for brevity; at
times, however, both are mentioned for dual emphasis.

Figure 5.1, from Gee and Ro (2009), depicts structural racism as the hidden base of
an iceberg. The visible part of the iceberg, the part we see, represents the overt racism that
manifests in blatant hate crimes and explicit discrimination—the explicitly racist treatment that may be relatively easy to recognize. The visible tip of the iceberg also contains
interpersonal discrimination driven by implicit bias—that is, prejudicial ways of treating
people of color of which the perpetrators are unaware. The base of the iceberg, the part

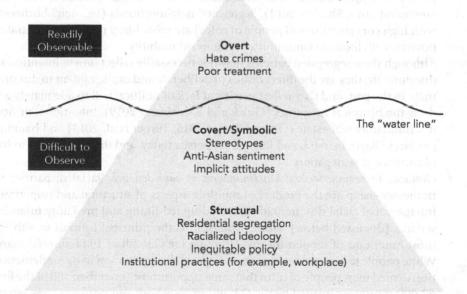

FIGURE 5.1 The racism iceberg. *Source*: Gee, G. C., and A. Ro. 2009. "Racism and discrimination." In *Asian American Communities and Health: Context, Research, Policy and Action*, edited by
C. Trinh-Shevrin, N. S. Islam, and M. J. Rey, 364–402. San Francisco, CA: Jossey-Bass. Copyright ©
2009 by John Wiley & Sons, Inc. All rights reserved.

we usually do not see, represents systemic or structural racism—the societal structures (laws, policies, institutions, practices, norms, and attitudes) that impose and perpetuate barriers to opportunities (e.g., well-paying jobs with benefits, safe neighborhoods with good schools, and access to high-quality health care) that promote health and well-being. Systemic and structural racism—and the ways in which they systematically place people of color at disadvantage in multiple domains that affect health—may be more difficult to recognize; often, it may be seen as the way things must be done and assumed to be unchangeable. Examples of systemic racism include the following:

- *Racial residential segregation* is a particularly clear example of the enduring nature of systemic or structural racism. More than 50 years after the passage of the Fair Housing Act outlawed racial discrimination in housing, the United States remains a highly segregated society. U.S. Census data from 2013 to 2017 show that nationally, the median metropolitan "dissimilarity index"—a measure comparing two groups of people and indicating the percentage of one group that would need to move in order for the two groups to be fully integrated—was 52.6, meaning that 52.6% of Black people would need to move in order to be fully integrated with White people (Governing 2019). Although this represents a decline in Black–White segregation in the United States, it is still considered high. Segregation varies widely by metropolitan area (Frey 2018). For example, for the same years, in cities such as Milwaukee, Chicago, and New York, at least three out of four Black residents would need to move to achieve full integration with Whites (Frey 2018). Segregation plays a major role in socioeconomic inequality. Black and Hispanic people of all incomes are more likely than Whites with similar incomes to live in neighborhoods with concentrated disadvantage (Reardon, Fox, and Townsend 2015; Sharkey 2014). Segregated neighborhoods (i.e., neighborhoods with high concentrations of people of color) are more likely to have concentrated poverty, with limited opportunities for upward mobility.
  Although these segregated patterns may not necessarily reflect *current* intention to discriminate, they are the direct results of deliberate and explicit intent to discriminate in the past, and they reflect persistent lack of political will to adequately address the historical inequities (Quick and Kahlenberg 2019). Intentional or not, discriminatory real estate (Oh and Yinger 2015; Turner et al. 2013) and banking practices (Bayer, Ferreira, and Ross 2014) persist today, and they contribute to the persistence of segregation.
- *Obstacles to homeownership: Discrimination in bank lending.* Racial disparities in homeownership are the product of multiple aspects of structural and sometimes interpersonal racial discrimination, including red-lining and predatory financial services (discussed below). Homeownership is the principal form of wealth for most Americans of modest means. Although the G.I. Bill of 1944 allowed many White people to become homeowners, flagrant discrimination in its implementation denied most people of color that same opportunity. Fewer than 100 of the first 67,000 mortgages insured by the G.I. Bill in New York and northern New Jersey, for example, were issued to non-White people (Katznelson 2005). Similarly, although low-interest Federal Housing Authority (FHA) loans made available by the National Housing Act in 1934 enabled many Whites to accumulate wealth

in the form of homeownership, ill-concealed racial discrimination often denied that opportunity to people of color. A study of seven large metropolitan real estate markets found that during the U.S. housing bubble of 2004–2008, African American and Latino borrowers were more likely to receive high-cost, subprime mortgage loans even when controlling for common indicators of creditworthiness and risk (Bayer, Ferreira, and Ross 2014).

- *Red-lining.* Beginning in the 1930s, guidelines established by the federal Home Owners' Loan Corporation (HOLC), later adopted by private banks, explicitly used neighborhood racial/ethnic composition (and income level) in determining and ranking the riskiness of mortgage lending (Swope and Hernández 2019). During decades when federal loan programs expanded homeownership among Whites, particularly in the growing suburbs, non-White and low-income areas were disproportionately "redlined"—a term referring to the red shading on HOLC maps of neighborhoods deemed "hazardous" for lending. Racial/ethnic differences in homeownership, home values, and credit scores in redlined areas persist to the present day (Aaronson, Hartley, and Mazumder 2017; Mitchell and Franco 2018).

- *Obstacles to economic well-being in general.* Predatory financial services—including payday lenders and check-cashing services that typically charge excessive fees and usurious interest rates—are known to disproportionately target communities of color (Faber 2016). These "fringe" financial services place heavy costs on and limit opportunities to build wealth for communities of color; predatory financial services are thus another important example of systemic or structural racism. Even when mainstream banking services are available, people of color are often subjected to higher costs associated with these services. Even small community banks in majority Black and interracial neighborhoods have higher minimum opening deposits and balances for checking accounts than banks in majority White neighborhoods. This means that greater shares of Black and Latino people's incomes must be sequestered in checking accounts to avoid fees (Faber and Friedline 2018). As also occurs with red-lining, these practices create obstacles to homeownership and to starting or expanding businesses. Like residential segregation, predatory financial services can harm health by constraining socioeconomic opportunities and can have self-perpetuating effects.

- *Environmental injustice.* Racially segregated communities of color have often experienced the damaging health effects of environmental injustice. They are disproportionately used as sites for sources of pollution, such as coal-fired power plants, and for hazardous waste disposal, with documented serious adverse effects on health (Cushing, Faust, et al. 2015; Morello-Frosch and Lopez 2006; Cushing, Morello-Frosch, et al. 2015). A telling example of environmental injustice occurred in Flint, Michigan, in 2014, with contamination of the water supply creating a crisis of lead poisoning among the city's children. The Flint water crisis, discussed later, reflected a legacy of residential racial segregation, concentrated poverty, disinvestment in city resources and infrastructure, and dismissal and inaction on behalf of those in power, with devastating, disproportionate impact on the largely Black residents of Flint. (See Chapter 7.)

- *Racially discriminatory policing and sentencing practices* and resulting inequities in incarceration rates are well documented (Wildeman and Wang 2017; Pettit and Western 2004; Western 2006). Although people of color represent 39% of the U.S. population, they comprise 60% of incarcerated persons (The Sentencing Project 2018). Black, American Indian, and Latino youth are 5, 3, and 1.65 times, respectively, more likely than White youth to be incarcerated (The Sentencing Project 2017a, 2017b, 2017c). At the rates of incarceration in 2001, researchers estimated that one in three Black men born that year would be incarcerated during his lifetime (Bonczar 2003). At the peak of U.S. incarceration rates in 2007, the rate for Black men who had not completed high school was 50 times the national average (Western and Simes 2019). Since that time, incarceration rates for Black people have declined; nonetheless, Black–White disparities in incarceration remain extreme (Western and Simes 2019), and the devastating impacts on the life trajectories of incarcerated people and their families persist. Mass incarceration has exacerbated racial disparities in income and wealth by stigmatizing young people of color, thereby denying them opportunities to obtain employment after release and restricting long-term economic options for them, their families, and their communities. The roots of mass incarceration can be traced to the Reagan-era "War on Drugs" during the 1980s, which aggressively criminalized drug use, with selective enforcement in poor communities of color. Mass incarceration of people of color was greatly accelerated during the 1990s by legislation passed during the Clinton administration.
- *Unequal access to quality education.* Given the powerful links between education, income, and health (World Health Organization Commission on Social Determinants of Health 2008), disparities in education translate into economic and health disparities across the life course. Schools' dependence on local property taxes results in schools in segregated areas often being poorly resourced and therefore underperforming (Owens 2017), making it difficult for children to escape from poverty as adults. Although this affects poor White people as well, it disproportionately affects Black people because systemic racism has resulted in higher rates of poverty, low income, and concentrated community poverty among the latter. Property tax revenue is lower in segregated areas because of racism-based obstacles to homeownership and wealth mentioned above. Because of resource constraints, schoolchildren in racially segregated neighborhoods are less likely to experience the academic and extracurricular enrichments available in largely White neighborhoods; their teachers may be unable to devote the time necessary to provide additional support needed by at-risk students (Williams and Collins 2001).

  The *school-to-prison pipeline* refers to the phenomenon in which children—mainly but not exclusively boys—of color are systematically disciplined more harshly in school than other children for behavioral problems that warrant counseling and support rather than punishment. "Zero tolerance" policies treat a range of nonviolent misbehaviors with severe punishments, including suspension and expulsion. Related policies include stationing police officers inside schools and/or calling the police into schools to deal with misbehavior by students of color. The involvement of police and suspensions/expulsions raise the risk of school dropout and incarceration. Low-income children of color—who are more likely to have suffered trauma and therefore to exhibit behavioral problems—are far more likely to be suspended or expelled than their White counterparts (Hirschfield 2008; Mallett 2016; Nelson and Lind 2015). Like many other discriminatory patterns, the school-to-prison pipeline is not based on written policies explicitly instructing school personnel to treat Black, Brown, and Indigenous children more harshly than others. Nevertheless, the effects are profoundly discriminatory and rooted in policies and attitudes that reflect systemic racism.

- *Racial discrimination in employment due to overt or implicit bias* can reflect systemic as well as interpersonal racism; it places people of color at a disadvantage that translates into disparities in earning potential, which can affect health. (See Chapter 2.) Although illegal since 1964, racial discrimination in hiring, pay, and promotions persists (Bonilla-Silva 2018; Pager and Shepherd 2008). Discriminatory procedures may be so firmly embedded in recruitment, hiring, and promotion practices—for example, preference for graduates of elite schools, or negative assumptions about people with certain kinds of race-/ethnicity-associated names, ways of speaking, or manners of dress—that people of color may not have a fair chance of being considered for their abilities.

- *Political disenfranchisement/disempowerment through systemic racism: Gerrymandering and voter suppression.* The legal right for all men to vote regardless of race was secured on paper in 1870 with the 15th amendment. Voter suppression of Black people was maintained, however, through violent, organized intimidation and onerous, selectively applied requirements in formerly Confederate states during the almost 100-year reign of Jim Crow laws. The 1964 Civil Rights Act outlawed the blatantly unequal application of voter registration requirements, but requirements that differentially and adversely affect people of color remain to this day. For example, voter identification laws and restrictions on early and absentee voting differentially affect people of color; restrictions on voting for felons disproportionately affect Black and other people of color because they are—unjustly—disproportionately likely to have been incarcerated.

  Gerrymandering is the systematic and deliberate redrawing of the boundaries of electoral districts for the express purpose of favoring the political party in power in subsequent elections. It makes some people's votes, often those of people of color, count less than the votes of others, depriving the affected voters of full representation. The practice has a long history—two centuries—in the United States and is still in effect today (Bentele and O'Brien 2013; Keyssar 2009; Solomon, Maxwell, and Castro 2019; Tausanovitch 2019; Uggen, Larson, and Shannon 2016).

- *The forcible internment of approximately 120,000 West Coast Japanese immigrants and their citizen children during World War II* is an example of structural racism. Discussed further later in this chapter, it was mandated by law—Executive Order 9066—signed by President Franklin Delano Roosevelt following the bombing of Pearl Harbor, as a national security measure. Neither German nor Italian immigrants were interned (Park 2008). Serious adverse health consequences of the internment have been documented (Jensen 1998).

- *Boarding schools for Indigenous American children* are another historical example of systemic racism. Throughout much of the 19th century and until 1978, thousands of school-age American Indian children in the United States and Canada were forcibly removed from their families and placed in generally harsh and often abusive boarding schools located far from their families. This was a deliberate federally funded effort to cut children off from their Native cultures so they would assimilate. Attendance at these schools has been tied to multiple adverse health consequences (although some attendees experienced some socioeconomic benefits) (Evans-Campbell et al. 2012; Feir 2016; Pember 2019). In 2021, the remains of 215 children were discovered in mass graves at one of these sites in Canada, and this issue is being investigated in the United States as well (U.S. Department of the Interior 2021).

5.4. HOW RACISM CAN DAMAGE HEALTH

How Racism Is Thought to Produce Inequities in Health:
A General Overview

Racism can damage the health of people of color through many different causal pathways. An extensive and growing body of scientific research indicates how diverse experiences of racism likely play a fundamental role in producing racial/ethnic disparities in health by setting in motion different causal pathways—that is, sequential chains of consecutive causes. These pathways can be complex and long, often playing out over lifetimes and even generations. The complexity and length of the causal pathways often make it difficult to detect their origins—that is, the underlying causes of the observed causes—the hidden but largest and most dangerous part of the iceberg.

Although the focus here is on how racism can damage the health of people of color, it is important to note that it may damage the health and well-being of virtually the entire society in which it operates. The evidence for this hypothesis comes from research on social inequality in general rather than on racism specifically; the case has been made that social inequality damages the health of societies overall, largely by undermining social cohesion (Wilkinson and Pickett 2009; McGhee 2021).

Based on the literature, Figure 5.2 depicts, in a greatly simplified way, a series of sequential general steps through which racism is thought to produce racial disparities in health. A number of the factors listed in Figure 5.2 could arguably be placed in more than one box. The first box on the left in Figure 5.2 represents the beginning of the causal pathways, with systemic racism, the unjust systems or structures that result in unfair treatment and differential access to resources and opportunities (the second box). In turn, the unfair treatment and differential access to resources and opportunities result not only in exposure to health-harming conditions (e.g., toxic environmental hazards and chronic stress) but also limited access to conditions that are health-promoting, such as good schools, a nutritious diet, green spaces, bicycle lanes, being able to afford a gym membership, and quality medical care; these are represented by the third box. These health-harming (or lack of health-promoting) exposures or experiences in turn more immediately trigger the biological mechanisms that produce ill health (the fourth box).

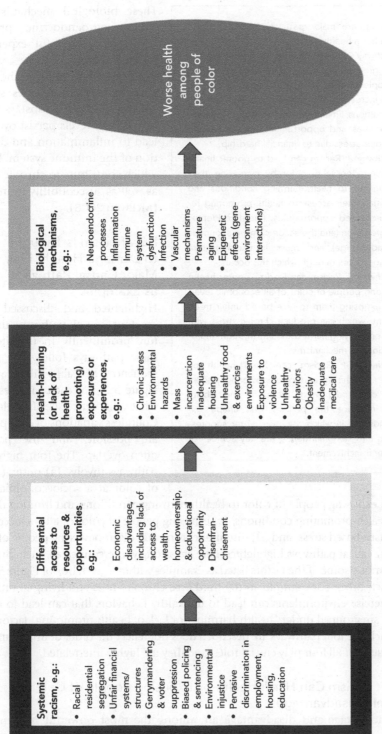

FIGURE 5.2 How racism is thought to damage health: A general overview of key sequential steps, from upstream to downstream influences.

The following are major pathways through which racism can harm health:

- *Pathway 1*: Racism can harm health by leading to greater economic disadvantage among people of color. This leads to poorer health by increasing exposures to health-harming conditions, limiting access to health-promoting resources and opportunities, and increasing chronic stress due to financial hardship.
- *Pathway 2*: Racism can lead to poorer health among people of color by increasing their exposure to health-harming conditions and limiting their access to health-promoting resources and opportunities. Racial residential segregation (and the accompanying economic disadvantage) and mass incarceration are major routes through which this occurs.
- *Pathway 3*: Racism can lead to poorer health among people of color of all economic levels by exposing them to race-based unfair treatment, which can produce chronic stress with accompanying harm to health through neuroendocrine mechanisms.
- *Pathway 4*: Racism can harm health by disenfranchising and disempowering people of color, depriving them of the ability to influence the policies that shape the conditions in which they live. Voter suppression and gerrymandering are key sources of disenfranchisement.

These biological mechanisms include neuroendocrine processes triggered by stressful experiences. When chronic, these stressful experiences can result in the body's production of hormones such as cortisol (and other substances) that can, if high levels persist over time, lead to inflammation and dysfunction of the immune system, both of which contribute to chronic disease as well as susceptibility to infection (McEwen 2008).

How Racism Is Thought to Damage Health: Four Major Causal Pathways as Examples

Highlighted and discussed below are four causal pathways that feature prominently in the literature; these pathways follow the general sequence of steps illustrated in Figure 5.2, but each involves somewhat different specific elements. Countless variations of each pathway are possible, and the pathways often overlap. The four highlighted pathways involve (a) putting people of color at a socioeconomic disadvantage, (b) exposing people of color to health-harming conditions and limiting their exposure to health-promoting conditions, (c) exposing people of color of all socioeconomic levels to racism-based stress, and (d) disenfranchising and disempowering people of color.

The four causal pathways highlighted here are strongly interconnected, including causally. Furthermore, some of the factors listed as examples within a given box of Figure 5.2 may influence each other. For example, in the third box, chronic stress and living in unhealthy food and exercise environments can lead to unhealthy behaviors that can lead to obesity, all of which are grouped under "health-harming (or lack of health-promoting) factors." The order in which the four pathways are described does not reflect the order of importance; evidence suggests that all four play crucial roles, and they are highly interrelated.

Pathway 1: Racism Can Harm Health by Exposing People of Color to Economic Disadvantage

Economic advantage and disadvantage are among the most powerful influences on health (World Health Organization Commission on Social Determinants of Health 2008;

McDonough et al. 1997; Martinson and Reichman 2016; Lantz et al. 1998; Hajat et al. 2010a, 2010b; Demakakos et al. 2016; Daly et al. 2002; Chetty et al. 2016; Case, Lubotsky, and Paxson 2002; Braveman et al. 2010; Braveman and Egerter 2008; Blumenshine et al. 2010). (See Chapter 2.) Lower levels of income, accumulated wealth, and education among people of color have repeatedly been shown to be major contributors to racial or ethnic disparities in health (Williams et al. 2016; Pollack et al. 2013; Adler and Rehkopf 2008; Braveman et al. 2005). Given the well-documented effects of economic conditions on health, racially discriminatory obstacles to economic resources and opportunities are a major pathway through which racism can harm health (Williams and Collins 2001; Williams, Lawrence, and Davis 2019; Bailey et al. 2017).

African Americans, American Indians/Alaska Natives, and Latinos are disproportionately represented among economically disadvantaged groups in the United States. Figure 5.3 shows striking racial/ethnic differences in median income for the largest ethnic groups; it is important to note that these aggregated figures can mask large disparities among smaller ethnic subgroups, distinguished by national origin or tribe (López, Ruiz, and Patten 2017; Kochhar and Cilluffo 2018). When official statistics fail to provide information on marginalized or excluded ethnic groups, such as Indigenous groups or disadvantaged subgroups of Asian Americans, this can render the marginalized groups invisible, adding to the likelihood that policies and programs will not address their needs.

Wealth varies by race even more than does income and may be more important for health. As a consequence of many aspects of racism—particularly the historic and contemporary policies and practices noted above that have made it difficult for people of color to accumulate wealth—accumulated financial assets vary even more by racial/

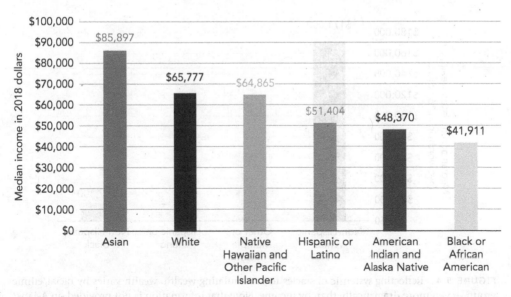

FIGURE 5.3 The median income of U.S. households varies markedly by racial/ethnic group. Households are categorized by the racial/ethnic group of the person in whose name a home is owned or rented. *Sources*: U.S. Census Bureau, 2018 American Community Survey and 2018 Puerto Rico Community Survey.

ethnic group than does income. Figure 5.4 shows that in 2016, the median wealth of White households was 10 times that of Black households and 8.3 times that of Latino households (Board of Governors of the Federal Reserve System 2016). Income measures earnings over a finite period of time—typically 2 weeks, 1 month, or 1 year—whereas wealth refers to the current monetary value of all of a person's or household's accumulated (including inherited) assets—such as the value of a home and other real estate, vehicles, jewelry, savings, stocks and other investments, and any other possessions with monetary value. Because it reflects financial resources accumulated over time, wealth may be a better measure of relative socioeconomic advantage than income; it may be more likely to capture one's economic conditions during childhood. Wealth is more difficult than income to measure, however, and thus is rarely measured in health research. Wealth provides security; it is a financial safety net to fall back on during times of temporary unemployment (such as experienced by so many people during the COVID-19 pandemic), unexpected medical expenses, or other unanticipated bills. Wealth also tends to better reflect a person's economic conditions during childhood. Conditions in childhood could have particularly strong effects on health throughout life, including adulthood (Kim et al. 2013; Blumenshine et al. 2010; Pervanidou and Chrousos 2011; Shonkoff et al. 2012; Sonu, Post, and Feinglass 2019; Corcoran 1995).

The lower incomes and wealth of African Americans, American Indians/Alaska Natives, and Latinos reflect historical and ongoing systemic discrimination in banking, education, housing, and hiring and promotions (Williams and Collins 2001; Pager and Shepherd 2008; Williams et al. 2019). The legacy of formerly legal discrimination

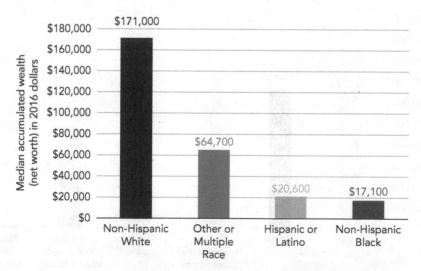

FIGURE 5.4 Reflecting systemic obstacles to accumulating wealth, wealth varies by racial/ethnic group—even more dramatically than by income. Note that information is not provided on Asians/Pacific Islanders, American Indians/Alaska Natives, or other groups, presumably included among "Other/Multiple Races." *Source*: Survey of Consumer Finances (Board of Governors of the Federal Reserve System, 2016).

continues to shape living and working conditions that systematically keep people of color at economic disadvantage (Williams and Collins 2001; Gee and Ford 2011; Williams et al. 2019).

People of color have experienced and continue to experience major racism-related obstacles to economic opportunity (Williams and Collins 2001; Swope and Hernández 2019; Pager and Shepherd 2008; Rothstein 2017; Katznelson 2005). The striking disparities in income—strongly correlated with disparities in health—between different racial and ethnic groups in the United States reflect a long history of de jure (by law) and de facto (by fact; in effect, based on deeply entrenched institutional practices rather than on law) discriminatory policies and practices rooted in systemic racism. Many were intentionally built into policies and laws that limited access to resources and opportunities. Enslaved people had no property rights. The end of outright slavery was followed by the brief period called Reconstruction during which significant advances were made in the rights, including property rights, of former slaves. Those advances were largely rolled back, however, beginning in 1877 when federal troops withdrew from occupying former Confederate states. This initiated almost 100 years of Jim Crow laws in those states, deliberately and systematically making it difficult for Black as well as Asian and Latino people to realize their rights and to accumulate wealth (Rothstein 2017). Low-interest G.I. and FHA loans (described previously) enabled many Whites to buy homes but were given to few Black people (Rothstein 2017). The "Great Recession" of 2007–2009 exacerbated already large racial or ethnic gaps in wealth that had been growing steadily for years: Although people in every racial/ethnic group experienced steep declines in wealth, people of color were disproportionately affected (Kochhar and Fry 2014), in part because African American and Latino borrowers were more likely to have high-cost, subprime mortgage loans, reflecting discriminatory lending practices (Bocian, Ernst, and Li 2008; Steil et al. 2018).

Racial/ethnic differences in economic resources are amplified by gender. Women of color have substantially less wealth compared both with men of the same racial group and with White women (Richard 2014). In 2007, for example, the median wealth levels for single Black, Latina, and White women were $100, $120, and $41,500, respectively, compared to $7,900, $9,730, and $43,800 for single Black, Latino, and White men (Chang 2010). These striking differences both by gender and by race are not explained by differences in educational attainment: Single White women *without* bachelor's degrees have $3,000 more wealth than single Black women *with* bachelor's degrees (Zaw et al. 2017).

Given the effects of socioeconomic conditions on health, unmeasured socioeconomic differences due to racism—such as differences in accumulated wealth, neighborhood socioeconomic conditions, or childhood circumstances—are likely to play a significant role in racial/ethnic disparities in health. Socioeconomic advantage and disadvantage, particularly in childhood, have powerful effects on health across the life course. These factors, however, are rarely measured in health studies. Despite this limitation, many studies claim to have "controlled for socioeconomic status" when they have measured only a small fraction of the socioeconomic factors likely to have affected health. Many conclude, without scientific justification, that an observed racial/ethnic difference in health must be due to underlying biological differences (Braveman et al. 2005). Economic disadvantage also may exacerbate disenfranchisement and disempowerment.

Pathway 2: Racism Exposes Many People of Color to Health-Damaging Conditions and Limits Their Access to Health-Promoting Resources and Opportunities

Another important causal pathway through which racism can harm health involves greater exposure to health-harming conditions and more limited access to health-promoting resources and opportunities. This disproportionately affects low-income people of color but may affect people of color of all socioeconomic levels. The forcible internment of Japanese immigrants and their citizen children during World War II, noted previously, exposed approximately 120,000 people to multiple health-harming environmental conditions, including crowding and extremes of cold, heat, and dust. Careers, businesses, and lives were disrupted and sometimes permanently lost (Park 2008). Increased rates of suicide, cardiovascular disease, and premature death were linked to the internment (Jensen 1998). Greater exposure to the novel coronavirus (because of residential crowding, dependence on public transportation, and potentially conditions in low-wage service jobs) is thought to be a likely important explanation for the disproportionate rates of COVID-19 affecting low-income Latino communities (Wood 2020; Macias Gil et al. 2020). Additional examples are discussed below.

Greater Exposure to Environmental Health Hazards

Racism can lead to poorer health through the disproportionate exposure of people of color to environmental hazards in their homes, neighborhoods, and workplaces as a result of poverty or racial residential segregation. Environmental injustice, defined as the systematically higher exposure of low-income communities (particularly those of color) to environmental hazards such as hazardous waste sites and poor quality water, has been well documented (Cushing, Faust, et al. 2015; Cushing, Morello-Frosch, et al. 2015; Morello-Frosch and Lopez 2006). In 2014, for example, dangerous lead levels were discovered in the water supply of Flint, Michigan. The contamination resulted from cost-savings measures by city officials. Many believe that both the contamination and officials' inadequate initial response reflected disregard for the well-being of Flint's predominantly Black low-income population (Michigan Civil Rights Commission 2017; Mohai 2018). In the 18 months of city inaction, the incidence of elevated blood lead levels in young children doubled, with likely serious implications for children's long-term health and life trajectories (Hanna-Attisha et al. 2015). Environmental injustice and racial segregation both reflect systemic racism. Segregation exposes people of color to both physical hazards and adverse social environments, such as the high levels of crime that often accompany concentrated poverty. People of color also are more likely to be exposed to hazardous substances at work, given the concentration of people of color in low-status employment (Murray 2003), reflecting inequities in education as well as in hiring.

Widespread and Recurring Racially Motivated Acts of Physical Violence

Although slavery has been outlawed in the United States for more than 150 years, it is important to understand racism in a historical context. There is increasing recognition of how historical trauma may harm health—how traumatic events even in the distant past can be sources of ongoing stress today. Epigenetic effects (gene–environment interactions) may, for example, explain how health effects of slavery could persist today. Traumatic experiences may have epigenetic effects that can be inherited from one generation to another (Thayer and Kuzawa 2011; Yehuda and Lehrner 2018). Epigenetic effects do not alter a person's DNA. They can be thought of as "on/off" switches that control whether one's DNA is expressed or suppressed.

Enslaving people is intrinsically violent; keeping people enslaved requires ongoing violence and/or the threat of it. Along with harsh working conditions and inadequate housing and nutrition, whipping and other brutal forms of physical punishment and torture were used with impunity by slaveholders. Slavery in the United States extended over a 250-year period that ended officially in 1865 at the end of the Civil War (or, arguably, in 1868 with passage of the Fourteenth Amendment to the U.S. Constitution). As noted previously, during the Jim Crow period, which lasted for almost 100 years following the end of Reconstruction after the Civil War, many laws, policies, and practices were established in former Confederate states with the express purpose of constraining the new rights of Black people; these were enforced through violence and terror, for example, by the Ku Klux Klan. Lynching is the premeditated, extrajudicial murder of a person or persons by a group. Lynching was used to punish Black people deemed to have "crossed a line" (typically by being insufficiently submissive to a White person or asserting their rights) and to intimidate other Black people. During the period between the end of Reconstruction and 1950, more than 4,000 lynchings have been documented, a likely undercount; although the vast majority of victims were Black, some Whites were also lynched for helping Black people (Equal Justice Initiative 2017).

Discriminatory Policing, Police Violence, and Mass Incarceration

Widespread racial bias in policing (Ross 2015; Spencer, Charbonneau, and Glaser 2016; Kahn and Martin 2016), sentencing (Kutateladze et al. 2014; Nellis 2016), and incarceration has been well documented (Nellis 2016; Burch 2015). Neighborhoods with many Black or Latino residents are more often the targets of intensive policing than predominantly White neighborhoods; neighborhoods with many residents of color are placed under ongoing surveillance and subjected to frequent stops without cause. For example, New York City's "stop and frisk" policy, most active during 2010–2013, but still in operation through 2017 (Astor 2020; Southall and Gold 2019), empowered police to stop anyone they thought might have committed *or be likely to commit* a crime; the latter was widely interpreted by police to mean any young man of color. Without any evidence that a crime had been committed, police would often search the "suspects" and treat them disrespectfully and often roughly, a humiliating and infuriating experience. A search could easily escalate into arrest—for example, for possessing small amounts of marijuana or other illicit substance that would not have been detected in predominantly White neighborhoods that were not subjected to frequent, arbitrary police searches. Between 2002 and 2017, New Yorkers were subject to more than 5 million police stops, most of which were of Black and Latino people (New York Civil Liberties Union 2019). Comprising just 5% of New York City's population, Black and Latino males between ages 14 and 24 years accounted for 38% of reported stops between

2014 and 2017 (New York Civil Liberties Union 2019). Although the number of stops in the city has dropped dramatically since the peak in 2011, young Black and Latino males continue to be stopped disproportionately, without evidence of their having committed crimes.

Between 2010 and 2014, Black Americans and American Indian/Alaska Natives were nearly three times and Latinos were nearly twice as likely as White Americans to be killed by police officers (Buehler 2016); similar disparities have been noted in other data sources (Edwards, Lee, and Esposito 2019; Bui, Coates, and Matthay 2018; "The Counted" 2016). Well-publicized shooting deaths by police of Black men, women, and children have sparked national and international outrage and greater awareness of implicit bias—that is, prejudice that is not conscious. The outrage has been compounded when, in many cases, the officers involved generally have not initially been charged with crimes or, when charged, have often been acquitted, despite incriminating evidence from bystander videos and/or police body cameras. Although killings by police represent the most extreme form of police violence (Cooper and Fullilove 2020), many more Americans experience nonfatal injuries at the hands of police, with similarly stark racial disparities (Feldman et al. 2016). Community-based surveys suggest that Latino (and queer and gender-nonconforming) people are likelier than others to be victims of police sexual violence (DeVylder et al. 2017). The widespread and persistent patterns reflect a pervasive lesser regard for the lives of people of color by the killer, the police, and the courts; they reflect a sense of impunity in the killers—that is, that the consequences of killing a person of color, if any, will not be severe.

Extreme racial disparities in incarceration rates, driven by discriminatory policing and sentencing, put people of color at greater risk of exposure to the health-harming conditions of incarceration. Black and Latino individuals are more likely to be sentenced to prison and receive longer sentences than White people who have committed similar crimes (Spohn 2000). Many researchers have concluded that Black people are more likely to be sentenced to death for similar crimes committed by White people (Ogletree and Sarat 2006). Incarcerated people, including youth in juvenile correctional facilities, are at considerable risk of experiencing violence, including sexual assault, and/or inadequate medical care while institutionalized (Beck et al. 2013; Mendel 2015; Modvig 2014; Wolff et al. 2007). In a 2017 survey of inmates across 83 prisons in 21 states, 63% of prisoners reported being denied needed health care (Incarcerated Workers Organizing Committee 2018). Given the large racial disparity in incarceration, mass incarceration likely plays a substantial role in race-based disparities in health (Wildeman and Wang 2017; Acker et al. 2019).

Racism Can Harm Health by Limiting the Access of People of Color to the Conditions Needed to Achieve Good Health

Racial residential segregation not only exposes people in segregated neighborhoods to health hazards but also deprives them of access to health-promoting conditions, such as a quality education and safe and appealing recreational spaces for physical activity. Schoolchildren in racially segregated neighborhoods are less likely to experience the academic and extracurricular enrichments available in largely White neighborhoods; their teachers may be unable to devote the time necessary to provide additional support needed by at-risk students (Williams and Collins 2001). Disparities in education generate disparities in health. (See Chapter 3.) These negative health impacts of segregation are not limited to people of color at greatest economic disadvantage; they also can affect middle-class people of color (Adelman 2004; Sharkey 2014).

Racism Can Harm Health (or at the Least Not Promote It) by Leading to Inequitable Access to and Quality of Health Care

Lack of access to quality health care can harm health, or deprive affected people of potential health benefit. Widespread and pervasive racially discriminatory practices affecting the receipt and quality of health care have been shown repeatedly to play a role in racial disparities in health (Feagin and Bennefield 2014; Yearby 2018). Historically, Black people have suffered greatly at the hands of White doctors and researchers (Washington 2006). One of the most infamous incidents of racist exploitation and mistreatment in health care is the Public Health Service Tuskegee Experiment, designed to study the natural course of untreated syphilis. The experiment followed nearly 400 Black men with syphilis for 40 years (1932–1972), deliberately withholding treatment and suppressing information about the men's diagnosis and need for treatment. The Tuskegee Experiment is emblematic of long-standing and widespread racial inequities in health care (Gamble 1997) that reflect deep-seated and pervasive beliefs and attitudes valuing Black people less than Whites. In 2003, the Institute (now National Academy) of Medicine's landmark report *Unequal Treatment* (Institute of Medicine Committee on Understanding and Eliminating Racial and Ethnic Disparities in Health Care 2003) documented widespread disparities in the medical care received by people of color compared with Whites; evidence collected since that report shows that significant disparities in care continue (Fiscella and Sanders 2016; Hoffman et al. 2016; Williams and Mohammed 2013).

Studies have repeatedly shown that doctors are more likely to prescribe pain medication for White patients than for Black patients with similar health conditions and clinical characteristics (Goyal et al. 2015; Anderson, Green, and Payne 2009; Green et al. 2003; Wyatt 2013). These disparities have been attributed to providers' biased beliefs and attitudes, of which the providers are often not aware (Shavers, Bakos, and Sheppard 2010). A study revealed that more than half of White medical students at a medical school believed—without scientific basis—that Black people have thicker skin than Whites. The students who believed this were less likely to prescribe adequate pain medication to Black patients than to clinically similar Whites (Hoffman et al. 2016). Compared with pregnant White women, pregnant Black women have received less advice—such as standard-of-care information about recommended weight gain and breastfeeding—from their prenatal care providers (Kogan, Kotelchuck, et al. 1994; Kogan, Alexander, et al. 1994; Cox et al. 2011), likely reflecting providers' assumptions about Black women's likelihood of using the information.

Access to medical care can be blocked by lack of insurance, and many providers do not accept patients covered by Medicaid, because the reimbursement is inadequate or because they choose not to serve low-income people or both. Even people with private insurance may have limited access to care if they cannot afford the often-sizable co-payments and deductibles required by many private insurers. In 2017, African American/Black and Hispanic/Latino people had the highest rates of not receiving needed prescription drugs because of cost (National Center for Health Statistics 2018).

Access to care also can be blocked when people avoid seeking health care because they do not trust providers or institutions to treat them fairly, competently, and with dignity, either based on their own or others' prior adverse experiences. Common fears include fear of being treated disrespectfully and fear of exploitation for research (Armstrong et al. 2013), as in the Tuskegee Experiment. Mistrust of and/or perceived lack of respect from health care providers or staff contribute to delays in care-seeking and non-adherence to treatment, both of which contribute to adverse health consequences, avoidable suffering, and significant costs.

Pathway 3: Racism Harms Health by Exposing People of Color to Higher Levels of Chronic Stress, Which Increases the Risk of Chronic Disease

> "Stress" (or more precisely being "stressed" or "stressed out") refers to a state in which the body's adaptive mechanisms are overwhelmed by challenges, setting in motion physiologic processes that can over time lead to chronic disease and premature aging (McEwen 2007). Stress, an experience, should be distinguished from a stressor, a condition or event that causes people to experience stress.

Figure 5.2 illustrates how racism can lead to poorer health outcomes among people of color through causal pathways involving stress. Chronic (i.e., prolonged over time) stress is known to have major adverse health consequences, involving inflammation and immune system dysfunction. Neuroscience has revealed that chronic stress, even at a relatively undramatic level, is particularly harmful to health; it appears to have more adverse consequences for health than a single dramatically stressful incident (McEwen 2008). Chronic stress experienced during childhood may be particularly damaging to health; effects can manifest across the entire life course, not just in childhood (Kim et al. 2013; Pervanidou and Chrousos 2011; Shonkoff et al. 2012; Sonu et al. 2019). (See Chapter 4.)

A large and growing body of evidence indicates the likely role of stress, including racism-related stress, in a range of important physical health outcomes, particularly chronic diseases such as heart disease and diabetes and potentially very low birthweight (Collins et al. 2000; Borrell et al. 2006; Krieger 2014). Experiences of stress can lead to poor health in two main ways: directly, by triggering physiologic mechanisms that damage health, and indirectly, by increasing the likelihood of health-harming behaviors.

Experiencing financial hardship or living in a racially segregated neighborhood can be stressful. Racial segregation, neighborhood social disadvantage, and poverty continue to be tightly linked. People of color are more likely to experience multiple stressors where they live, such as greater exposure to crime, police violence, substandard housing (with poor maintenance indoors and outdoors), and sometimes, because of concentrated poverty, desperate people around them. Inadequate services can compound these stressors, creating ongoing challenges to carrying out essential everyday tasks. Parents may worry about the quality of their children's education and prospects for future employment, both vital to escape poverty.

Experiencing racial discrimination is stressful. Experiencing racially discriminatory treatment has been shown repeatedly to be a significant stressor (Pascoe and Smart Richman 2009; Dominguez et al. 2008; Lewis, Cogburn, and Williams 2015; Collins et al. 2000; Borrell et al. 2006). To understand the toll that racism may take on the body, it is important to be aware of the wide range of experiences of racial discrimination that can be powerful stressors for people of color. Experiences of racial discrimination can take multiple forms, including not only overt or ambiguous incidents but also a range of psychological and emotional reactions. Even without experiencing incidents themselves, individuals may worry or be anxious about potential race-based discrimination against themselves or loved ones (Nuru-Jeter et al. 2009). Chronic vigilance or worry in anticipation or fear of potential discrimination—feeling that one must be constantly on guard— has been linked with adverse health outcomes including preterm birth (Lewis et al. 2015; Braveman et al. 2017). People may have ongoing concerns about encountering or confirming negative stereotypes about their social group (Steele and Aronson 1995). They may ruminate about past experiences of their own, their loved ones, or their racial/ ethnic group in general or they may believe they always must perform exceptionally to disprove prejudicial assumptions (Box 5.2). Diverse stressful psychological reactions to any of these concerns or experiences may occur; the reactions may take the form of worry, anger, or self-doubt, and these reactions can have adverse health consequences (Dominguez et al. 2008; Lewis et al. 2015; Williams and Mohammed 2013; Pascoe and Smart Richman 2009).

How Stress, Including Racism-Related Stress, Damages Health

Racism-related stress can trigger a chain of physiologic mechanisms with health-damaging effects (Allen et al. 2019; D. Lee et al. 2018; Busse, Yim, Campos, and Marshburn 2017; Tomfohr, Pung, and Dimsdale 2016; Busse, Yim, and Campos 2017). Neuroscience has made tremendous strides in understanding the physiologic mechanisms that can be

---

BOX 5.2   **The Hidden Costs of Upward Mobility for People of Color: Chronic Stress**

Perhaps counterintuitively, some studies have found that socioeconomically better-off Black women were *more* likely than their socioeconomically worse-off counterparts to report pervasive worry about experiencing discrimination (Braveman et al. 2017; Colen et al. 2018; Nuru-Jeter et al. 2009). This unexpected finding may shed light on a perplexing result reported in other research as well: Among Black people, greater socioeconomic advantage does not necessarily translate into expected improvements in health (Braveman et al. 2015; Colen et al. 2006; Collins and Butler 1997; Foster et al. 2000; McGrady et al. 1992). One theory is that Black people with higher incomes or educational attainment could in fact worry *more* about racial discrimination— and experience greater racism-related stress—than their socioeconomically less-advantaged Black counterparts. This could happen, perhaps, because more socioeconomically advantaged Black people may interact more frequently and closely with Whites, particularly at work. They may be more likely to be in the minority in their workplaces and potentially where they shop, study, and obtain services (Myers, Lewis, and Parker-Dominguez 2003); they may also feel an ongoing need to prove themselves against negative stereotypes. Cole and Omari (2003) discussed the "hidden costs of upward mobility" for middle-class African Americans, including encountering glass ceilings to advancement at work, potential alienation from other African Americans, and frequent demands for financial support from less well-off family and friends, all of which could be stressful.

"A large and growing body of evidence indicates that experiences of racial discrimination are an important type of psychosocial stressor that can lead to adverse changes in health status and altered behavioral patterns that increase health risks" (Williams and Mohammed 2013, p. 1).

triggered by stressful experiences. The body's response to stress begins when a stressful experience activates certain areas of the brain. Both acute (short-term, temporary) and chronic (repeated, sustained, long-term) stress produce responses of multiple physiologic systems, including cognitive, neuroendocrine, cardiovascular, immune, and metabolic systems (McEwen 2008). Many different mediators of the stress response have been identified, including cortisol (McEwen 2008). These mediators may have both protective and damaging effects on the body, depending on many factors, including the context, the timing in a person's life cycle, and the duration of exposure to stressors. Acute stress may not necessarily harm the body. It appears, however, that chronic stress can exact a heavy toll, setting in motion mechanisms involving inflammation and immune system dysfunction, which can lead to cardiovascular disease, diabetes, and other chronic disease (McEwen 2008) and potentially preterm birth (Dunkel Schetter 2011), a leading cause of infant mortality. The inflammation and immune system dysfunction caused by chronic stress may not produce visible health effects for decades, however, making it very difficult to study. The term *allostatic load* refers to the wear and tear on the body due to the body's attempts to adapt in the face of chronic stress that overwhelms its capacity. The physiologic consequences of chronic stress may be transmitted across generations; as noted previously, epigenetic effects may explain how the stressful and health-damaging experiences of one generation (e.g., enslaved people) can be inherited across generations (Thayer and Kuzawa 2011; Yehuda and Lehrner 2018).

Stress also can lead to health-damaging behaviors. Few of us have never engaged in unhealthy behaviors when experiencing stress. Attempts to cope with stressors often include behaviors such as overeating or eating unhealthy foods ("comfort foods"), excessive alcohol intake, inadequate physical activity, smoking, and drug abuse (McEwen 2008). Children who experience stressful circumstances, particularly on a daily basis, are more likely later in life to adopt—and less likely to discontinue—risky health behaviors such as smoking, drug use and excessive alcohol intake and abuse of alcohol or drugs (Hughes et al. 2017; Rehkopf et al. 2016; Loudermilk et al. 2018; R. Lee and Chen 2017) that may function as coping mechanisms. Racially segregated neighborhoods are disproportionately targeted with advertising that promotes alcohol and tobacco use, particularly among minority youth (J. Lee et al. 2015; Martino et al. 2018). These neighborhoods also often lack some of the resources (e.g., parks, bike lanes, recreation centers, and healthy food environments) that could encourage healthier coping strategies (Grasser et al. 2013; Hirsch et al. 2014; Golden et al. 2019; Sherk et al. 2018; Erickson et al. 2012; Leventhal and Dupéré 2019; Putnam 1993; Kawachi, Subramanian, and Kim 2008; Carpiano 2008).

Pathway 4: Racism Can Damage the Health of People of Color by Disenfranchising and Disempowering Them, Depriving Them of the Right to Vote or the Extent to Which Their Vote Counts

Racism can damage health by disenfranchising and disempowering people of color, for example, through policies that create gerrymandering (defined previously) and voter suppression. Voter suppression intentionally creates or exacerbates obstacles to voting through written or unwritten policies and practices imposing requirements such as a poll tax or literacy test, mandating that prospective voters provide documents that may be more difficult for low-income people to produce readily, deliberately closing accessible polling places and placing them where they will be inaccessible to people of color, or creating confusion about the location or hours of polling sites.

Voter suppression and gerrymandering are policies that affect health indirectly by depriving people of the ability to influence policies that affect them—for example, policies addressing economic disadvantage, environmental injustice, policing and sentencing bias, and funding for services. Disenfranchisement deprives people of the ability to address unfair policies affecting all of the other pathways noted above (economic disadvantage, health-harming exposures, and chronic stress).

5.5. OTHER FORMS OF DISCRIMINATION ALSO CAN DAMAGE HEALTH

Health can be adversely affected by discrimination related to a wide array of personal characteristics in addition to race or ethnic group, including a person's immigration status, national origin, religion, gender and gender identity, disability status, and/or sexual orientation. Many people experience discrimination based on multiple characteristics—for example, being a lesbian Latina woman or a formerly incarcerated Black man with a physical disability; experiencing discrimination based on multiple stigmatized characteristics, sometimes referred to as *intersectionality*, can have particularly negative effects. The effects may not be simply additive but, rather, synergistic. The nature of the general pathways through which these kinds of discrimination influence health may be qualitatively similar to many of those discussed above but may have compound effects.

Regardless of who is targeted, all types of discrimination involve unfair treatment and different degrees of social exclusion, rejection, or marginalization of people based on their being identified as belonging to a particular social group. Social exclusion in any form is likely to produce a range of effects that pose risks to health. First, social exclusion places targeted individuals at a social disadvantage, excluding them from the benefits (e.g., access to opportunities for education, employment, and social support) typically associated with full participation in society. Awareness of being excluded or marginalized can result in psychological distress. As discussed above, physiologic responses to stress over time involve potentially harmful neuroendocrine and vascular mechanisms with prolonged exposure to stressors over time, these mechanisms can lead to inflammation and dysregulation of the immune system, which in turn increase a person's risk of a range of adverse birth outcomes (Rubens et al. 2014; Yao et al. 2014; Knight and Smith 2016) or chronic diseases that typically manifest in adulthood (McEwen 2007). For example, the birth outcomes of Arabic-named women (and not other groups of women) in California were observed to worsen after 9/11; researchers attributed this to the stress of experiencing the anti-Arab sentiment that arose after 9/11 (Lauderdale 2006).

As with race-based discrimination, internalizing negative views about one's group with resulting loss of self-esteem can increase the risk of unhealthy behaviors (Williams and Mohammed 2013; Kwate and Meyer 2011). Internalized racism may also have more direct adverse physiologic effects (Euteneuer 2014).

Discrimination in general, including racial/ethnic and other forms of unfair treatment, is often accompanied by limited economic and/or social opportunities. Because of the powerful role of socioeconomic resources in health, this places victims at both socioeconomic and health disadvantage (see discussion of the connection between socioeconomic disadvantage and health disadvantage in Chapter 2). For example, people with disabilities often face obstacles to earning income and building wealth, which in turn constitute obstacles to their achieving the highest level of health possible for them. Compared to those without disabilities, people with disabilities are more than twice as likely to live in poverty, less likely to be employed, and less likely to have a bank account—further limiting their opportunities to build credit and savings (Goodman and Morris 2017). These effects can be particularly damaging for Black people, who in every age group are more likely to have a disability than their White or Latino counterparts (Goodman et al. 2017). Similarly, disparities in pay, advancement, and caregiving roles associated with gender-based discrimination continue to limit women's opportunities for generating income and building wealth. Discrimination against women also can be seen in the refusal of some employers to cover a full range of reproductive health care services.

Discrimination based on characteristics other than race can also adversely affect people's health by limiting their ability to receive timely, quality health care. Health care professionals are seldom trained in the competencies needed to best serve people living with disabilities (National Council on Disability 2009). As a group, people living with disabilities are also more likely to lack insurance coverage—and thus financial access—for needed health services such as prescription medications, medical equipment, long-term and specialty care, and assistive technologies (National Council on Disability 2009). A survey by a respected national civil rights organization found that approximately 56% of lesbian, gay, and bisexual people and 70% of transgender people reported experiencing discrimination (e.g., harsh language, refusal of care, and physical roughness) in their interactions with health care providers (Lambda Legal Defense and Education Fund 2014). Transgender persons frequently avoid seeking medical care due to fears of being mistreated (Safer et al. 2016).

5.6. STRATEGIES TO ADDRESS RACISM OR MITIGATE ITS HARMFUL EFFECTS ON HEALTH

As discussed in this chapter, racism, and particularly systemic racism, has deep roots. It has persisted across centuries even as some societal gains in greater racial equity have been made. This section makes recommendations for action to reduce and ultimately eliminate racism, particularly systemic racism. These recommendations are based on the author's interpretation of widely held knowledge, including but not limited to sources cited earlier in the chapter.

Examples of General and Specific Strategies for Action

Box 5.3 presents several examples of general approaches that appear to be useful based on current knowledge of the causal pathways through which racism harms health; these are followed by examples of specific approaches that have been implemented in

| BOX 5.3 | General Strategies for Dismantling Racism |

As part of a multipronged strategy, approaches to dismantling racism may take many different forms, including the following:

- Enacting new laws or policies that will counter racism, particularly systemic racism.
- Enforcing existing laws and policies, which requires sustained attention and funding. Enacting laws and policies that are more just and eliminating unjust laws and policies are necessary but insufficient. Without enforcement, deeply entrenched and widespread practices, beliefs, and attitudes will continue to allow de facto discriminatory practices to continue even after written laws and policies have been changed.
- Identifying and eliminating existing laws, policies, and practices that enable and perpetuate systemic racism, regardless of their intent.
- Preventing voter suppression, which denies people a voice, thereby reducing their power to dismantle racism.
- Advocacy and education are crucial components of virtually any strategy to dismantle systemic racism.

Advocacy and education include building and maintaining public support for dismantling racism. Advocacy and education are needed to promote the values of fairness, justice, diversity, inclusion, and equal opportunities for all to achieve health and well-being. Preschool and kindergarten–college education are crucial opportunities to promote these values. Civil society (including, for example, civil rights, faith-based, health and health care, academic, business, and nonprofit organizations) has a crucial role to play in keeping equity on the agenda as a priority. Civil society can advocate for changes in policies and laws, support enforcement, and identify what is and what is not working and the changes needed in strategy. The examples below demonstrate that changes, including systemic or structural changes, can be achieved when many individuals, organizations, and leaders are mobilized.

- Helping reduce or repair the damages caused by racism—for example, through reparations—will not eliminate it. Healing wounds is, however, an aspect of pursuing equity.

the past with the goal of dismantling systemic racism, which, as an upstream cause, the upstream cause that sets multiple health-damaging causal chains in motion. The specific examples listed here are deliberately weighted toward national or state laws, policies, and systems because of their potential for impact on systemic racism and on a larger scale. Local governments (cities or counties) and individual public and private institutions also should undertake systemic changes to address racism within their domains of influence.

Upstream actions also are favored because, from an ethical point of view, strategies that would reduce and ultimately eliminate racism are preferable over strategies that would only mitigate its harmful effects on health. From a practical perspective as well, upstream approaches that would remove the fundamental cause of harm are likely to be more effective and potentially more efficient on a long-term basis than those aimed at damage control rather than prevention.

Examples of -Strategies Addressing Racism

Laws enacted to prohibit discrimination (Box 5.4)

- The Civil Rights Act of 1964 prohibited race-based discrimination in schools, employment, and public places.

| BOX 5.4 | Impacts of Laws Prohibiting Discrimination |

• After passage of the 1964 Civil Rights Act, the desegregation of public hospitals, particularly in Mississippi, led to dramatically improved access to medical care for Black mothers and infants. From 1965 to 1971, declines in the Black infant mortality rate related to the 1964 law produced the narrowest gap between Black and White infant mortality rates in the post-World War II era (Almond, Chay, and Greenstone 2007).

• The Civil Rights Act of 1964 and the Voting Rights Act of 1965 were associated with opening up broader economic opportunities for Black women, which were accompanied by measurable economic and social gains in the late 1960s and the 1970s. These economic and social gains were accompanied by declines in disparities in life expectancy between White and Black women (Kaplan, Ranjit, and Burgard 2008).

• The Voting Rights Act of 1965 prohibited discrimination in voting.
• The Fair Housing Act (also called the Civil Rights Act) of 1968 strengthened the 1964 Act with regard to discrimination in housing.

Strengthening the enforcement of anti-discrimination laws

• Intervention by federal (and, less frequently, state) officials to protect people from physical harm when they exercise their civil rights—for example, by protecting children and youth of color who are attending a previously segregated school or university. Such interventions have been crucial in efforts to desegregate schools and universities.
• Organized actions to end voter suppression, including litigation, demonstrations, placing attorneys or other personnel at poll sites to witness and deter acts of suppression, and assisting people with transportation to polling sites.

Affirmative action/diversity/equity/inclusion efforts have aimed to address centuries of exclusion of people of color from employment, promotions, and admissions to schools and universities. Affirmative action involves giving thoughtful consideration to qualified candidates who in the past may have been rejected based on their race or ethnic group; this typically involves considering the obstacles faced by candidates of color when assessing their strengths and potential to succeed. In response to extensive challenges to affirmative action initiatives—which frequently have cast such initiatives as discriminatory against Whites and/or Asians—many institutions have reframed their relevant efforts (often under the banner of diversity, equity, and inclusion) as pursuing greater diversity and inclusion to the benefit of everyone (Box 5.5).

5.7. CONCLUSION

One—albeit not the only—cause of the persistence of systemic racism has been a lack of awareness of it on the part of those who do not suffer it. There is a widespread lack of awareness of the often hidden but most deadly part of the iceberg and the damages that it inflicts by placing major obstacles to health and well-being in the way of people of color. Those obstacles include infringements on voting rights; biased treatment by police and courts; and denial of equal access to quality education, good jobs, housing, bank loans,

BOX 5.5	Building Awareness and Attempting to Change Attitudes: An Adjunct, Not a Substitute, for Systemic and Structural Approaches

One widely encountered approach to addressing racism attempts to change the discriminatory attitudes of White people toward people of color, typically through interventions such as organizational retreats or workshops. A central underlying assumption is that changing people's attitudes by raising their awareness of their own implicit (unconscious) racial biases will lead to changes in their behavior that will help "undo racism." Expert consultants lead retreats and trainings for employees and/or leadership staff. Some police departments have voluntarily undergone this type of training (James 2017). This approach is often appealing because it is relatively brief and inexpensive and requires no

systemic or structural changes. Because widely prevalent beliefs and attitudes are part of systemic racism, approaches making people more aware of racism and the harm it inflicts deserve consideration. Awareness can be raised of systemic as well as interpersonal racism; greater awareness among the public and leaders is important to achieve systemic change. Data assessing the impact of these approaches are scarce, however, and it seems reasonable to question the sustained effects of a limited, brief training experience, particularly if it is not repeatedly reinforced over a longer period of time. This approach may, however, be a useful adjunct to efforts to change systems, policies, and structures.

and health-promoting neighborhoods. Because systemic racism permeates all sectors and geographic areas, effective strategies will require actions in multiple sectors, at levels from local to national. No single strategy by itself is likely to be effective. Eliminating systemic racism will require multiple strategies that reinforce each other.

Although changing awareness is crucial, it is not enough without changing the systems and structures in which systemic racism is embedded. Changing laws, policies, and practices also is necessary but not sufficient without enforcement. History has made it clear that for the foreseeable future, real change will require strong, adequately funded enforcement strategies.

Dismantling systemic racism requires changing laws, policies, systems, practices, and beliefs in ways that will be effective, endure over the long term, and affect many people, rather than implementing piecemeal, time-limited programs. This is not easy to do. It is far easier to enact initiatives that only mitigate the harmful effects of systemic racism while leaving the unfair systems and structures in place or to engage in actions that do not produce sustained or fundamental change.

Advocacy and education are among the forms that action can take. Virtually all effective, sustained actions to dismantle systemic racism require advocacy and education—including increasing public awareness and influencing public opinion. Because dismantling systemic racism must call for systemic and structural change, effective strategies will necessarily require the sustained support of policymakers, organized civil society groups, and concerned residents.

Progress toward ending racism will require continuing and deepening the study of racism, both revealing the harms it has caused and continues to cause and identifying promising actions to end it. The findings must be used to educate the public and policymakers and to guide further action. The knowledge gained from study and experience must be disseminated widely; it must describe what systemic racism is, the shocking damage it has inflicted and continues to inflict, and why dismantling it must be a priority. Awareness must include understanding of how White people have—intentionally or not—benefited from systemic racism and how achieving a more just society will benefit all of us. This awareness should not be confused with guilt; it should move us forward. Moving forward will require identifying for the public and policymakers the links between racism and inequities in health and well-being as they arise in multiple arenas that attract public attention—for example, during the COVID pandemic and in relation to climate change.

Effective strategies will activate people to vote; learn; speak out to their children, families, friends, and co-workers; and organize in their neighborhoods, towns, states, and nationally. They will move people to support, join, and become leaders of organizations pushing for change. Moving forward will require awareness and commitment from individuals, private organizations, and government, including at the national level, to stay the course over the long term. It will require the strong and enduring commitment of leaders—for example, in government, business, health and health care, education, housing, transportation, and environment and climate change. It will require vigilance over time to ensure enforcement of policies to dismantle racism, particularly systemic racism, and to detect and actively oppose any new efforts that would exacerbate racism.

Dismantling racism, particularly systemic racism, will not be easy to accomplish, given how widespread and deeply entrenched systemic racism remains in our nation. Examples presented in this chapter demonstrate, however, that important advances have been made in the past. We can learn much from the past—both about the horrifying harms caused by systemic racism and about approaches that hold promise for moving us toward a more equitable and healthy society for everyone.

5.8. KEY POINTS

- Racism is a system of oppression—of treating some people adversely based on their perceived race or ethnic group and justifying the adverse treatment by valuing them differently.
- Race is primarily a social, not a biological, construct.
- Racism can take many different forms. Systemic (structural) racism is the most upstream form—the laws, policies, entrenched practices, and pervasive beliefs that foster, condone, and perpetuate prejudicial treatment based on race. Systemic racism is often so embedded in familiar structures that it may not be as readily visible as interpersonal discrimination—that is, prejudicial treatment of an individual(s) by another individual(s) based on race. Systemic racism produces interpersonal discrimination.
- Racism is an upstream (fundamental) cause of differences in the environments, experiences, resources, and opportunities that shape health and disease. It acts through multiple causal pathways.
- Among the many pathways through which racism is likely to affect health are pathways generating stress, which can harm health long term by leading to inflammation and immune system dysregulation, thereby increasing risks of chronic disease in adulthood such as heart disease, stroke, and diabetes.
- Systemic or structural racism is the fundamental, upstream cause of most racial disparities in health. Strategies focusing only on increasing awareness of racism

are unlikely to be effective without also dismantling the systemic and structural barriers themselves.

5.9. QUESTIONS FOR DISCUSSION

1. What are the different causal pathways through which racism could harm health?
2. What is systemic or structural racism? Interpersonal racism (interpersonal racial discrimination)? What is the relationship between systemic and interpersonal racism? What are some historical and contemporary examples of each?
3. When did the concept of race first emerge and why? How—in what historical contexts—has race been used to justify treating people differently? How is it being used in contemporary times?
4. Why is "Latino" or "Hispanic" not considered a race in official U.S. population statistics, whereas Black/African/African American, Asian, and White/European are? Is the distinction justified? What are the social and policy implications?
5. What could be done to reduce and ultimately eliminate racism?

ACKNOWLEDGMENTS

Elaine Arkin made significant contributions to this chapter, particularly the final section. Susan Egerter, PhD, and Miranda Brillante, MPH, also made valuable contributions.

This chapter builds on material written by the author and colleagues in the following issue briefs published by the Robert Wood Johnson Foundation:

- Braveman, P., E. Arkin, D. Proctor, T. Kauh, and N. Holm. 2021. *Systemic Racism Is a Health Equity Issue*. Princeton, NJ: Robert Wood Johnson Foundation.
- Braveman, P., J. Acker, E. Arkin, D. Proctor, A. Gillman, L. A. McGeary, and G, Mallya. 2018. *Wealth Matters for Health Equity*. Princeton, NJ: Robert Wood Johnson Foundation.
- Braveman, P., L. Gottlieb, D. Francis, E. Arkin, and J. Acker. 2019. *What Can the Health Care Sector Do to Advance Health Equity?* Princeton, NJ: Robert Wood Johnson Foundation.
- Acker, J., P. Braveman, E. Arkin, L. Leviton, J. Parsons, and G. Hobor. 2019. *Mass Incarceration Threatens Health Equity in America*. Princeton, NJ: Robert Wood Johnson Foundation.

REFERENCES

Aaronson, D., D. Hartley, and B. Mazumder. 2017. "The effects of the 1930s HOLC "redlining" maps." Working Paper No. 2017-12. Chicago, IL: Federal Reserve Bank of Chicago.

Abuelezam, N. N., A. M. El-Sayed, and S. Galea. 2018. "The health of Arab Americans in the United States: An updated comprehensive literature review." *Front Public Health* 6: 262.

Acker, J., P. Braveman, E. Arkin, L. Leviton, J. Parsons, and G. Hobor. 2019. "Mass incarceration threatens health equity in America." Executive Summary. Princeton, NJ: Robert Wood Johnson Foundation.

Adakai, M., M. Sandoval-Rosario, F. Xu, T. Aseret-Manygoats, M. Allison, K. J. Greenlund, and K. E. Barbour. 2018. "Health disparities among American Indians/Alaska Natives—Arizona, 2017." *MMWR Morb Mortal Wkly Rep* 67(47): 1314–1318.

Adelman, R. M. 2004. "Neighborhood opportunities, race, and class: The Black middle class and residential segregation." *City Community* 3(1): 43–63. https://doi.org/10.1111/j.1535-6841.2004.00066.x.

Adler, N. E., and D. H. Rehkopf. 2008. "US disparities in health: Descriptions, causes, and mechanisms." *Annu Rev Public Health* 29: 235–252.

Allen, A. M., M. D. Thomas, E. K. Michaels, A. N. Reeves, U. Okoye, M. M. Price, R. E. Hasson, S. L. Syme, and D. H Chae. 2019. "Racial discrimination, educational attainment, and biological dysregulation among midlife African American women." *Psychoneuroendocrinology* 99: 225–235.

Almond, D. V., K. Y. Chay, and M. Greenstone. 2007. Civil rights, the war on poverty, and black-white convergence in infant mortality in the rural South and Mississippi. Massachusetts Institute of Technology, Department of Economics. Working Paper No. 07-04.

Anderson, K. O., C. R. Green, and R. Payne. 2009. "Racial and ethnic disparities in pain: Causes and consequences of unequal care." *J Pain* 10(12): 1187–1204. https://doi.org/10.1016/j.jpain.2009.10.002.

Arias, E., and J. Xu. 2019. United States life tables: 2017. In *National Health Statistics Reports*. Hyattsville, MD: National Center for Health Statistics, 68(7): 1–66.

Arias, E., J. Xu, and M. A. Jim. 2014. "Period life tables for the non-Hispanic American Indian and Alaska Native population, 2007–2009." *Am J Public Health* 104(Suppl 3): S312–S319.

Armstrong, K., M. Putt, C. H. Halbert, D. Grande, J. S. Schwartz, K. Liao, N. Marcus, M. B. Demeter, and J. A. Shea. 2013. "Prior experiences of racial discrimination and racial differences in health care system distrust." *Med Care* 51(2): 144–150. https://doi.org/10.1097/MLR.0b013e31827310a1.

Astor, M. 2020. "Why did Bloomberg turn against stop-and-frisk? When he ran for President." *The New York Times* Accessed December 2, 2020. https://www.nytimes.com/2020/02/19/us/politics/michael-bloomberg-stop-and-frisk.html?action=click&module=RelatedLinks&pgtype=Article.

Bailey, Z. D., N. Krieger, M. Agénor, J. Graves, N. Linos, and M. T. Bassett. 2017. "Structural racism and health inequities in the USA: Evidence and interventions." *Lancet* 389(10077): 1453–1463.

Bayer, P., F. Ferreira, and S. L. Ross. 2014. Race, ethnicity and high-cost mortgage lending (No. w20762). National Bureau of Economic Research.

Beck, A., M. Berzofsky, R. Caspar, and C. Krebs. 2013. "Sexual victimization in prisons and jails reported by inmates, 2011–12." U.S. Department of Justice. https://bjs.ojp.gov/content/pub/pdf/svpjri1112.pdf

Bentele, K. G., and E. E. O'Brien. 2013. "Jim Crow 2.0? Why states consider and adopt restrictive voter access policies." *Perspect Politics* 11(4): 1088–1116. https://doi.org/10.1017/S1537592713002843.

Blumenshine, P., S. Egerter, C. J. Barclay, C. Cubbin, and P. A. Braveman. 2010. "Socioeconomic disparities in adverse birth outcomes: A systematic review." *Am J Prev Med* 39(3): 263–272. https://doi.org/10.1016/j.amepre.2010.05.012.

Board of Governors of the Federal Reserve System. 2016. "Survey of consumer finances." https://www.federalreserve.gov/econres/scfindex.htm.

Bocian, D. G., K. S. Ernst, and W. Li. 2008. "Race, ethnicity and subprime home loan pricing." *J Econ Bus* 60(1): 110–124. https://doi.org/10.1016/j.jeconbus.2007.10.001.

Bonczar, T. P. 2003. "Prevalence of imprisonment in the US population, 1974–2001." Bureau of Justice Statistics. https://bjs.ojp.gov/content/pub/pdf/piusp01.pdf.

Bonilla-Silva, E. 2018. *Racism Without Racists: Color-Blind Racism and the Persistence of Racial Inequality in America*. 5th ed. Lanham, MD: Rowman & Littlefield.

Borrell, L. N., C. I. Kiefe, D. R. Williams, A. V. Diez-Roux, and P. Gordon-Larsen. 2006. "Self-reported health, perceived racial discrimination, and skin color in African

Americans in the CARDIA study." *Soc Sci Med* 63(6): 1415–1427.

Boswell, T. E. 1986. "A split labor market analysis of discrimination against Chinese immigrants, 1850–1882." *Am Sociol Rev* 51(3): 352–371. https://doi.org/10.2307/2095307.

Braveman, P., and T. P. Dominguez. 2021. "Abandon 'race.' Focus on racism." *Front Public Health* 9(1318). https://doi.org/10.3389/fpubh.2021.689462.

Braveman, P., and S. Egerter. 2008. *Overcoming Obstacles to Health: Report from the Robert Wood Johnson Foundation to the Commission to Build a Healthier America*. Princeton, NJ: Robert Wood Johnson Foundation.

Braveman, P., K. Heck, S. Egerter, T. P. Dominguez, C. Rinki, K. S. Marchi, and M. Curtis. 2017. "Worry about racial discrimination: A missing piece of the puzzle of Black–White disparities in preterm birth?" *PLoS One* 12(10): e0186151.

Braveman, P. A., C. Cubbin, S. Egerter, D. R. Williams, and E. Pamuk. 2010. "Socioeconomic disparities in health in the United States: What the patterns tell us." *Am J Public Health* 100(Suppl 1): S186–S196. https://doi.org/10.2105/AJPH.2009.166082.

Braveman, P. A., C. Cubbin, S. Egerter, S. Chideya, K. S. Marchi, M. Metzler, and S. Posner. 2005. "Socioeconomic status in health research: One size does not fit all." *JAMA* 294(22): 2879–2888.

Braveman, P. A., K. Heck, S. Egerter, K. S. Marchi, T. P. Dominguez, C. Cubbin, K. Fingar, J. A. Pearson, and M. Curtis. 2015. "The role of socioeconomic factors in Black–White disparities in preterm birth." *Am J Public Health* 105(4): 694–702.

Buehler, J. W. 2016. "Racial/ethnic disparities in the use of lethal force by US police, 2010–2014." *Am J Public Health* 107(2): 295–297. https://doi.org/10.2105/AJPH.2016.303575.

Bui, A. L., M. M. Coates, and E. C. Matthay. 2018. "Years of life lost due to encounters with law enforcement in the USA, 2015–2016." *J Epidemiol Community Health* 72(8): 715. https://doi.org/10.1136/jech-2017-210059.

Burch, T. 2015. "Skin color and the criminal justice system: Beyond Black–White disparities in sentencing." *J Empirical Legal Stud* 12(3): 395–420. https://doi.org/10.1111/jels.12077.

Busse, D., I. S. Yim, and B. Campos. 2017. "Social context matters: Ethnicity, discrimination and stress reactivity." *Psychoneuroendocrinology* 83: 187–193. https://doi.org/10.1016/j.psyneuen.2017.05.025.

Busse, D., I. S. Yim, B. Campos, and C. K. Marshburn. 2017. "Discrimination and the HPA axis: Current evidence and future directions." *J Behav Med* 40(4): 539–552. https://doi.org/10.1007/s10865-017-9830-6.

Carpiano, R. M. 2008. "Actual or potential neighborhood resources for health." In *Social Capital and Health*, edited by I. Kawachi, S. V. Subramanian, and D. Kim, 83–93. New York, NY: Springer.

Case, A., D. Lubotsky, and C. Paxson. 2002. "Economic status and health in childhood: The origins of the gradient." *Am Econ Rev* 92(5): 1308–1334.

Chang, M. 2010. *Lifting as We Climb: Women of Color, Wealth, and America's Future*. Oakland, CA: Insight Center for Community Economic Development.

Chetty, R., M. Stepner, S. Abraham, S. Lin, B. Scuderi, N. Turner, A. Bergeron, and D. Cutler. 2016. "The association between income and life expectancy in the United States, 2001–2014." *JAMA* 315(16): 1750–1766. https://doi.org/10.1001/jama.2016.4226.

Cole, E. R., and S. R. Omari. 2003. "Race, class and the dilemmas of upward mobility for African Americans." *J Soc Issues* 59(4): 785–802.

Colen, C. G., A. T. Geronimus, J. Bound, and S. A. James. 2006. "Maternal upward socioeconomic mobility and Black–White disparities in infant birthweight." *Am J Public Health* 96(11): 2032–2039.

Colen, C. G., D. M. Ramey, E. C. Cooksey, and D. R. Williams. 2018. "Racial disparities in health among nonpoor African Americans and Hispanics: The role of acute and chronic discrimination." *Soc Sci Med* 199: 167–180.

Collins, J. W., Jr., and A. G. Butler. 1997. "Racial differences in the prevalence of small-for-dates infants among college-educated women." *Epidemiology* 8(3): 315–317.

Collins, J. W., Jr., R. J. David, R. Symons, A. Handler, S. N. Wall, and L. Dwyer. 2000.

"Low-income African-American mothers' perception of exposure to racial discrimination and infant birth weight." *Epidemiology* 11(3): 337–339.

Cooper, H. L. F., and M. T. Fullilove. 2020. *From Enforcers to Guardians: A Public Health Primer on Ending Police Violence.* Baltimore, MD: Johns Hopkins University Press.

Cooper, R. S., J. S. Kaufman, and R. Ward. 2003. "Race and genomics." *N Engl J Med* 348(12): 1166–1170. https://doi.org/10.1056/NEJMsb022863.

Corcoran, M. 1995. "Rags to rags: Poverty and mobility in the United States." *Annu Rev Sociol* 21(1): 237–267. https://doi.org/10.1146/annurev.so.21.080195.001321.

Cox, R. G., L. Zhang, M. E. Zotti, and J. Graham. 2011. "Prenatal care utilization in Mississippi: Racial disparities and implications for unfavorable birth outcomes." *Matern Child Health J* 15(7): 931–942. https://doi.org/10.1007/s10995-009-0542-6.

Cushing, L., J. Faust, L. M. August, R. Cendak, W. Wieland, and G. Alexeeff. 2015. "Racial/ethnic disparities in cumulative environmental health impacts in California: Evidence from a statewide environmental justice screening tool (CalEnviroScreen 1.1)." *Am J Public Health* 105(11): 2341–2348. https://doi.org/10.2105/AJPH.2015.302643.

Cushing, L., R. Morello-Frosch, M. Wander, and M. Pastor. 2015. "The haves, the have-nots, and the health of everyone: The relationship between social inequality and environmental quality." *Annu Rev Public Health* 36(1): 193–209. https://doi.org/10.1146/annurev-publhealth-031914-122646.

Daly, M. C., G. J. Duncan, P. McDonough, and D. R. Williams. 2002. "Optimal indicators of socioeconomic status for health research." *Am J Public Health* 92(7): 1151–1157. https://doi.org/10.2105/ajph.92.7.1151.

Demakakos, P., J. P. Biddulph, M. Bobak, and M. G. Marmot. 2016. "Wealth and mortality at older ages: A prospective cohort study." *J Epidemiol Community Health* 70(4): 346–353. https://doi.org/10.1136/jech-2015-206173.

DeVylder, J. E., H. Y. Oh, B. Nam, T. L. Sharpe, M. Lehmann, and B. G. Link. 2017. "Prevalence, demographic variation and psychological correlates of exposure to police victimisation in four US cities." *Epidemiol Psychiatr Sci* 26(5): 466–477.

Dominguez, T. P., C. Dunkel-Schetter, L. M. Glynn, C. Hobel, and C. A. Sandman. 2008. "Racial differences in birth outcomes: The role of general, pregnancy, and racism stress." *Health Psychol* 27(2): 194.

Dunkel Schetter, C. 2011. "Psychological science on pregnancy: Stress processes, biopsychosocial models, and emerging research issues." *Annu Rev Psychol* 62:531–558. https://doi.org/10.1146/annurev.psych.031809.130727.

Duster, T. 2005. "Race and reification in science." *Science* 307(5712): 1050. https://doi.org/10.1126/science.1110303.

Edwards, F., H. Lee, and M. Esposito. 2019. "Risk of being killed by police use of force in the United States by age, race–ethnicity, and sex." *Proc Natl Acad Sci USA* 116(34): 16793–16798. https://doi.org/10.1073/pnas.1821204116.

Ely, D. M., and A. K. Driscoll. 2019. Infant mortality in the United States, 2017: Data from the period linked birth/infant death file. Natl Vital Stat Rep 68(10): 1–20.

Equal Justice Initiative. 2017. *Lynching in America: Confronting the Legacy of Racial Terror.* 3rd edition. Montgomery, AL: Equal Justice Initiative.

Erickson, P. G., L. Harrison, S. Cook, M.-M. Cousineau, and E. M. Adlaf. 2012. "A comparative study of the influence of collective efficacy on substance use among adolescent students in Philadelphia, Toronto, and Montreal." *Addict Res Theory* 20(1): 11–20. https://doi.org/10.3109/16066359.2010.530710.

Euteneuer, F. 2014. "Subjective social status and health." *Curr Opin Psychiatry* 27(5): 337–343. https://doi.org/10.1097/yco.0000000000000083.

Evans-Campbell, T., K. L. Walters, C. R. Pearson, and C. D. Campbell. 2012. "Indian boarding school experience, substance use, and mental health among urban two-spirit American Indian/Alaska natives." *Am J Drug Alcohol Abuse* 38(5): 421–427. https://doi.org/10.3109/00952990.2012.701358.

Executive Office of the President, Office of Management and Budget. 1997. "Revisions to the standards for the classification of federal data on race and ethnicity." *Fed Reg* 62(210): 58782.

Faber, J. W. 2016. "Cashing in on distress: The expansion of fringe financial institutions during the Great Recession." *Urban Affairs Rev* 54(4): 663–696. https://doi.org/10.1177/1078087416684037.

Faber, J. W., and T. Friedline. 2018. *The racialized costs of banking*. Washington, DC: New America.

Feagin, J., and Z. Bennefield. 2014. "Systemic racism and U.S. health care." *Soc Sci Med* 103: 7–14. https://doi.org/10.1016/j.socscimed.2013.09.006.

Feir, D. L. 2016. "The long-term effects of forcible assimilation policy: The case of Indian boarding schools." *Can J Econ* 49(2): 433–480. https://doi.org/10.1111/caje.12203.

Feldman, J. M., J. T. Chen, P. D. Waterman, and N. Krieger. 2016. "Temporal trends and racial/ethnic inequalities for legal intervention injuries treated in emergency departments: US men and women age 15–34, 2001–2014." *J Urban Health* 93(5): 797–807.

Fiscella, K., and M. R. Sanders. 2016. "Racial and ethnic disparities in the quality of health care." *Annu Rev Public Health* 37: 375–394.

Foster, H. W., L. Wu, M. B. Bracken, K. Semenya, J. Thomas, and J. Thomas. 2000. "Intergenerational effects of high socioeconomic status on low birthweight and preterm birth in African Americans." *J Natl Med Assoc* 92(5): 213.

Frey, W. 2018. "Black–White segregation edges downward since 2000, census shows." The Brookings Institution. Accessed May 7, 2020. https://www.brookings.edu/blog/the-avenue/2018/12/17/black-white-segregation-edges-downward-since-2000-census-shows.

Gamble, V. N. 1997. "Under the shadow of Tuskegee: African Americans and health care." *Am J Public Health* 87(11): 1773–1778. https://doi.org/10.2105/ajph.87.11.1773.

Gee, G. C., and C. L. Ford. 2011. "Structural racism and health inequities: Old issues, new directions." *Du Bois Rev* 8(1): 115–132. https://doi.org/10.1017/S1742058X11000130.

Gee, G. C., and A. Ro. 2009. "Racism and discrimination." In Asian American Communities and Health: Context, Research, Policy and Action, edited by C. Trinh-Shevrin, N. S. Islam, and M. J. Rey, 364–402. San Francisco, CA: Jossey-Bass.

Golden, S. D., T.-M. Kuo, A. Y. Kong, C. D. Baggett, L. Henriksen, and K. M. Ribisl. 2019. "County-level associations between tobacco retailer density and smoking prevalence in the USA, 2012." *Prev Med Rep* 17: 101005. https://doi.org/10.1016/j.pmedr.2019.101005.

Goodman, N., and M. Morris. 2017. *Banking Status and Financial Behaviors of Adults with Disabilities: Findings from the 2015 FDIC National Survey of Unbanked and Underbanked Households*. Washington, DC: National Disability Institute.

Goodman, N., M. Morris, K. Boston, and D. Walton. 2017. *Financial Inequality: Disability, Race, and Poverty in America*. Washington, DC: National Disability Institute.

Gordon, N. P., T. Y. Lin, J. Rau, and J. C. Lo. 2019. "Aggregation of Asian-American subgroups masks meaningful differences in health and health risks among Asian ethnicities: An electronic health record based cohort study." *BMC Public Health* 19(1): 1551.

Gover, A. R., S. B. Harper, and L. Langton. 2020. "Anti-Asian hate crime during the COVID-19 pandemic: Exploring the reproduction of inequality." *Am J Crim Justice* 45(4): 647–667. https://doi.org/10.1007/s12103-020-09545-1.

Governing. 2019. "Residential segregation data for U.S. metro areas." Accessed May 7, 2020. https://www.governing.com/gov-data/education-data/residential-racial-segregation-metro-areas.html.

Goyal, M. K., N. Kuppermann, S. D. Cleary, S. J. Teach, and J. M. Chamberlain. 2015. "Racial disparities in pain management of children with appendicitis in emergency departments." *JAMA Pediatr* 169(11): 996–1002.

Grasser, G., D. Van Dyck, S. Titze, and W. Stronegger. 2013. "Objectively measured walkability and active transport and weight-related outcomes in adults: A systematic review." *Int J Public Health* 58(4): 615–625. https://doi.org/10.1007/s00038-012-0435-0.

Graves, J. L., Jr., and A. H. Goodman. 2021. *Racism, Not Race: Answers to Frequently Asked Questions*: New York, NY: Columbia University Press.

Green, C. R., K. O. Anderson, T. A. Baker, L. C. Campbell, S. Decker, R. B. Fillingim, D. A. Kalauokalani, et al. 2003. "The unequal burden of pain: Confronting racial and ethnic disparities in pain." *Pain Med* 4(3): 277–294. https://doi.org/10.1046/j.1526-4637.2003.03034.x.

Hajat, A., J. S. Kaufman, K. M. Rose, A. Siddiqi, and J. C. Thomas. 2010a. "Do the wealthy have a health advantage? Cardiovascular disease risk factors and wealth." *Soc Sci Med* 71(11): 1935–1942. https://doi.org/10.1016/j.socscimed.2010.09.027.

Hajat, A., J. S. Kaufman, K. M. Rose, A. Siddiqi, and J. C. Thomas. 2010b. "Long-term effects of wealth on mortality and self-rated health status." *Am J Epidemiol* 173(2): 192–200. https://doi.org/10.1093/aje/kwq348.

Hanna-Attisha, M., J. LaChance, R. C. Sadler, and A. C. Schnepp. 2015. "Elevated blood lead levels in children associated with the Flint drinking water crisis: A spatial analysis of risk and public health response." *Am J Public Health* 106(2): 283–290. https://doi.org/10.2105/AJPH.2015.303003.

Hirsch, J. A., K. A. Moore, P. J. Clarke, D. A. Rodriguez, K. R. Evenson, S. J. Brines, M. A. Zagorski, and A. V. Diez Roux. 2014. "Changes in the built environment and changes in the amount of walking over time: Longitudinal results from the Multi-Ethnic Study of Atherosclerosis." *Am J Epidemiol* 180(8): 799–809. https://doi.org/10.1093/aje/kwu218.

Hirschfield, P. J. 2008. "Preparing for prison? The criminalization of school discipline in the USA." *Theoretical Criminol* 12(1): 79–101. https://doi.org/10.1177/1362480607085795.

Hoffman, K. M., S. Trawalter, J. R. Axt, and M. N. Oliver. 2016. "Racial bias in pain assessment and treatment recommendations, and false beliefs about biological differences between Blacks and Whites." *Proc Natl Acad Sci USA* 113(16): 4296–4301. https://doi.org/10.1073/pnas.1516047113.

Holland, A. T., and L. P. Palaniappan. 2012. "Problems with the collection and interpretation of Asian-American health data: Omission, aggregation, and extrapolation." *Ann Epidemiol* 22(6): 397–405. https://doi.org/10.1016/j.annepidem.2012.04.001.

Huang, K.-Y., E. Calzada, S. Cheng, and L. Miller Brotman. 2012. "Physical and mental health disparities among young children of Asian immigrants." *J Pediatr* 160(2): 331–336.e1. https://doi.org/10.1016/j.jpeds.2011.08.005.

Hughes, H. K., E. C. Matsui, M. M. Tschudy, C. E. Pollack, and C. A. Keet. 2017. "Pediatric asthma health disparities: Race, hardship, housing, and asthma in a national survey." *Acad Pediatr* 17(2): 127–134. https://doi.org/10.1016/j.acap.2016.11.011.

Ignatiev, N. 2009. *How the Irish became White*: Routledge.

Incarcerated Workers Organizing Committee. 2018. *Cruel and Unusual: A National Prisoner Survey of Prison Food and Health Care Quality*. Washington, DC: Incarcerated Workers Organizing Committee.

Institute of Medicine Committee on Understanding and Eliminating Racial and Ethnic Disparities in Health Care. 2003. *Unequal Treatment: Confronting Racial and Ethnic Disparities in Health Care*, edited by B. D. Smedley, A. Y. Stith, and A. R. Nelson. Washington, DC: National Academies Press.

James, T. 2017, December 23. "Can cops unlearn their unconscious biases?" *The Atlantic*. https://www.theatlantic.com/politics/archive/2017/12/implicit-bias-training-salt-lake/548996.

Jensen, G. M. 1998. "The experience of injustice: Health consequences of the Japanese American internment." *Diss Abstr Int A Humanities Soc Sci* 58(7-A): 2718.

Jones, C. P., B. I. Truman, L. D. Elam-Evans, C. A. Jones, C. Y. Jones, R. Jiles, S. F. Rumisha, and G. S. Perry. 2008. "Using 'socially assigned race' to probe White advantages in health status." *Ethnic Dis* 18(4): 496–504.

Kahn, K. B., and K. D. Martin. 2016. "Policing and race: Disparate treatment, perceptions, and policy responses." *Soc Issues Policy Rev* 10(1): 82–121. https://doi.org/10.1111/sipr.12019.

Kaplan, G. A., N. Ranjit, and S. A. Burgard. 2008. "Lifting gates—lengthening lives: Did civil rights policies improve the health of African-American women in the 1960's and 1970's?" In *Making Americans Healthier, Social and Economic Policy as Health Policy*, edited by R. F. Schoeni, J. S. House, G. A. Kaplan, and H. Pollack, 145–169. New York, NY: Russell Sage Foundation.

Karklis, L., and E. Badger. 2015, November 4. "Every term the Census has used to describe America's racial and ethnic groups since 1790." *The Washington Post.* https://www.was hingtonpost.com/news/wonk/wp/2015/11/ 04/every-term-the-census-has-used-to-descr ibe-americas-racial-groups-since-1790.

Katznelson, I. 2005. *When Affirmative Action Was White: An Untold History of Racial Inequality in Twentieth-Century America.* New York, NY: Norton.

Kawachi, I., S. V. Subramanian, and D. Kim. 2008. "Social capital and health." In *Social Capital and Health,* edited by I. Kawachi, S. V. Subramanian, and D. Kim, 1–26. New York, NY: Springer.

Keyssar, A. 2009. *The right to vote: The contested history of democracy in the United States.* New York, NY: Basic Books.

Kim, P., G. W. Evans, M. Angstadt, S. S. Ho, C. S. Sripada, J. E. Swain, I. Liberzon, and K. L. Phan. 2013. "Effects of childhood poverty and chronic stress on emotion regulatory brain function in adulthood." *Proc Natl Acad Sci USA* 110(46): 18442–18447. https://doi. org/10.1073/pnas.1308240110.

Knight, A. K., and A. K. Smith. 2016. "Epigenetic biomarkers of preterm birth and its risk factors." *Genes* 7(4): 15.

Kochhar, R., and A. Cilluffo. 2018. *Income Inequality in the U.S. Is Rising Most Rapidly Among Asians.* Washington, DC: Pew Research Center.

Kochhar, R., and Fry, R. 2014. *Wealth Inequality Has Widened Along Racial, Ethnic Lines Since End of Great Recession.* Washington, DC: Pew Research Center.

Kogan, M. D., G. R. Alexander, M. Kotelchuck, D. A. Nagey, and B. W. Jack. 1994. "Comparing mothers' reports on the content of prenatal care received with recommended national guidelines for care." *Public Health Rep* 109(5): 637–646.

Kogan, M. D., M. Kotelchuck, G. R. Alexander, and W. E. Johnson. 1994. "Racial disparities in reported prenatal care advice from health care providers." *Am J Public Health* 84(1): 82–88. https://doi.org/10.2105/ajph.84.1.82.

Krieger, N. 1987. "Shades of difference: Theoretical underpinnings of the medical controversy on Black/White differences in the United States, 1830–1870." *Int J Health Services* 17(2): 259–278.

Krieger, N. 2014. "Discrimination and health inequities." *Int J Health Services* 44(4): 643–710.

Kutateladze, B. L., N. R. Andiloro, B. D. Johnson, and C. C. Spohn. 2014. "Cumulative disadvantage: Examining racial and ethnic disparity in prosecution and sentencing." *Criminology* 52(3): 514–551. https://doi.org/ 10.1111/1745-9125.12047.

Kwate, N. O. A., and I. H. Meyer. 2011. "On sticks and stones and broken bones: Stereotypes and African American health." *Du Bois Rev* 8(1): 191–198. https://doi.org/10.1017/ S1742058X11000014.

Lambda Legal Defense and Education Fund. 2014. *When Health Care Isn't Caring: Lambda Legal's Survey on Discrimination Against LGBT People and People Living with HIV.* New York, NY: Lambda Legal Defense and Education Fund.

Lantz, P. M., J. S. House, J. M. Lepkowski, D. R. Williams, R. P. Mero, and J. Chen. 1998. "Socioeconomic factors, health behaviors, and mortality: Results from a nationally representative prospective study of US adults." *JAMA* 279(21): 1703–1708. https://doi.org/ 10.1001/jama.279.21.1703.

Lauderdale, D. S. 2006. "Birth outcomes for Arabic-named women in California before and after September 11." *Demography* 43(1): 185–201.

Lazo, M., U. Bilal, and R. Perez-Escamilla. 2015. "Epidemiology of NAFLD and type 2 diabetes: Health disparities among persons of Hispanic origin." *Curr Diabetes Rep* 15(12): 116. https://doi.org/10.1007/s11892-015-0674-6.

Le, H., S. Hirota, J. Liou, T. Sitlin, C. Le, and T. Quach. 2017. "Oral health disparities and inequities in Asian Americans and Pacific Islanders." *Am J Public Health* 107(Suppl 1): S34–S35. https://doi.org/10.2105/ ajph.2017.303838.

Lee, D. B., M. K. Peckins, J. E. Heinze, A. L. Miller, S. Assari, and M. A. Zimmerman. 2018. "Psychological pathways from racial discrimination to cortisol in African American males and females." *J Behav Med* 41(2): 208–220. https://doi.org/10.1007/s10 865-017-9887-2.

Lee, E. 2002. "Enforcing the borders: Chinese exclusion along the U.S. borders with Canada and Mexico, 1882–1924." *J Am Hist* 89(1): 54–86. https://doi.org/10.2307/2700784.

Lee, J. G., L. Henriksen, S. W. Rose, S. Moreland-Russell, and K. M. Ribisl. 2015. "A systematic review of neighborhood disparities in point-of-sale tobacco marketing." *Am J Public Health* 105(9): e8–e18. https://doi.org/10.2105/AJPH.2015.302777.

Lee, R. D., and J. Chen. 2017. "Adverse childhood experiences, mental health, and excessive alcohol use: Examination of race/ethnicity and sex differences." *Child Abuse Negl* 69: 40–48. https://doi.org/10.1016/j.chiabu.2017.04.004.

Leventhal, T., and V. Dupéré. 2019. "Neighborhood effects on children's development in experimental and nonexperimental research." *Annu Rev Dev Psychol* 1: 149–176. https://doi.org/10.1146/annurev-devpsych-121318-085221.

Lewis, T. T., C. D. Cogburn, and D. R. Williams. 2015. "Self-reported experiences of discrimination and health: Scientific advances, ongoing controversies, and emerging issues." *Annu Rev Clin Psychol* 11(11): 407–440.

López, G., N. G. Ruiz, and E. Patten. 2017. *Key Facts About Asian Americans, a Diverse and Growing Population*. Washington, DC: Pew Research Center.

Loudermilk, E., K. Loudermilk, J. Obenauer, and M. A. Quinn. 2018. "Impact of adverse childhood experiences (ACEs) on adult alcohol consumption behaviors." *Child Abuse Negl* 86: 368–374. https://doi.org/10.1016/j.chiabu.2018.08.006.

Macias Gil, R., J. R. Marcelin, B. Zuniga-Blanco, C. Marquez, T. Mathew, and D. A. Piggott. 2020. "COVID-19 pandemic: Disparate health impact on the Hispanic/Latinx population in the United States." *J Infect Dis* 222(10): 1592–1595. https://doi.org/10.1093/infdis/jiaa474.

Mallett, C. A. 2016. "The school-to-prison pipeline: A critical review of the punitive paradigm shift." *Child Adolesc Soc Work J* 33(1): 15–24. https://doi.org/10.1007/s10560-015-0397-1.

Martino, S., R. L Collins, S. A. Kovalchik, C. M. Setodji, E. J. D'Amico, K. Becker, W. G. Shadel, and A. A. Tolpadi. 2018. "Drinking it in: The impact of youth exposure to alcohol advertising." RAND Corporation. https://doi.org/10.7249/RB10015.

Martinson, M. L., and N. E. Reichman. 2016. "Socioeconomic inequalities in low birth weight in the United States, the United Kingdom, Canada, and Australia." *Am J Public Health* 106(4): 748–754. https://doi.org/10.2105/ajph.2015.303007.

McDonough, P., G. J. Duncan, D. Williams, and J. House. 1997. "Income dynamics and adult mortality in the United States, 1972 through 1989." *Am J Public Health* 87(9): 1476–1483.

McEwen, B. S. 2007. "Physiology and neurobiology of stress and adaptation: Central role of the brain." *Physiol Rev* 87 (3):873–904.

McEwen, B. S. 2008. "Central effects of stress hormones in health and disease: Understanding the protective and damaging effects of stress and stress mediators." *Eur J Pharmacol* 583(2–3): 174–185. https://doi.org/10.1016/j.ejphar.2007.11.071.

McGhee, H. C. 2021. *The Sum of Us: What Racism Costs Everyone and How We Can Prosper Together*. New York, NY: One World.

McGrady, G. A., J. F. C. Sung, D. L. Rowley, and C. J. R. Hogue. 1992. "Preterm delivery and low birth weight among first-born infants of Black and White college graduates." *Am J Epidemiol* 136(3): 266–276.

Mendel, R. A. 2015. *Maltreatment of Youth in US Juvenile Corrections Facilities*. Baltimore, MD: Annie E. Casey Foundation.

Michigan Civil Rights Commission. 2017. *The Flint Water Crisis: Systemic Racism Through the Eyes of Flint*. Lansing, MI: Michigan Civil Rights Commission.

Mitchell, B., and J. Franco. 2018. "HOLC 'redlining' maps: The persistent structure of segregation and economic inequality." National Community Reinvestment Coalition. https://ncrc.org/holc.

Modvig, J. 2014. "Violence, sexual abuse and torture in prisons." In *Prisons and Health*, edited by S. Enggist, L. Møller, G. Galea, and C. Udesen, 19–26. Geneva, Switzerland: World Health Organization.

Mohai, P. 2018. "Environmental justice and the Flint water crisis." *Michigan Soc Rev* 32: 1–41.

Morello-Frosch, R., and R. Lopez. 2006. "The riskscape and the color line: Examining the role of segregation in environmental health disparities." *Environ Res* 102(2): 181–196. https://doi.org/10.1016/j.envres.2006.05.007.

Murray, L. R. 2003. "Sick and tired of being sick and tired: Scientific evidence, methods, and research implications for racial and ethnic disparities in occupational health." *Am J Public Health* 93(2): 221–226. https://doi.org/10.2105/ajph.93.2.221.

Myers, H. F., T. T. Lewis, and T. Parker-Dominguez. 2003. "Stress, coping and minority health." In *Handbook of Racial and Ethnic Minority Psychology*, edited by G. Bernal, J. E. Trimble, A. K. Burlew, and F. T. L. Leong, 377–400. Thousand Oaks, CA: Sage.

National Center for Health Statistics. 2018. "Health, United States, 2018." Centers for Disease Control and Prevention. Accessed December 1, 2020. https://www.cdc.gov/nchs/data/hus/hus18.pdf

National Council on Disability. 2009. *The Current State of Health Care for People with Disabilities*. Washington, DC: National Council on Disability.

Nellis, A. 2016. *The Color of Justice: Racial and Ethnic Disparity in State Prisons*. Washington, DC: The Sentencing Project.

Nelson, L., and D. Lind. 2015. *The School to Prison Pipeline, Explained*. Washington, DC: Justice Policy Institute.

New York Civil Liberties Union. 2019. "Stop-and-frisk in the de Blasio era." https://www.nyclu.org/sites/default/files/field_documents/20190314_nyclu_stopfrisk_singles.pdf

Nguyen, T. T., S. Criss, P. Dwivedi, D. Huang, J. Keralis, E. Hsu, L. Phan, et al. 2020. "Exploring U.S. shifts in anti-Asian sentiment with the emergence of COVID-19." *Int J Environ Res Public Health* 17(19): 7032. https://doi.org/10.3390/ijerph17197032.

Nuru-Jeter, A., T. P. Dominguez, W. P. Hammond, J. Leu, M. Skaff, S. Egerter, C. P. Jones, and P. Braveman. 2009. "'It's the skin you're in': African-American women talk about their experiences of racism. An exploratory study to develop measures of racism for birth outcome studies." *Matern Child Health J* 13(1): 29–39. https://doi.org/10.1007/s10995-008-0357-x.

Ogletree, C., Jr, and A. Sarat. 2006. *From Lynch Mobs to the Killing State: Race and the Death Penalty in America*. The Charles Hamilton Houston Institute Series on Race and Justice, Vol. 6. New York, NY: New York University Press.

Oh, S. J., and J. Yinger. 2015. "What have we learned from paired testing in housing markets?" *Cityscape* 17(3): 15–60.

Owens, A. 2017. "Income segregation between school districts and inequality in students' achievement." *Sociol Educ* 91(1): 1–27.

Pager, D., and H. Shepherd. 2008. "The sociology of discrimination: Racial discrimination in employment, housing, credit, and consumer markets." *Annu Rev Sociol* 34(1): 181–209. https://doi.org/10.1146/annurev.soc.33.040406.131740.

Park, Y. 2008. "Facilitating injustice: Tracing the role of social workers in the World War II internment of Japanese Americans." *Soc Service Rev* 82: 447–483. https://doi.org/10.1086/592361.

Pascoe, E. A., and L. Smart Richman. 2009. "Perceived discrimination and health: A meta-analytic review." *Psychol Bull.* 135(4): 531.

Pember, M. A. 2019. "Death by civilization." *The Atlantic*. https://www.theatlantic.com/education/archive/2019/03/traumatic-legacy-indian-boarding-schools/584293/

Pervanidou, P., and G. P. Chrousos. 2011. "Stress and obesity/metabolic syndrome in childhood and adolescence." *Int J Pediatr Obes* 6(Suppl 1): 21–28. https://doi.org/10.3109/17477166.2011.615996.

Petersen, E. E., N. L. Davis, D. Goodman, S. Cox, C. Syverson, K. Seed, C. Shapiro-Mendoza, W. M. Callaghan, and W. Barfield. 2019. "Racial/ethnic disparities in pregnancy-related deaths—United States, 2007–2016." *MMWR Morb Mortal Wkly Rep* 68(35): 762–765. https://doi.org/10.15585/mmwr.mm6835a3.

Pettit, B., and B. Western. 2004. "Mass imprisonment and the life course: Race and class inequality in US incarceration." *Am Sociol Rev* 69(2): 151–169.

Pollack, C. E., C. Cubbin, A. Sania, M. Hayward, D. Vallone, B. Flaherty, and P. A. Braveman. 2013. "Do wealth disparities contribute to health disparities within racial/ethnic groups?" *J Epidemiol Community Health* 67(5): 439–445.

Pratt, B. M., L. Hixson, and N. A. Jones. 2015. "Measuring race and ethnicity across the decades: 1790–2010." https://www.census.gov/newsroom/blogs/random-samplings/2015/11/measuring-race-and-ethnicity-across-the-decades-1790-2010.html.

Putnam, R. D. 1993. "The prosperous community: Social capital and public life." *Am Prospect* (13): 35–42.

Quick, K., and R. D. Kahlenberg. 2019. *Attacking the Black–White Opportunity Gap That Comes from Residential Segregation*. New York, NY: The Century Foundation.

Reardon, S. F., L. Fox, and J. Townsend. 2015. "Neighborhood income composition by household race and income, 1990–2009." *Ann Am Acad Polit Soc Sci* 660(1): 78–97.

Rehkopf, D. H., I. Headen, A. Hubbard, J. Deardorff, Y. Kesavan, A. K. Cohen, D. Patil, L. D. Ritchie, and B. Abrams. 2016. "Adverse childhood experiences and later life adult obesity and smoking in the United States." *Ann Epidemiol* 26(7): 488–492.e5. https://doi.org/10.1016/j.annepidem.2016.06.003.

Richard, K. 2014, October. "The wealth gap for women of color." Center for Global Policy Solutions. http://globalpolicysolutions.org/wp-content/uploads/2014/10/Wealth-and-women-of-color.pdf.

Roediger, D. R. 2006. *Working Toward Whiteness: How America's Immigrants Became White: The Strange Journey from Ellis Island to the Suburbs*. New York, NY: Hachette.

Rosenberg, N. A., J. K. Pritchard, J. L. Weber, H. M. Cann, K. K. Kidd, L. A. Zhivotovsky, and M. W. Feldman. 2002. "Genetic structure of human populations." *Science* 298(5602): 2381–2385.

Ross, C. T. 2015. "A multi-level Bayesian analysis of racial bias in police shootings at the county-level in the United States, 2011–2014." *PLoS One* 10(11): e0141854. https://doi.org/10.1371/journal.pone.0141854.

Rossen, L. M., L. S. Womack, D. L. Hoyert, R. N. Anderson, and S. F. G. Uddin. 2020. "The impact of the pregnancy checkbox and misclassification on maternal mortality trends in the United States, 1999–2017." *Vital Health Stat 3*(44): 1–61.

Rothstein, R. 2017. *The Color of Law: A Forgotten History of How Our Government Segregated America*. New York, NY: Liveright.

Rubens, C. E., Y. Sadovsky, L. Muglia, M. G. Gravett, E. Lackritz, and C. Gravett. 2014. "Prevention of preterm birth: Harnessing science to address the global epidemic." *Sci Transl Med* 6(262): 262sr5.

Safer, J. D., E. Coleman, J. Feldman, R. Garofalo, W. Hembree, A. Radix, and J. Sevelius. 2016. "Barriers to healthcare for transgender individuals." *Curr Opin Endocrinol Diabetes Obes* 23(2): 168–171. https://doi.org/10.1097/MED.0000000000000227.

Shah, S. M., C. Ayash, N. A. Pharaon, and F. M. Gany. 2008. "Arab American immigrants in New York: Health care and cancer knowledge, attitudes, and beliefs." *J Immigr Minor Health* 10(5): 429–436. https://doi.org/10.1007/s10903-007-9106-2.

Sharkey, P. 2014. "Spatial segmentation and the Black middle class." *Am J Sociol* 119(4): 903–954.

Shavers, V. L., A. Bakos, and V. B. Sheppard. 2010. "Race, ethnicity, and pain among the U.S. adult population." *J Health Care Poor Underserved* 21(1): 177–220. https://doi.org/10.1353/hpu.0.0255.

Sherk, A., T. Stockwell, T. Chikritzhs, S. Andréasson, C. Angus, J. Gripenberg, H. Holder, et al. 2018. "Alcohol consumption and the physical availability of take-away alcohol: Systematic reviews and meta-analyses of the days and hours of sale and outlet density." *J Stud Alcohol Drugs* 79(1): 58–67. https://doi.org/10.15288/jsad.2018.79.58.

Shirer, W. L. 1991. *The Rise and Fall of the Third Reich: A History of Nazi Germany*. New York, NY: Random House.

Shonkoff, J. P., A. S. Garner, B. S. Siegel, M. I. Dobbins, M. F. Earls, A. S. Garner, L. McGuinn, J. Pascoe, and D. L. Wood. 2012. "The lifelong effects of early childhood adversity and toxic stress." *Pediatrics* 129(1): e232–e246. https://doi.org/10.1542/peds.2011-2663.

Smedley, A. 2007. *Race in North America: Origin and Evolution of a Worldview*. Boulder, CO: Westview.

Solomon, D., C. Maxwell, and A. Castro. 2019. *Systematic Inequality and American Democracy*. Washington, DC: Center for American Progress.

Sonu, S., S. Post, and J. Feinglass. 2019. "Adverse childhood experiences and the onset of chronic disease in young adulthood." *Prev Med* 123: 163–170. https://doi.org/10.1016/j.ypmed.2019.03.032.

Southall, A., and M. Gold. 2019. "Why 'stop-and-frisk' inflamed Black and Hispanic neighborhoods." *The New York Times*. Accessed December 2, 2020. https://www.nytimes.com/2019/11/17/nyregion/bloomberg-stop-and-frisk-new-york.html.

Spencer, K. B., A. K. Charbonneau, and J. Glaser. 2016. "Implicit bias and policing." *Soc Pers Psychol Compass* 10(1): 50–63. https://doi.org/10.1111/spc3.12210.

Spohn, C. C. 2000. "Thirty years of sentencing reform: The quest for racially neutral sentencing process." National Criminal Justice Reference Service. Accessed December 2, 2020. https://www.ncjrs.gov/App/Publications/abstract.aspx?ID=185535.

Steele, C. M., and J Aronson. 1995. "Stereotype threat and the intellectual test performance of African Americans." *J Pers Social Psychol* 69(5): 797.

Steil, J. P., L. Albright, J. S. Rugh, and D. S. Massey. 2018. "The social structure of mortgage discrimination." *Housing Stud* 33(5): 759–776. https://doi.org/10.1080/02673037.2017.1390076.

Strandjord, C. 2009. "Filipino resistance to anti-miscegenation laws in Washington state." Accessed February 11, 2021. https://depts.washington.edu/depress/filipino_anti_miscegenation.shtml

Swope, C. B., and D. Hernández. 2019. "Housing as a determinant of health equity: A conceptual model." *Soc Sci Med* 243: 112571. https://doi.org/10.1016/j.socscimed.2019.112571.

Tausanovitch, A. 2019. *Voter-Determined Districts: Ending Gerrymandering and Ensuring Fair Representation*. Washington, DC: Center for American Progress.

Thayer, Z. M., and C. W. Kuzawa. 2011. "Biological memories of past environments: Epigenetic pathways to health disparities." *Epigenetics* 6(7): 798–803. https://doi.org/10.4161/epi.6.7.16222.

"The Counted: People killed by police in the United States." 2016. *The Guardian*. Accessed May 25, 2020. https://www.theguardian.com/us-news/ng-interactive/2015/jun/01/the-counted-police-killings-us-database.

The Sentencing Project. 2017a. "Black disparities in youth incarceration." https://www.sentencingproject.org/publications/black-disparities-youth-incarceration

The Sentencing Project. 2017b. "Latino disparities in youth incarceration." https://www.sentencingproject.org/publications/latino-disparities-youth-incarceration.

The Sentencing Project. 2017c. "Native disparities in youth incarceration." https://core.ac.uk/download/pdf/141922676.pdf.

The Sentencing Project. 2018. "Fact sheet: Trends in U.S. corrections." https://www.sentencingproject.org/wp-content/uploads/2021/07/Trends-in-US-Corrections.pdf.

Tomfohr, L. M., M. A. Pung, and J. E. Dimsdale. 2016. "Mediators of the relationship between race and allostatic load in African and White Americans." *Health Psychol* 35(4): 322–332. https://doi.org/10.1037/hea0000251.

Turner, M. A., R. Santos, D. K. Levy, D. Wissoker, C. L. Aranda, R. Pitingolo, and the Urban Institute. 2013. *Housing Discrimination Against Racial and Ethnic Minorities 2012*. Washington, DC: U.S. Department of Housing and Urban Development.

Uggen, C., R. Larson, and S. Shannon. 2016. "6 million lost voters: State-level estimates of felony disenfranchisement, 2016." Sentencing Project. https://www.sentencingproject.org/publications/6-million-lost-voters-state-level-estimates-felony-disenfranchisement-2016.

U.S. Department of the Interior. 2021. "Secretary Haaland announces federal Indian boarding school initiative." https://www.doi.gov/pressreleases/secretary-haaland-announces-federal-indian-boarding-school-initiative.

Uzogara, E. E., and J. S. Jackson. 2016. "Perceived skin tone discrimination across contexts: African American women's reports." *Race Soc Probl* 8(2): 147–159. https://doi.org/10.1007/s12552-016-9172-y.

Velasco-Mondragon, E., A. Jimenez, A. G. Palladino-Davis, D. Davis, and J. A. Escamilla-Cejudo. 2016. "Hispanic health in the USA: A scoping review of the literature." *Public Health Rev* 37(1): 31.

Vidal-Ortiz, S. 2008. "People of color." In Encyclopedia of *Race, Ethnicity*, and *Society*, edited by R. T. Schaefer, 1037–1039. Thousand Oaks, CA: Sage.

Washington, H. A. 2006. *Medical Apartheid: The Dark History of Medical Experimentation on Black Americans from Colonial Times to the Present*. New York, NY: Doubleday.

Western, B. 2006. *Punishment and Inequality in America*. New York, NY: Russell Sage Foundation.

Western, B., and J. Simes. 2019. "Criminal justice." In Stanford Center on Poverty and Inequality. https://inequality.stanford.edu/sites/default/files/Pathways_SOTU_2019_CriminalJustice.pdf.

Wheeler, S. M., and A. S. Bryant. 2017. "Racial and ethnic disparities in health and health care." *Obstet Gynecol Clin North Am* 44(1): 1–11. https://doi.org/10.1016/j.ogc.2016.10.001.

White, K., J. A. Lawrence, N. Tchangalova, S. J. Huang, and J. L. Cummings. 2020. "Socially-assigned race and health: A scoping review with global implications for population health equity." *Int J Equity Health* 19(1): 25. https://doi.org/10.1186/s12939-020-1137-5.

Wildeman, C., and E. A. Wang. 2017. "Mass incarceration, public health, and widening inequality in the USA." *Lancet* 389(10077): 1464–1474. https://doi.org/10.1016/S0140-6736(17)30259-3.

Wilkinson, R. G, and K. Pickett. 2009. The Spirit Level: Why More Equal Societies Almost Always Do Better. London, UK: Lane.

Williams, D. R. 2001. "Ethnicity, race, and health." In *International Encyclopedia of the Social & Behavioral Sciences*, edited by N. J. Smelser and P. B. Baltes, 4831–4838. Oxford, UK: Pergamon.

Williams, D. R., and C. Collins. 2001. "Racial residential segregation: A fundamental cause of racial disparities in health." *Public Health Rep* 116(5): 404–416. https://doi.org/10.1093/phr/116.5.404.

Williams, D. R., J. A. Lawrence, and B. A. Davis. 2019. "Racism and health: Evidence and needed research." *Annu Rev Public Health* 40(1): 105–125. https://doi.org/10.1146/annurev-publhealth-040218-043750.

Williams, D. R., and S. A. Mohammed. 2009. "Discrimination and racial disparities in health: Evidence and needed research." *J Behav Med* 32: 20–47.

Williams, D. R., and S. A. Mohammed. 2013. "Racism and health I: Pathways and scientific evidence." *Am Behav Sci* 57(8): 1152–1173. https://doi.org/10.1177/0002764213487340.

Williams, D. R., N. Priest, and N. B. Anderson. 2016. "Understanding associations among race, socioeconomic status, and health: Patterns and prospects." *Health Psychol* 35(4): 407–411. https://doi.org/10.1037/hea0000242.

Witherspoon, D. J., S. Wooding, A. R. Rogers, E. E. Marchani, W. S. Watkins, M. A. Batzer, and L. B. Jorde. 2007. "Genetic similarities within and between human populations." *Genetics* 176(1): 351–359.

Wolff, N., C. L. Blitz, J. Shi, J. Siegel, and R. Bachman. 2007. "Physical violence inside prisons: Rates of victimization." *Criminal Justice Behav* 34 (5): 588–599.

Wood, D. 2020. "As pandemic deaths add up, racial disparities persist—And in some cases worsen." NPR. Accessed December 1, 2020. https://www.npr.org/sections/health-shots/2020/09/23/914427907/as-pandemic-deaths-add-up-racial-disparities-persist-and-in-some-cases-worsen.

World Health Organization Commission on Social Determinants of Health. 2008. "Closing the gap in a generation: Health equity through action on the social determinants of health." *Lancet* 372(9650): 1661–1669.

Wormser, R. 2014. *The Rise and Fall of Jim Crow: The Companion to the PBS Television Series*. New York, NY: St. Martin's Press.

Wyatt, R. 2013. "Pain and ethnicity." *AMA J Ethics* 15 (5):449–54.

Yao, Y., A. M. Robinson, F. C. R. Zucchi, J. C. Robbins, O. Babenko, O. Kovalchuk, I. Kovalchuk, D. M. Olson, and G. A. S. Metz. 2014. "Ancestral exposure to stress epigenetically programs preterm birth risk and adverse maternal and newborn outcomes." *BMC Med* 12(1): 121.

Yearby, R. 2018. "Racial disparities in health status and access to healthcare: The continuation of inequality in the United States due to structural racism." *Am J Econ Sociol* 77(3-4): 1113–1152. https://doi.org/10.1111/ajes.12230.

Yehuda, R., and A. Lehrner. 2018. "Intergenerational transmission of trauma effects: Putative role of epigenetic mechanisms." *World Psychiatry* 17(3): 243–257. https://doi.org/10.1002/wps.20568.

Yi, S. S., S. C. Kwon, R. Sacks, and C. Trinh-Shevrin. 2016. "Commentary: Persistence and health-related consequences of the model minority stereotype for Asian Americans." *Ethnicity Dis* 26(1): 133–138. https://doi.org/10.18865/ed.26.1.133.

Yudell, M., D. Roberts, R. DeSalle, and S. Tishkoff. 2016. "Taking race out of human genetics." *Science* 351(6273): 564. https://doi.org/10.1126/science.aac4951.

Zaw, K., J. Bhattacharya, A. Price, D. Hamilton, and W. Darity, Jr. 2017. *Women, Race & Wealth.* Durham, NC/Oakland, CA: Samuel Duois Cook Center on Social Equity/Insight Center for Community Economic Development.

Zhang, W. 2019. "Standing up against racial discrimination: Progressive Americans and the Chinese Exclusion Act in the late nineteenth century." *Phylon* 56(1): 8–32.

CHAPTER 6

Early Childhood Experiences Shape Health Throughout Life

6.1. HOW DO ECONOMIC AND SOCIAL CONDITIONS EARLY IN LIFE SHAPE CHILDREN'S HEALTH AND DEVELOPMENT, AFFECTING THEIR HEALTH AS ADULTS?

Overview

Few people would doubt that childhood experiences are important, but many may be surprised that the social and economic conditions we experience in early childhood—defined here as the first 5 years of life—are among the most powerful forces that shape our health throughout life. During the past 20 years, accumulated knowledge has revealed that family income, wealth, education, neighborhood resources, and other social and economic factors affect health at every stage of life; the effects on young children, however, are particularly dramatic (Center on the Developing Child 2010; Shonkoff, Slopen, and Williams 2021). The first few years of life are critical for establishing a child's path toward—or away from—good health and well-being across the entire life span.

Not all parents have the same resources to help their children grow up healthy. ("Parent" is used here to refer to any primary guardian or caregiver, including a grandparent or foster parent when appropriate.) Parents' education and income levels can create—or limit—opportunities to provide their children with nurturing and stimulating environments and to model healthy behaviors. By limiting socioeconomic opportunities for people of color, racism plays a major role in limiting opportunities for some parents to provide health-promoting environments for their children. (See Chapter 5) These opportunities and obstacles, along with their health impacts, often compound over time and can be transmitted across generations as children grow up and become parents themselves.

A large body of evidence, reviewed here, ties experiences in early childhood directly or indirectly with health and well-being throughout life. Whereas favorable conditions early in life can launch a child on pathways toward optimal health and well-being, adverse experiences in early childhood can set off a vicious cycle leading to both social

The Social Determinants of Health and Health Disparities. Paula Braveman, Oxford University Press. © Oxford University Press 2023.
DOI: 10.1093/oso/9780190624118.003.0006

and health disadvantage in adulthood and, in turn, to more disadvantage for the next generation, continuing the cycle (Friedman et al. 2015). Evidence also indicates that policies and programs can help turn potentially vicious cycles into paths toward health by intervening early. Although the effects of these interventions appear largest for the most socially disadvantaged children, children in families of all socioeconomic levels experience benefits.

Children's Economic and Social Conditions Can Affect Their Health

The association between socioeconomic factors and child health is evident from birth. Factors such as nutrition, housing quality, and safety at home and in the community—all linked with family economic resources—are strongly associated with child health. For example, research shows that children's nutrition varies with parents' income and education and can have lasting effects on health throughout life (Patrick and Nicklas 2005). Both household budget constraints and greater exposure to convenience stores and fast-food outlets can thwart parents' efforts to provide nutritious food to their children (Drewnowski and Specter 2004; Black, Moon, and Baird 2014). As a result, many children in food-insecure homes are obese (Vargas, Stines, and Granado 2017). Obesity in childhood strongly predicts adult obesity and the accompanying long-term risks of chronic disease, disability, and premature death. Low-income children are more likely to be exposed to lead-based paint, most commonly found in substandard housing in lower income neighborhoods; this can lead to irreversible neurological damage. Socioeconomic characteristics of neighborhoods, which, because of racism, are often correlated with racial/ethnic composition of residents, also are associated with differences in air quality (Hajat, Hsia, and O'Neill 2015), pedestrian safety (Lee et al. 2015; DiMaggio 2015), and crime rates (Friedson and Sharkey 2015). African American, American Indian/Alaskan Native, and Latino children are far more likely to live in impoverished households than are Asian American or White children (U.S. Census Bureau 2018), putting them at heightened risk for all of the adverse exposures associated with poverty.

Children in impoverished families often face multiple adverse conditions at the same time, and they experience the cumulative effects of adversity over time (Evans 2004). The combined effects of the adverse experiences can take a particularly heavy toll on children's health, partly by causing chronic stress that overwhelms one's ability to cope (Evans and Kim 2013), sometimes referred to as "toxic stress" (Center on the Developing Child 2010; Shonkoff and Garner 2012). Physiologic effects of chronic stress in early childhood can include inflammation and altered immune function; these may contribute to depression, anxiety, cancer, diabetes, hypertension, and cardiovascular disease later in life (Center on the Developing Child 2010; Shonkoff and Garner 2012). (See Chapter 4.)

Children in African American, American Indian, and Latino families of all economic levels are often disadvantaged by systemic or structural racism. *Systemic* or *structural racism* refers to systems and structures—laws, other policies, and entrenched practices and beliefs—that systematically and repeatedly put people of color at a disadvantage; this can happen even when no individual now consciously intends to discriminate. Racial residential segregation is an illustrative example. Discriminatory housing and banking practices historically have relegated residents of largely minority areas to poorer housing and environmental quality, inferior schools, and obstacles to building wealth. Thus, segregated areas with high concentrations of people of color are often particularly underresourced. Discriminatory policing and sentencing place Black children at increased risk of having a parent incarcerated (or being incarcerated themselves) and therefore unable to contribute economically to their family's livelihood during and (because of stigmatization) following incarceration. The inequitable opportunities for good health experienced by children of color reflect not only greater exposure to health hazards but also more limited opportunities to benefit from the positive health-promoting conditions in more advantaged neighborhoods. These health consequences can accumulate across lifetimes and generations (Friedman et al. 2015). As a result, young children can suffer the effects of racism experienced by their parents years or even decades ago (Black et al. 2014). For example, poverty experienced by young children often reflects their parents' lack of economic and educational opportunities due to racial discrimination in their parents' childhood and young adulthood (Gee, Walsemann, and Brondolo 2012). (See Chapter 5.)

Economic and Social Conditions Also Affect Children's Development, Often Through Their Effects on Parents

Scientific advances in recent decades have demonstrated how economic and social experiences in the first few years of life shape infants' and toddlers' development, creating physiological as well as emotional and behavioral foundations—adverse or favorable—for health throughout life. Studies have tracked children's cognitive, behavioral, and physical development over time, along with environmental factors and parents' and other caregivers' interactions with children; some of these studies have followed children into adulthood. The results consistently link children's early development with economic and social advantages or disadvantages in the home (Center on the Developing Child 2010; Evans and Kim 2013; Shonkoff and Garner 2012; Hackman et al. 2015; Shonkoff et al. 2021; Boyce and Hertzman 2018).

Studies have repeatedly shown that parents' economic resources can affect the quality and stability of their relationships with their infants and that parent–infant relationships affect the cognitive stimulation that children receive, thus influencing their emotional and behavioral development (Center on the Developing Child 2010; Evans and Kim 2013; Shonkoff and Garner 2012; Boyce and Hertzman 2018; Shonkoff et al. 2021). The effect of family socioeconomic circumstances on children's language development is evident as early as 18 months (Fernald, Marchman, and Weisleder 2013). Children in families of middle, as well as low, socioeconomic status are at a disadvantage compared with their better-off counterparts (Fernald et al. 2013). Results of a large national study of children entering kindergarten showed that higher family income was associated with children having the academic and social skills necessary for kindergarten. Compared with children in the highest income families, children in the lowest income families were least likely to have the needed skills, but children in middle-income families also performed less well, both socially and academically, than the most affluent children (Barnett, Brown, and Shore 2004).

What explains these socioeconomic gaps in child development? And what are the implications for policy? Maternal depression is more prevalent among low-income mothers, and it can inhibit mother–infant bonding and reduce maternal ability to cognitively stimulate an infant or young child (Center on the Developing Child 2009; Conners-Burrow et al. 2014). Higher income and/or educational attainment of parents have been associated with more stimulation of and responsiveness to infants and young children, which are directly linked to brain development (Center on the Developing Child 2010; Evans and Kim 2013; Shonkoff and Garner 2012). On average, children from families of lower socioeconomic status are exposed to fewer words and less complex and diverse speech and they are engaged in fewer back-and-forth conversations in the home than children from more advantaged backgrounds (Hart and Risley 1995; Huttenlocher et al. 2007; Hoff 2003; Rowe 2012; Gilkerson et al. 2017; Romeo et al. 2018; Merz et al. 2020). Rich early language environments lead to better language and cognitive development, which in turn predicts school performance and, ultimately, economic and social opportunities in adulthood.

Educational differences in parents' awareness of children's early developmental needs probably play a role as well, although they are certainly not the only factor. Research also shows that higher income generally means lower levels of chronic, overwhelming stress in the home, as well as greater resources to cope with stressors—both of which can affect how parents interact with their children (Evans and Kim 2013). Financial hardship creates stress that can impede the ability of even highly motivated parents to provide the supportive and stimulating home environments needed in early childhood for optimal lifelong health and development (Masarik and Conger 2017). The chronic stress of facing ongoing demands with limited economic resources can create cognitive overload for parents, making it even more difficult for them to cope with parenting challenges (Mani et al. 2013; Vasquez and Howard-Field 2016; Oshri et al. 2019). All of these factors can adversely affect their children's future health.

Racial discrimination—including unconscious or "implicit" biases and often hidden discrimination built into laws, institutions, and policies—can create chronic stress for parents of color of all income and education levels. Among people of color with limited schooling and/or economic resources, this stress can add to the health-harming effects of poverty (Williams 1999; Clark et al. 1999). Experiences of racial discrimination have been shown to trigger physiologic mechanisms involved in the body's response to stressors in general (Clark et al. 1999; Adam et al. 2015; Lewis et al. 2010; Korous, Causadias, and Casper 2017; Busse et al. 2017). These mechanisms can be triggered not only by overt or dramatic incidents (e.g., being attacked physically) but also by chronic experiences (e.g., social dynamics at work or being followed by employees in stores because of stereotypical assumptions that people of particular races are likely to shoplift) that are less dramatic but pervasive (McEwen 2007). Chronic stress due to any cause, including racial discrimination, may make it more difficult for parents to provide optimal stimulation and support, despite strong motivation. (See Chapters 4 and 5.)

In addition to stress, racism can negatively affect early childhood development in many other ways. It can limit parents' wealth and educational attainment, for example, by relegating people of color to living in neighborhoods with little opportunity to escape poverty and build wealth. In addition, as a result of bias, children of color are more likely than others to be expelled from preschool for behavioral issues—often arising from experiences of trauma—that warrant supportive social and mental health services rather than punishment (Gilliam 2005; Meek and Gilliam 2016). Excluding these very young children from preschool can compromise their cognitive and socioemotional development, limiting their future economic opportunities and affecting their lifelong health. Racially discriminatory criminal justice practices that have produced mass incarceration of men of color have deprived many children of their father's involvement in their early life and have had devastating economic consequences for families and communities (Banks 2004; Nellis 2016).

Children's Development Shapes Their Educational Success and Therefore Their Economic and Social Well-Being as Adults

The first few years of life are crucial in establishing the path—including the opportunities and obstacles along the way—that a child will follow toward economic and social well-being in adulthood. Without intervention, the gaps in cognitive and behavioral skills that are apparent when children enter school generally do not close. In fact, these gaps can grow even larger as disadvantaged children progress more slowly than children from higher income and better educated families. A large national study by the U.S. Department of Education showed that children at higher social risk (e.g., because of poverty) not only had lower reading and math scores in kindergarten but also experienced smaller gains in both of these areas by the end of third grade compared with children who had fewer family risk factors (National Center for Education Statistics 2017). In turn, poor academic performance in elementary school is linked with subsequently dropping out of high school (Lee-St. John et al. 2018), which increases the risk of using illicit drugs and being arrested, fired from employment, receiving food stamps (Supplemental Nutrition Assistance Program [SNAP] benefits), and having poor health by age 27 years (Lansford et al. 2016).

Children's Development Shapes Their Health Throughout Life

Our health as adults is powerfully influenced by how we developed—physically, cognitively, and emotionally—as children. Research has strongly linked brain, cognitive, and behavioral development early in life with an array of important health and health-related outcomes later in life, including cardiovascular disease, hypertension, diabetes, obesity, smoking, drug use, and depression (Center on the Developing Child 2010; Evans and Kim 2013; Shonkoff and Garner 2012). These conditions account for a major portion of preventable morbidity and premature mortality in the United States. Inadequate stimulation and nurturing by adults and experiences of toxic stress are thought to play important roles in suboptimal development—for example, by leading to changes in brain architecture and in physiologic systems controlling responses to stress (Shonkoff and Garner 2012). Early cognitive, emotional, and behavioral developmental damage related to toxic stress can lead to difficulties paying attention and poor impulse control, which can hamper educational success and subsequent economic and social well-being—and health—during adulthood (Moffitt et al. 2011; Jones, Greenberg, and Crowley 2015). Damage to cognitive, emotional, and behavioral development in early childhood also increases the risk of engaging in unhealthy behaviors that can adversely affect health throughout life (Jones, Greenberg, and Crowley 2015; Moffitt et al. 2011; Conti and Heckman 2010). Self-regulation—the capacity to control one's own emotions and behaviors—is thought to play a key role in these relationships (Center on the Developing Child 2010; Blair and Raver 2016).

6.2. WHAT IS KNOWN ABOUT WHAT WORKS?

Although many studies have shown that social and economic disadvantage early in life can limit opportunities for good health across the life span, a growing body of research indicates that early childhood interventions have the potential to interrupt the inequitable cycle linking young children's experiences of social and economic disadvantage with health disadvantage throughout their lives. A range of knowledge-based programs and policies can help improve children's prospects for lifelong health and well-being. Accumulated knowledge supports a comprehensive approach to intervention. Isolated programs generally have had limited effects; effective solutions will require programs and policies across multiple domains—for example, education, housing, employment development, and mental health. Even for programs and policies that have been studied extensively, more research is needed to determine how they can be most effectively and efficiently implemented, particularly on a large scale.

Early Care and Education Programs Have Been Linked with Lifelong Health

Evidence from more than 40 years of research links both short- and long-term health and health-related outcomes with a range of early care and education programs (Campbell et al. 2014; Conti, Heckman, and Pinto 2016; Duffee et al. 2017; Michalopoulos et al. 2019). These center- or home-based programs are typically designed to provide young children with experiences that buffer or protect against the negative effects of the social and economic challenges they may face in their homes and neighborhoods. Health benefits of these types of interventions include lower rates of adverse outcomes such as maternal and child mortality, child emergency department visits, child maltreatment, and adolescent mental health problems, as well as improved health-related behaviors such as better eating habits, reduced substance use in adolescence, and better use of preventive health services such as screenings and immunizations (Conti, Heckman, and Pinto 2016; Duffee et al. 2017; Michalopoulos et al. 2019; Olds et al. 2014; Cannon et al. 2017). Experimental and observational studies have also linked early care and education with favorable health outcomes by demonstrating their impact on later social outcomes that have well-established health consequences. These outcomes include teen pregnancy, school performance, intelligence quotient (IQ), receipt of special education services, educational attainment, employment (of the child's mother and of the child as an adult), income in adulthood, receipt of public assistance, delinquency and criminal behavior, arrests, and incarceration (Karoly, Kilburn, and Cannon 2005; De Haan and Leuven 2019; Reynolds et al. 2007, 2017; Miller 2015).

The positive impacts of early care and education are not confined to a particular social group; they are apparent across different socioeconomic groups. Evaluations of center-based programs including children from families of different income levels have shown favorable impacts among all participants, including middle-class children (Yoshikawa et al. 2013). For disadvantaged children, high-quality child care, education, and family support programs appear to act as buffers against physical and psychosocial adversity both by providing stability and stimulation for the children and by strengthening parents' abilities to meet their children's developmental and health needs at home (Shonkoff and Fisher 2013).

Despite greater need, access to promising interventions is often limited among the socioeconomically disadvantaged families whose children would benefit most. Available child care services range from care provided by untrained and unlicensed individual caregivers to care at licensed centers run by staff trained in promoting early childhood development. For low-income families, settings with unlicensed and untrained caregivers are often the only affordable and accessible option. Head Start is the oldest and largest federally funded early care and education program serving low-income children and their families. Due to limited availability, however, only 54% of children who were eligible for Head Start and 5% of infants and toddlers who were eligible for Early Head Start were enrolled in 2016 (The Children's Defense Fund 2018).

Despite promising findings from a number of studies, there are major methodological challenges in studying the health effects of early care and education programs. Because childhood is a time of generally good health, the direct health benefits of such interventions can be difficult to demonstrate. The signs and symptoms of chronic disease—for example, heart disease, stroke, and diabetes—rarely become evident until middle to late adulthood, and few studies have had sufficient resources to follow program participants and comparison groups for such long durations. Much of the evidence, therefore, has not linked early childhood interventions directly with health; rather, it has required "connecting the dots" between early childhood interventions and later social outcomes—such as educational attainment, economic self-sufficiency, or incarceration—with well-documented links to health.

In addition, although randomized experimental studies are generally considered more rigorous than nonrandomized observational studies, they usually require more resources and sometimes are not feasible or ethical. Given the expense and difficulty of conducting studies that are both randomized and longitudinal, much of our knowledge about the effects of early care and education has been drawn from evaluations of a relatively limited number of intensive programs that have been constrained by small sample sizes, participant attrition over time, and concerns about replicability (Conti, Heckman, and Pinto 2016; Englund et al. 2014; Shonkoff 2016). For example, a 2014 study found biomedical evidence that participants in a high-quality early care and education program had lower risks of heart disease and diabetes as adults, but its small sample size and high loss to follow-up limited the conclusiveness of its findings (Campbell et al. 2014). Larger scale programs, such as Head Start, have often had less consistent or less dramatic results, particularly when participants are followed over time. Some Head Start programs, however, have shown both short- and long-term—although not necessarily intermediate-term—positive effects (Duncan and Magnuson 2013). Head Start's initial impact on learning has been shown to vary substantially by geographic context as well as children's baseline skills, with lower-performing children and children from homes in which English is not the primary language experiencing the greatest gains (Morris et al. 2018).

Overall, the results of these studies support the need both to intervene and to conduct larger and more rigorous longitudinal studies of outcomes strongly linked to adult health from a wide range of promising programs. Although many positive health and health-related outcomes of center-based early care and education have been documented, more research is needed to identify the specific program components that are crucial to success. Current evidence suggests, however, that the effectiveness of these programs depends on a range of factors, including well-trained and responsive caregivers, small class sizes with high teacher–child ratios, safe and adequate physical environments, an age-appropriate curriculum focused on enhancing cognitive and social–emotional development, and comprehensive family engagement activities. There is little doubt, however, that early childhood intervention is worthwhile; rather, the questions are about the most effective and efficient approaches.

Supporting Children Requires Supporting Families

Children live with adults. Even when children are in full-time center-based programs, most of their time is spent at home, where persistent stress and limited resources can make it difficult for their parents to provide them with sufficiently stable and nurturing care (Center on the Developing Child 2010). Many successful early care and education programs therefore have included not only education and stimulation for children but also support for parents to help them improve their children's experiences at home. Services for parents often include referrals to social services and center-based activities designed to help them improve their parenting skills. Some programs do considerably more, such as helping parents continue their education, find work or job training, and enhance their self-efficacy and life skills (Chase-Lansdale and Brooks-Gunn 2014; Cannon et al. 2017). Some programs provide this support through home visits from paraprofessionals or registered nurses (Duffee et al. 2017). In others, pediatric primary care sites serve as entry points for parental services that can benefit children, such as take-home play activities that facilitate positive parenting behaviors (Shah et al. 2017); dietary counseling (Resnicow et al. 2015); and referrals to social workers, mental health professionals, or other community resources (Beck et al. 2018). The American Academy of Pediatrics has issued a policy statement urging providers to screen for maternal depression, parental substance abuse, domestic violence, and other family- and community-level factors that put children at risk for toxic stress and also to complement such screenings with "a greater focus on those interventions and community investments that reduce external threats to healthy brain growth" (Garner and Shonkoff 2012, p. 224). A growing number of communities are coordinating early care and education with health and support services for children and families. Although most programs target mothers, some also recognize the need to provide more support for fathers—for example, by providing parenting training, assistance with child support and related legal issues, and guidance for developing and maintaining healthy relationships with their partners and other coparents (Robin Dion, Zaveri, and Holcomb 2015).

Although parental leave is not often considered to be an early childhood intervention, flexible schedules and paid time off for working parents have been associated with significant reductions in adverse outcomes, including maternal stress and depression, low birth weight, and post-neonatal and early childhood mortality (Ruhm 2000; Burtle and Bezruchka 2016; Petts 2017). One way parental leave may promote early childhood development is by reducing obstacles to positive parent–child interactions and breastfeeding, both of which have been linked with improved neurocognitive development (Takeuchi et al. 2015; Hughes and Devine 2019; Eidelman et al. 2012). Breastfeeding is also associated with lower frequency and severity of childhood diseases such as respiratory infections and asthma (Eidelman et al. 2012). Parental leave can also have long-term benefits for children, including higher educational attainment and earnings in adulthood, especially when mothers have limited schooling (Carneiro, Loken, and Salvanes 2015). The United States is the only affluent country that, at the national level, does not guarantee paid time off after a birth or adoption (Raub et al. 2018); low- and middle-wage workers are far less likely to have paid parental leave than higher earners (U.S. Bureau of Labor Statistics 2018).

Broad Policies Addressing Social and Economic Disadvantage During Childhood

Poverty, discrimination, and their consequences are key obstacles to thriving during early childhood. Among affluent nations, the United States has one of the highest rates of both child and overall poverty (Organisation for Economic Co-operation and Development 2019). With few exceptions, the United States also has the worst health outcomes during childhood and throughout life up to 75 years of age (Woolf and Aron 2013). Other countries have seen declining child poverty and improved health outcomes across the life course after implementing deliberate social policies with a strong focus on early childhood. While keeping in mind unique features of the U.S. context, we can learn from the experiences of other countries with far less child poverty—for example, through policies providing government-guaranteed child support in the event of absent or delayed payments from noncustodial parents (Thévenon et al. 2018). We can also build on promising homegrown approaches to reduce child poverty and/or its deleterious consequences, such as the Earned Income Tax Credit (EITC) (Hoynes and Patel 2018), the Child Tax Credit (CTC) (Chetty, Friedman, and Rockoff 2011), and raising minimum wages (Allegreto et al. 2018).

Although ensuring income support for struggling families is crucial, additional supports—including improved access to high-quality child care, housing, nutritional support, and medical and mental health care—are also likely to be needed. Current knowledge about the links between housing and health indicates the crucial role that affordable housing initiatives can play in addressing the adverse health consequences of inadequate living conditions experienced by many children in low-income families. Research has documented many infant, child, and maternal health benefits of the Special Supplemental Nutrition Program for Women, Infants, and Children (WIC) (Colman et al. 2012) and SNAP (formerly called "food stamps") (Almond, Hoynes, and Schanzenbach 2010; Fox et al. 2004; Kreider et al. 2012). It is also worth considering how Medicare and Social Security have transformed the lives of the elderly and their families—and ways in which those successes might inform interventions for young children. Reducing poverty and strengthening supports and services for families are crucial, but they will not be sufficient without committed efforts to end structural inequities that disproportionately burden and marginalize people of color.

The Business Case for Investing in Early Childhood

Many programs and policies that seek to promote early childhood health and development have been evaluated, with varying levels of rigor. A 2017 RAND report systematically assessed 115 programs for which suitable health data were available; economic outcomes were also formally evaluated for 25 of these programs (Cannon et al. 2017). That report is the most comprehensive and up-to-date assessment of early childhood programs. More research is needed to identify the most effective and efficient approaches under varying conditions. Based on current knowledge, however, it is reasonable to expect large returns—in both human and economic terms—on investment in promising early childhood policies and programs. This will, however, require long-term investments, with benefits that may not be measurable for years or even decades—a reality that can be politically problematic for policymakers facing pressure to demonstrate short-term outcomes of spending.

Current knowledge indicates that addressing early childhood conditions will not only have favorable effects on disadvantaged children but also is likely to benefit the overall U.S. economy. For example, a larger investment in early childhood is likely to benefit the overall U.S. economy by producing healthier, better educated, and therefore more productive adults in the future. Children who participate in high-quality, early childhood programs are more likely to have the necessary skills—such as emotional regulation, abstract reasoning, problem-solving, and communication—to meet the demands of tomorrow's workforce. Children who have participated in center-based early care and education are more likely to be healthy and have higher earnings as adults, and they are less likely to commit crime and receive public assistance (Campbell et al. 2014; De Haan and Leuven 2019; Reynolds et al. 2007, 2017; Muennig et al. 2011). Several major national business organizations (e.g., the Committee for Economic Development, PNC Financial Services Group, and the Business Roundtable) and prominent economists (e.g., Arthur Rolnick and Rob Grunewald of the Federal Reserve Bank of Minneapolis and Nobel laureate James Heckman of the University of Chicago) have called for universal preschool as both a wise financial investment and an essential means of achieving a productive—which requires healthy and educated—U.S. workforce for the future (Grunewald and Rolnick 2006; Heckman et al. 2010; The PNC Financial Services Group 2017; Committee for Economic Development 2012).

The Nurse–Family Partnership, a nationwide home visiting program, was estimated to have prevented 684,000 crimes committed by youth and 36,000 youth arrests, and also to have reduced Temporary Assistance for Needy Families, SNAP, and Medicaid spending by $3 billion from 1996 to 2013; by comparison, the program costs for that time span totaled $1.6 billion (Miller 2015). Each dollar spent on a pregnant woman in WIC has been estimated to save approximately $2.48 in societal costs (including medical, educational, and economic productivity costs) due to the program's success in preventing preterm births (Nianogo et al. 2019).

Estimates of the expected rate of economic return on investment (i.e., the amount of economic savings that can be expected from investing a given amount of money) in center-based early care and education programs have ranged from $2.88 to $17.07 for every $1 spent, depending on the program and the length of follow-up (Karoly et al. 2005). These returns are projected to result from savings due to, for example, "less need for special education services, improved high school graduation rates, higher earnings, and less criminal activity in adulthood" (Karoly 2016, p. 37). A paper by Heckman and others (2010) estimated rates of economic return between 7% and 10%, which is higher than the historical return on capital investment. RAND senior economist Lynn Karoly recently stated that such estimates might be too high. Consistent with Bartik et al. (2016), who estimated benefit-to-cost ratios for the Tulsa, Oklahoma, pre-kindergarten program, Karoly (2016) argues that expected returns of $3 to $4 for every dollar spent may be more realistic, and these returns are still impressive. Programs that target disadvantaged children and families, as well as universal programs, have been associated with favorable economic returns (Cannon et al. 2017).

Experience has revealed that investments in early childhood must focus not only on providing early care and education services but also on ensuring that children grow up in health-promoting homes, schools, and neighborhoods, which requires addressing both poverty and systemic and structural racism. Although difficult to quantify, the lifelong health impacts of strategies to reduce (and/or buffer the effects of) childhood poverty are likely to be substantial. Low-income children whose families benefit from expanded state or federal EITCs, for example, are more likely to attend college. In addition, for children in families with incomes less than $25,000, receiving $3,000 a year in additional income before age 6 years is associated with 135 more working hours a year and a 17% increase in annual earnings in adulthood (Duncan and Magnuson 2011). Both college attendance and earnings in adulthood have been repeatedly linked with better health. (See Chapters 2 and 3.)

6.3. EXAMPLES OF EARLY CHILDHOOD INTERVENTIONS

As discussed above, many early childhood programs have been studied. More research is needed, however, to determine how they can be most effectively and efficiently implemented on a large scale across diverse settings. Examples of a range of programs and policies are briefly described here, primarily to acquaint the reader with the most widely known interventions and provide a sense of the broad scope of strategies. Some broad policies are noted here, such as the EITC, that do not target early childhood but are likely to have strong effects on families with young children. The interventions are grouped as center-based early care and education programs, home visiting programs, broad economic and social policies/programs, initiatives to strengthen systems, and efforts at clinical sites, recognizing that there is overlap in a number of cases.

> *Center-based early care and education programs* improve children's cognitive, socioemotional, and physical development, particularly when accompanied by significant supports for parents.(Note: Some center-based programs have included home visiting components)
> - The High/Scope Perry Preschool Project in Ypsilanti, Michigan, was a preschool experiment from 1963 to 1967 for 58 low-income African American children. The intervention consisted of daily classroom instruction by certified teachers and weekly home visits. Data were collected annually for ages 3–11 years and then later at ages 14, 15, 19, 27, and 40 years. Results showed that participants consistently outperformed controls on measures of educational attainment,

economic performance, family relationships, and health, and they were significantly less likely to commit crimes (Schweinhart 2004). High/Scope remains well known for its low child–teacher ratios (averaging 6:1) and emphasis on active learning; its curriculum is used in many preschools today.

- The Carolina Abecedarian Project was a preschool intervention targeting disadvantaged children in North Carolina from 1972 to 1985. A total of 57 low-income children were randomly assigned to receive full-time education from infancy through age 5 years. In addition to a game-based cognitive and language development curriculum, families received on-site pediatric health care, nutritional supplements, disposable diapers, and social work services. Studies conducted through age 35 years demonstrated long-lasting advantages, including greater educational attainment and employment, fewer depressive symptoms, and better physical health than controls (Campbell et al. 2014).

- Head Start, created in 1965, is the oldest federally funded program that provides low-income families with early learning and other support, such as health, nutrition, and other services determined by needs assessments. The program, operating in all 50 states, the District of Columbia, Puerto Rico, and the U.S. territories, encompasses Head Start center-based preschool programs and Early Head Start programs serving infants, toddlers, and pregnant women through home visiting, center-based care, and child care. The goal of Head Start is to promote development, good parenting, and parental self-sufficiency. Studies suggest that Head Start decreases preschool achievement gaps in language, literacy, and math. The Head Start Impact Study documents particularly notable performance gains among children facing unique academic challenges, such as dual language learners and children living with disabilities (Puma et al. 2010). Although some of these advantages appear to fade out by third grade, research has linked Head Start participation with long-term benefits known to predict better health, including lower rates of high school dropout and criminal activity (Cannon et al. 2017; Puma et al. 2012).

- Educare is a national network of year-round preschools. Educare promotes school readiness among low-income children from birth to age 5 years through parent–child engagement and instruction. The program is funded through public–private partnerships and currently operates in 20 sites, each serving 140–200 children (The Center for High Impact Philanthropy 2017). Evaluations show that Educare children have more extensive vocabularies and have better letter, number, and color recognition than their non-Educare peers. Educare-enrolled children also develop stronger social skills, including self-confidence, persistence, and emotional regulation (Yazejian et al. 2017). The Educare Chicago Follow-up Study found that children's socioemotional and concept development gains did not fade out at the end of third grade (Educare Learning Network 2017; Yazejian and Bryant 2012).

- Healthy Start is a large, long-standing (since 1991) center-based multistate federal program focused on community-based efforts to reduce infant mortality. Healthy Start is not generally thought of as an early childhood initiative. It could, however, be viewed as an effort to address upstream factors that influence not only infant mortality but also access to the resources and opportunities that shape early childhood and early childhood development.

Home visiting programs serving pregnant and/or postpartum mothers and their infants/toddlers through visits to the home by professionals and/or paraprofessionals to provide timely help with physical and cognitive development

- The Nurse–Family Partnership connects registered nurses with low-income, first-time mothers to conduct ongoing home visits from pregnancy through age 2 years. Visits focus on improving pregnancy outcomes by promoting favorable health-related behaviors, competent caregiving, pregnancy planning, education, and employment. Research suggests the program has reduced preterm birth and very low birth weight, child abuse and neglect, and arrests and convictions (Karoly et al. 2005; Holmes and Rutledge 2016; Thorland and Currie 2017). In addition, program participants were more likely to initiate and maintain breastfeeding and receive immunizations (Thorland et al. 2017). The Nurse–Family Partnership is supported by federal, state, and local agencies, as well as by the Robert Wood Johnson Foundation and other philanthropies. The program currently serves 34,405 families nationwide and has worked with 286,387 families since replication began in 1996 (Nurse–Family Partnership 2018).
- Healthy Families America (HFA), launched in 1992, is a nationally recognized home visiting program for families with low incomes or a history of child and substance abuse, mental health problems, or domestic violence. Families receive weekly visits until their child is 6 months old; later visit frequency is determined by families' needs (Healthy Families America 2015a). Implementation varies widely by region in terms of services, populations served, and quality, reflected by substantial variation in program effectiveness. However, many rigorous evaluations of well-established iterations of the program link HFA participation with greater maternal educational attainment and, reduced substance use, low birth weight, and child abuse. Children in HFA also experience improvements in cognitive and behavioral development (Healthy Families America 2015b; Jacobs et al. 2016; LeCroy and Davis 2016; Easterbrooks et al. 2017; Green, Sanders, and Tarte 2017). HFA currently serves approximately 100,000 families in more than 550 sites across 38 states, Washington, DC, and five U.S. territories. (U.S. Department of Health and Human Services 2018).

Initiatives to strengthen systems of care and education for young children by promoting coordination across multiple programs and sectors

- The Early Childhood Comprehensive Systems Collaborative Innovation and Improvement Network (ECCS CoIIN), funded by the Maternal and Child Health Bureau of the federal Health Resources and Service Administration, is a multiyear effort to improve early childhood systems across 12 states. The CoIIN strategy brings together multidisciplinary teams of federal, state, and local leaders through collaborative learning and quality improvement activities to reduce developmental disparities and enhance age-appropriate developmental skills in 3-year-olds. The grant program allowed recipients to select up to five place-based communities within their state to participate in efforts to improve the developmental skills of 3-year-olds by 25% by July 2021 (Health Resources and Services Administration 2017; National Institute for Children's Health Quality 2019).

- The Early Childhood Leadership Commission (ECLC) of Colorado, established in 2010, is a state advisory council composed of 20 early childhood advocates and leaders, including parents, early childhood professionals, and staff of Head Start, as well as school districts, local municipalities, foundations, other nonprofits, businesses, and numerous state agencies. ECLC aims to align and monitor programs and services for young children and their families, make policy recommendations, and improve the accessibility and quality of resources for pregnant women and children ages 0–8 years. ECLC's seventh annual report highlighted achievements including (among many others) working with more than 100 partners to align and strengthen Colorado's early childhood systems, building infrastructure to support a high-quality early childhood workforce, and launching a website for early childhood professionals to share and align their work (Early Childhood Leadership Commission 2018).

Efforts at pediatric care sites to refer parents to social services or to promote positive parent–child interaction and family stability
- HealthySteps, administered by the global nonprofit ZERO TO THREE, is transforming pediatric primary care by promoting the well-being of parents and children. HealthySteps specialists are integrated into primary care teams and are available to answer parents' questions about developmental milestones and parenting challenges before, during, and after their health care visit. When needed, specialists also provide home visiting, referrals to community resources, information about parent support groups, and written materials. Participation has been linked with higher rates of timely screenings and vaccines, positive parenting practices, and increased parent–child engagement in early literacy activities (HealthySteps 2017, 2019). HealthySteps was judged effective on many outcomes in a meta-analysis evaluating 48 studies in which 24 different interventions were described (Peacock-Chambers, Ivy, and Bair-Merritt 2017). In 2018, HealthySteps served more than 37,000 children across 120 pediatric and family care sites in 15 states. HealthySteps sites receive a mix of public and private funding, including from Medicaid, the Children's Health Insurance Program, private payer reimbursements, and local foundations.
- Reach Out and Read, pioneered in 1989, trains pediatric providers to encourage parents to read aloud to their children. Reach Out and Read has been linked to higher rates of parents reading to their children, increased brain stimulation and vocabulary growth among children, enhanced language development by 3–6 months, and more well-child visits (Needlman et al. 2019; Reach Out and Read 2014). A review concluded that pediatric practice-based literacy interventions in general were consistently associated with more parental reading out loud and better child language outcomes (Peacock-Chambers et al. 2017). Funded by philanthropies and government agencies, the program has

been implemented by 32,700 pediatric providers at 6,000 health care locations nationwide, serving approximately 4.7 million children and distributing more than 7 million books annually (Reach Out and Read 2019).

Broad economic and social policies/programs, such as tax credits, affordable and fair housing initiatives, community development, nutritional supports for low-income families, and initiatives to eliminate racial discrimination: Although not exclusively focused on early childhood, such efforts may substantially reduce the economic and social disadvantages that underlie health disadvantage that begins in early childhood and continues throughout life.

- The CTC, enacted in 1997 and expanded since 2001, is a federal tax credit that aims to help working families offset the costs of raising children. The Tax Cuts and Jobs Act of 2017 expanded eligibility to families earning at least $2,500 annually (down from a $3,000 minimum under previous law) and increased the maximum credit from $1,000 to $2,000. The CTC phases out at higher levels of income (beginning at $200,000, or $400,000 for married parents filing jointly) than the EITC, helping not only low- and moderate-income families but also middle-income and well-to-do families. Working families can receive a refund of 15% of their earnings above $2,500, up to the maximum refund of $1,400 per child. Although most of the benefits of the CTC therefore go to higher-income households, the CTC lifted 1.6 million children out of poverty and lessened poverty for an additional 6.7 million children in 2017 (Center on Budget and Policy Priorities 2019).
- WIC, created in 1972, provides supplemental food and nutrition education, as well as screening and referrals to health, welfare, and other social services, to low-income pregnant and postpartum women and their children up to age 5 years. Participants must have at least one medical or dietary condition that meets WIC's criteria for nutritional risk, such as anemia, underweight, history of pregnancy complications, or an unhealthy diet. The program is currently administered in approximately 47,000 local agencies, including schools, hospitals, public housing sites, and community centers. WIC served 6.9 million participants each month in 2018, including almost half of all infants born in the United States (U.S. Department of Agriculture Food and Nutrition Service 2017). In 2009, the government revised the types of foods that could be purchased with WIC vouchers to align more closely with the latest nutrition science. That change was associated with a reversal of the rapid increase in obesity prevalence observed among WIC participants from 2000 to 2014 (Daepp et al. 2019). Research suggests that infants born to WIC-participating women are more likely to be vaccinated and receive the recommended number of well-child visits (Bersak and Sonchak 2018).
- A range of other social policies/programs that have lifted families out of poverty include the EITC, SNAP, paid parental leave, child care subsidy programs, children's saving accounts, and full child support pass-through and disregard policies. These initiatives are discussed in more detail in Chapter 2.

6.4. KEY POINTS

- A life course perspective recognizes that health at any stage of life is influenced by experiences during prior life stages and particularly that adult health is powerfully shaped by childhood experiences.
- Although health is a product of experiences throughout life, early childhood conditions (material and psychosocial) appear to be particularly crucial. Favorable conditions early in life can launch a child on pathways toward optimal health and well-being. Conversely, adverse experiences in early childhood can set off a vicious cycle leading to both social and health disadvantage in adulthood and, in turn, to more disadvantage for the next generation, continuing the cycle.
- The first 5 years of life seem particularly important for lifelong health. Favorable or unfavorable exposures (e.g., poverty, economic insecurity, food insecurity, a parent with mental illness, an incarcerated parent, and abuse or neglect) or absence of sufficient stimulation during critical/sensitive periods for brain development can set a child on a path toward ill health throughout life.
- Poverty in early childhood is a threat to lifelong health in many ways, including exposures to poor nutrition and environmental hazards such as air pollution and toxic waste. In addition, chronic stress due to facing daily demands with inadequate economic resources can make it more difficult for parents to provide adequate stimulation for brain development, despite strong motivation.
- Although children who have experienced economic adversity appear to benefit the most from early childhood interventions such as center-based care and education or home visiting, children from middle-class families also experience substantial benefits.
- Psychosocial adversity (e.g., family disruption, domestic violence, and child abuse) in early childhood is associated with adverse adult outcomes; insufficient attention has been given to the conditions, such as low income, that produce or exacerbate adverse psychosocial events in families with young children.

6.5. QUESTIONS FOR DISCUSSION

1. In what ways can physical and social conditions experienced in early childhood influence a person's health in later adulthood?
2. How strong is the evidence base connecting early childhood experiences with adult health?
3. What are some of the scientific obstacles to directing major resources toward improving early childhood conditions and reducing disparities in the conditions needed for healthy development? What about the political obstacles? Which are greater—the scientific or political barriers?
4. How could racism affect early childhood? How could racism affect the life of a child too young to be aware of racism?
5. How could the health effects of racism experienced in early childhood be similar to and how could they be different from the health effects of poverty experienced by a White child during the same stage of life?

ACKNOWLEDGMENTS

Portions of this chapter build on material from the following sources:

Braveman P., J. Acker, E. Arkin, J. Bussel, K. Wehr, and D. Proctor. 2018. *Early Childhood Is Critical to Health Equity*. Princeton, NJ: Robert Wood Johnson Foundation.

Braveman P., S. Egerter, K. Arena, & R. Aslam. 2014. *Early Childhood Experiences Shape Health and Well-Being Throughout Life*. Princeton, NJ: Robert Wood Johnson Foundation.

Braveman P., T. Sadegh-Nobari, & S. Egerter. 2011. *Early Childhood Experiences: Laying the Foundation for Health Across a Lifetime*. Princeton, NJ: Robert Wood Johnson Foundation.

Julia Acker and Nicole Holm contributed to the research.

REFERENCES

Adam, E. K., J. A. Heissel, K. H. Zeiders, J. A. Richeson, E. C. Ross, K. B. Ehrlich, D. J. Levy, et al. 2015. "Developmental histories of perceived racial discrimination and diurnal cortisol profiles in adulthood: A 20-year prospective study." *Psychoneuroendocrinology* 62: 279–291. doi:10.1016/j.psyneuen.2015.08.018.

Allegreto, S., A. Godoey, C. Nadler, and M. Reich. 2018. *The New Wave of Local Minimum Wage Policies: Evidence from Six Cities*. Berkeley, CA: Center on Wage and Employment Dynamics, Institute for Research on Labor and Employment, University of California, Berkeley.

Almond, D., H. W. Hoynes, and D. W. Schanzenbach. 2010. "Inside the war on poverty: The impact of food stamps on birth outcomes." *Rev Econ Stat* 93(2): 387–403. doi:10.1162/REST_a_00089.

Banks, C. 2004. "Racial discrimination in the criminal justice system." In *Criminal Justice Ethics: Theory and Practice*, 98–125. Thousand Oaks, C: Sage.

Barnett, W. S., K. Brown, and R. Shore. 2004, April. "The universal vs. targeted debate: Should the United States have preschool for all?" *Preschool Policy Matters*. https://nieer.org/wp-content/uploads/2016/08/6.pdf

Bartik, T., W. Gormley, J. Belford, and S. Anderson. 2016. "A benefit–cost analysis of the Tulsa universal pre-K program" (Working Paper No. 16-261). Kalamazoo, MI: Upjohn Institute.

Beck, A. F., A. J. Cohen, J. D. Colvin, C. M. Fichtenberg, E. W. Fleegler, A. Garg, L. M. Gottlieb, et al. 2018. "Perspectives from the Society for Pediatric Research: Interventions targeting social needs in pediatric clinical care." *Pediatr Res* 84(1): 10–21. doi:10.1038/s41390-018-0012-1.

Bersak, T., and L. Sonchak. 2018. "The impact of WIC on infant immunizations and health care utilization." *Health Serv Res* 53(Suppl 1): 2952–2969. doi:10.1111/1475-6773.12810.

Black, C., G. Moon, and J. Baird. 2014. "Dietary inequalities: What is the evidence for the effect of the neighbourhood food environment?" *Health Place* 27: 229–242. doi:10.1016/j.healthplace.2013.09.015.

Blair, C., and C. C. Raver. 2016. "Poverty, stress, and brain development: New directions for prevention and intervention." *Acad Pediatr* 16 (3 Suppl): S30–S36. doi:10.1016/j.acap.2016.01.010.

Boyce, T. W., and C. Hertzman. 2018. "Early childhood health and the life course: The state of the science and proposed research priorities: A background paper for the MCH Life Course Research Network." In *Handbook of Life Course Health Development*, edited by N. Halfon, C. B. Forrest, R. M. Lerner, and E. M. Faustman, 61–93. Cham, Switzerland: Springer

Burtle, A., and S. Bezruchka. 2016. "Population health and paid parental leave: What the United States can learn from two decades of research." *Healthcare* 4(2): 30. doi:10.3390/healthcare4020030.

Busse, D., I. S. Yim, B. Campos, and C. K. Marshburn. 2017. "Discrimination and the HPA axis: Current evidence and future directions." *J Behav Med* 40(4): 539–552. doi:10.1007/s10865-017-9830-6.

Campbell, F., G. Conti, J. J. Heckman, S. H. Moon, R. Pinto, E. Pungello, and Y. Pan. 2014. "Early childhood investments substantially boost adult health." *Science* 343(6178): 1478–1485. doi:10.1126/science.1248429.

Cannon, J. S., M. R. Kilburn, L. A. Karoly, T. Mattox, A. N. Muchow, and M. Buenaventura. 2017. "Investing early: Taking stock of outcomes and economic returns from early childhood programs." *RAND Health Q* 7(4): 6.

Carneiro, P., K. V. Loken, and K. G. Salvanes. 2015. "A flying start? Maternity leave benefits and long-run outcomes of children." *J Polit Econ* 123(2): 365–412. doi:10.1086/679627.

Center on Budget and Policy Priorities. 2019. "Policy basics: The Child Tax Credit." https://www.cbpp.org/research/federal-tax/the-child-tax-credit

Center on the Developing Child. 2009. *Maternal Depression Can Undermine the Development of Young Children: Working Paper No. 8.* Cambridge, MA: Harvard University Press. www.developingchild.harvard.edu

Center on the Developing Child. 2010. *The Foundations of Lifelong Health Are Built in Early Childhood.* Cambridge, MA: Harvard University Press.

Chase-Lansdale, L., and J. Brooks-Gunn. 2014. "Two-generation programs in the twenty-first century." *Future Child* 24(1): 13–39. doi:10.1353/foc.2014.0003.

Chetty, R., J. N. Friedman, and J. Rockoff. 2011. "New evidence on the long-term impacts of tax credits: IRS Statistics of Income White Paper." Paper presented at the 104th Annual Conference on Taxation, New Orleans, LA.

Clark, R., N. B. Anderson, V. R. Clark, and D. R. Williams. 1999. "Racism as a stressor for African Americans. A biopsychosocial model." *Am Psychol* 54(10): 805–816. doi:10.1037//0003-066x.54.10.805.

Colman, S., I. Nichols-Barrer, J. E. Redline, B. Devaney, S. V. Ansell, and T. Joyce. 2012. "Effects of the Special Supplemental Nutrition Program for Women, Infants, and Children (WIC): A review of recent research." Alexandria, VA: U.S. Department of Agriculture, Food and Nutrition Service, Office of Research and Analysis.

Committee for Economic Development. 2012. *Unfinished Business: Continued Investment in Child Care and Early Education Is Critical to Business and America's Future.* Washington, DC: Policy and Impact Committee of the Committee for Economic Development.

Conners-Burrow, N. A., P. Bokony, L. Whiteside-Mansell, D. Jarrett, S. Kraleti, L. McKelvey, and A. Kyzer. 2014. "Low-level depressive symptoms reduce maternal support for child cognitive development." *J Pediatr Health Care* 28(5): 404–412. doi:10.1016/j.pedhc.2013.12.005.

Conti, G., and J. J. Heckman. 2010. "Understanding the early origins of the education–health gradient: A framework that can also be applied to analyze gene–environment interactions." *Perspect Psychol Sci* 5(5): 585–605. doi:10.1177/1745691610383502.

Conti, G., J. J. Heckman, and R. Pinto. 2016. "The effects of two influential early childhood interventions on health and healthy behaviour." *Econ J* 126(596): F28–F65. https://doi.org/10.1111/ecoj.12420.

Daepp, M. I. G., S. L. Gortmaker, Y. C. Wang, M. W. Long, and E. L. Kenney. 2019. "WIC food package changes: Trends in childhood obesity prevalence." *Pediatrics* 143(5): e20182841.

De Haan, M., and E. Leuven. 2019. "Head Start and the distribution of long-term education and labor market outcomes." *J Labor Econ* 38(3): 727–765. doi:10.1086/706090.

DiMaggio, C. 2015. "Small-area spatiotemporal analysis of pedestrian and bicyclist injuries in New York City." *Epidemiology* 26(2): 247–254. doi:10.1097/ede.0000000000000222.

Drewnowski, A., and S. E. Specter. 2004. "Poverty and obesity: The role of energy density and energy costs." *Am J Clin Nutr* 79(1): 6–16. doi:10.1093/ajcn/79.1.6.

Duffee, J., A. Mendelsohn, A. Kuo, L. Legano, and M. Earls. 2017. "Early childhood home visiting." *Pediatrics* 140: e20172150. doi:10.1542/peds.2017-2150.

Duncan, G. J., and K. Magnuson. 2011, Winter. "The long reach of early childhood poverty." *Pathways*, 22–27.

Duncan, G. J., and K. Magnuson. 2013. "Investing in preschool programs." *J Econ*

Perspect 27(2): 109–132. doi:10.1257/jep.27.2.109.

Early Childhood Leadership Commission. 2018. "Annual report." Early Childhood Leadership Commission. Colorado.

Easterbrooks, A., J. Chaudhuri, R. Fauth, M. Contreras, C. Kotake, D. Moosmanm, R. Katz, et al. 2017. *The Massachusetts Healthy Families Evaluation–2 Early Childhood (MHFE-2EC): Follow-Up Study of a Randomized, Controlled Trial of a Statewide Home Visiting Program for Young Parents*. Medford, MA: Eliot–Pearson Department of Child Study and Human Development, Department of Urban and Environmental Policy and Planning, Tufts Interdisciplinary Evaluation Research.

Educare Learning Network. 2017. *Educare Learning Network Research and Evaluation Summary*. Chicago, IL: Educare Learning Network.

Eidelman, A. I., R. J. Schanler, M. Johnston, S. Landers, L. Noble, K. Szucs, and L. Viehmann. 2012. "Breastfeeding and the use of human milk." *Pediatrics* 129(3): 496–506. doi:10.1542/peds.2011-3552.

Englund, M. M., B. White, A. J. Reynolds, L. J. Schweinhart, and F. A. Campbell. 2014. "Health outcomes of the Abecedarian, Child–Parent Center, and HighScope Perry Preschool programs." In *Health and Education in Early Childhood: Predictors, Interventions, and Policies*, edited by A. Reynolds, A. Rolnick, & J. Temple (Eds.), 257–291. New York, NY: Cambridge University Press.

Evans, G. W. 2004. "The environment of childhood poverty." *Am Psychol* 59(2): 77–92. doi:10.1037/0003-066x.59.2.77.

Evans, G. W., and P. Kim. 2013. "Childhood poverty, chronic stress, self-regulation, and coping." *Child Dev Perspect* 7(1): 43–48. https://doi.org/10.1111/cdep.12013.

Fernald, A., V. A. Marchman, and A. Weisleder. 2013. "SES differences in language processing skill and vocabulary are evident at 18 months." *Dev Sci* 16(2): 234–248. doi:10.1111/desc.12019.

Fox, M. K., W. L. Hamilton, and B. H. Lin. 2004. "Effects of food assistance and nutrition programs on nutrition and health. Vol. 3: Literature review." Food Assistance and Nutrition Research Report No. 19-3.

Washington, DC: Food and Rural Economics Division, Economic Research Service, U.S. Department of Agriculture.

Friedman, E. M., A. S. Karlamangla, T. L. Gruenewald, B. Koretz, and T. E. Seeman. 2015. "Early life adversity and adult biological risk profiles." *Psychosom Med* 77(2): 176–185. doi:10.1097/psy.0000000000000147.

Friedson, M., and P. Sharkey. 2015. "Violence and neighborhood disadvantage after the crime decline." *Ann Am Acad Polit Soc Sci* 660(1): 341–358. doi:10.1177/0002716215579825.

Garner, A. S., and J. P. Shonkoff. 2012. "Early childhood adversity, toxic stress, and the role of the pediatrician: Translating developmental science into lifelong health." *Pediatrics* 129(1): e224–e231. doi:10.1542/peds.2011-2662.

Gee, G. C., K. M. Walsemann, and E. Brondolo. 2012. "A life course perspective on how racism may be related to health inequities." *Am J Public Health* 102(5): 967–974. doi:10.2105/AJPH.2012.300666.

Gilkerson, J., J. A. Richards, S. F. Warren, J. K. Montgomery, C. R. Greenwood, D. Kimbrough Oller, J. H. L. Hansen, and T. D. Paul. 2017. "Mapping the early language environment using all-day recordings and automated analysis." *Am J Speech Lang Pathol* 26(2): 248–265. doi:10.1044/2016_ajslp-15-0169.

Gilliam, W. S. 2005. "Prekindergarteners left behind: Expulsion rates in state prekindergarten programs." FCD Policy Brief Series No. 3. New York, NY: Foundation for Child Development.

Green, B. L., M. B. Sanders, and J. Tarte. 2017. "Using administrative data to evaluate the effectiveness of the Healthy Families Oregon home visiting program: 2-year impacts on child maltreatment & service utilization." *Child Youth Serv Rev* 75: 77–86. https://doi.org/10.1016/j.childyouth.2017.02.019.

Grunewald, R., and A. Rolnick. 2006. "A proposal for achieving high returns on early childhood development." Federal Reserve Bank of Minneapolis. https://www.minneapolisfed.org/~/media/files/publications/studies/earlychild/highreturn.pdf?la=en

Hackman, D. A., R. Gallop, G. W. Evans, and M. J. Farah. 2015. "Socioeconomic status and executive function: Developmental trajectories and mediation." *Dev Sci* 18(5): 686–702. doi:10.1111/desc.12246.

Hajat, A., C. Hsia, and M. S. O'Neill. 2015. "Socioeconomic disparities and air pollution exposure: A global review." *Curr Environ Health Rep* 2(4): 440–450. doi:10.1007/s40572-015-0069-5.

Hart, B., and T. R. Risley. 1995. *Meaningful Differences in the Everyday Experience of Young American Children*. Baltimore, MD: Brookes.

Health Resources and Services Administration. 2017. "Maternal & child health: Collaborative Improvement & Innovation Networks (CoIINs)." Health Resources & Services Administration. https://mchb.hrsa.gov/maternal-child-health-initiatives/collaborative-improvement-innovation-networks-coiins.

Healthy Families America. 2015a. "Our Approach." hhttps://www.healthyfamilies america.org/our-approach/.

Healthy Families America. 2015b. "Healthy Families America: Rigorous evidence." https://static1.squarespace.com/static/55cce f2ae4b0fc9c2b64f3a1/t/589ce970e6f2e1bd3 c82696a/1486678385338/HFA%2BRigor ous%2BEvidence.r2.9.16.pdf.

HealthySteps. 2017. "The model." https://www. healthysteps.org/the-model.

HealthySteps. 2019. "HealthySteps: The evidence base." https://www.healthysteps.org/the-evidence.

Heckman, J. J., S. H. Moon, R. Pinto, P. A. Savelyev, and A. Yavitz. 2010. "The rate of return to the High/Scope Perry Preschool program." *J Public Econ* 94(1–2): 114–128. doi:10.1016/j.jpubeco.2009.11.001.

Hoff, E. 2003. "The specificity of environmental influence: Socioeconomic status affects early vocabulary development via maternal speech." *Child Dev* 74(5): 1368–1378. doi:10.1111/1467-8624.00612.

Holmes, M., and R. Rutledge. 2016. *Evaluation of the Nurse Family Partnership in North Carolina*. Charlotte, NC: The Duke Endowment.

Hoynes, H. W., and A. J. Patel. 2018. "Effective policy for reducing poverty and inequality? The Earned Income Tax Credit and the distribution of income." *J Hum Resour* 53(4): 859–890. doi:10.3368/jhr.53.4.1115.7494R1.

Hughes, C., and R. T. Devine. 2019. "For better or for worse? Positive and negative parental influences on young children's executive function." *Child Dev* 90(2): 593–609. doi:10.1111/cdev.12915.

Huttenlocher, J., M. Vasilyeva, H. R. Waterfall, J. L. Vevea, and L. V. Hedges. 2007. "The varieties of speech to young children." *Dev Psychol* 43(5): 1062–1083. doi:10.1037/0012-1649.43.5.1062.

Jacobs, F., M. A. Easterbrooks, J. Goldberg, J. Mistry, E. Bumgarner, M. Raskin, N. Fosse, and R. Fauth. 2016. "Improving adolescent parenting: Results from a randomized controlled trial of a home visiting program for young families." *Am J Public Health* 106(2): 342–349. doi:10.2105/AJPH.2015.302919.

Jones, D. E., M. Greenberg, and M. Crowley. 2015. "Early social–emotional functioning and public health: The relationship between kindergarten social competence and future wellness." *Am J Public Health* 105(11): 2283–2290. doi:10.2105/AJPH.2015.302630.

Karoly, L. A. 2016. "The economic returns to early childhood education." *Future Children* 26(2): 37–55. doi:10.1353/foc.2016.0011.

Karoly, L. A., M. R. Kilburn, and J. S. Cannon. 2005. *Early Childhood Interventions: Proven Results, Future Promise*. Santa Monica, CA: RAND Corporation.

Korous, K. M., J. M. Causadias, and D. M. Casper. 2017. "Racial discrimination and cortisol output: A meta-analysis." *Soc Sci Med* 193: 90–100. doi:10.1016/j.socscimed.2017.09.042.

Kreider, B., J. V. Pepper, C. Gundersen, and D. Jolliffe. 2012. "Identifying the effects of SNAP (food stamps) on child health outcomes when participation is endogenous and misreported." *J Am Stat Assoc* 107(499): 958–975. doi:10.1080/01621459.2012.682828.

Lansford, J. E., K. A. Dodge, G. S. Pettit, and J. E. Bates. 2016. "A public health perspective on school dropout and adult outcomes: A prospective study of risk and protective factors from age 5 to 27 years." *J Adolesc Health* 58(6): 652–658. doi:10.1016/j.jadohealth.2016.01.014.

LeCroy, C. W., and M. F. Davis. 2016. "Randomized trial of Healthy Families Arizona: Quantitative and qualitative outcomes." *Res Soc Work Pract* 27(7): 747–757. doi:10.1177/1049731516632594.

Lee, J., M. Abdel-Aty, K. Choi, and H. Huang. 2015. "Multi-level hot zone identification for pedestrian safety." *Accid Anal Prev* 76: 64–73. doi:10.1016/j.aap.2015.01.006.

Lee-St. John, T. J., M. E. Walsh, A. E. Raczek, C. E. Vuilleumier, C. Foley, A. Heberle, E. Sibley, and E. Dearing. 2018. "The long-term impact of systemic student support in elementary school: Reducing high school dropout." *AERA Open* 4(4): 2332858418799085. doi:10.1177/2332858418799085.

Lewis, T. T., A. E. Aiello, S. Leurgans, J. Kelly, and L. L. Barnes. 2010. "Self-reported experiences of everyday discrimination are associated with elevated C-reactive protein levels in older African-American adults." *Brain Behav Immun* 24(3): 438–443. doi:10.1016/j.bbi.2009.11.011.

Mani, A., S. Mullainathan, E. Shafir, and J. Zhao. 2013. "Poverty impedes cognitive function." *Science* 341(6149): 976–980. doi:10.1126/science.1238041.

Masarik, A. S., and R. D. Conger. 2017. *Stress and Child Development: A Review of the Family Stress Model*. New York, NY: Elsevier.

McEwen, B. S. 2007. "Physiology and neurobiology of stress and adaptation: Central role of the brain." *Physiol Rev* 87(3): 873–904. doi:10.1152/physrev.00041.2006.

Meek, S. E., and W. S. Gilliam. 2016. "Expulsion and suspension in early education as matters of social justice and health equity." NAM Perspectives discussion paper. Washington, DC: National Academy of Medicine.

Merz, E. C., E. A. Maskus, S. A. Melvin, X. He, and K. G. Noble. 2020. "Socioeconomic disparities in language input are associated with children's language-related brain structure and reading skills." *Child Dev* 91(3): 846–860. doi:10.1111/cdev.13239.

Michalopoulos, C., K. Faucetta, C. J. Hill, X. A. Portilla, L. Burrell, H. Lee, A. Duggan, and V. Knox. 2019. "Impacts on family outcomes of evidence-based early childhood home visiting: Results from the Mother and Infant Home Visiting Program evaluation." OPRE Report No. 2019-07. Washington, DC: Office of Planning, Research, and Evaluation, Administration for Children and Families, U.S. Department of Health and Human Services.

Miller, T. R. 2015. "Projected outcomes of nurse–family partnership home visitation during 1996–2013, USA." *Prev Sci* 16(6): 765–777. doi:10.1007/s11121-015-0572-9.

Moffitt, T. E., L. Arseneault, D. Belsky, N. Dickson, R. J. Hancox, H. Harrington, R. Houts, et al. 2011. "A gradient of childhood self-control predicts health, wealth, and public safety." *Proc Natl Acad Sci USA* 108(7): 2693–2698. doi:10.1073/pnas.1010076108.

Morris, P. A., M. Connors, A. Friedman-Krauss, D. C. McCoy, C. Weiland, A. Feller, L. Page, H. Bloom, and H. Yoshikawa. 2018. "New findings on impact variation from the Head Start Impact Study: Informing the scale-up of early childhood programs." *AERA Open* 4(2): 2332858418769287. doi:10.1177/2332858418769287.

Muennig, P., D. Robertson, G. Johnson, F. Campbell, E. P. Pungello, and M. Neidell. 2011. "The effect of an early education program on adult health: The Carolina Abecedarian Project randomized controlled trial." *Am J Public Health* 101(3): 512–516. doi:10.2105/AJPH.2010.200063.

National Center for Education Statistics. 2017. "Risk factors and academic outcomes in kindergarten through third grade." https://nces.ed.gov/programs/coe/pdf/coe_tgd.pdf.

National Institute for Children's Health Quality. 2019. "Initiatives: Early Childhood Comprehensive Systems Collaborative Improvement and Innovation Network (ECCS CoIIN). https://www.nichq.org/project/early-childhood-comprehensive-systems-collaborative-improvement-and-innovation-network-eccs.

Needlman, R. D., B. P. Dreyer, P. Klass, and A. L. Mendelsohn. 2019. "Attendance at well-child visits after Reach Out and Read." *Clin Pediatr* 58(3): 282–287. doi:10.1177/0009922818822975.

Nellis, A. 2016. "The color of justice: Racial and ethnic disparity in state prisons." The Sentencing Project. https://www.sentencingproject.org/publications/color-of-justice-racial-and-ethnic-disparity-in-state-prisons.

Nianogo, R. A., M. C. Wang, R. Basurto-Davila, T. Z. Nobari, M. Prelip, O. A. Arah, and S.

E. Whaley. 2019. "Economic evaluation of California prenatal participation in the Special Supplemental Nutrition Program for Women, Infants and Children (WIC) to prevent preterm birth." *Prev Med* 124: 42–49. doi:10.1016/j.ypmed.2019.04.011.

Nurse–Family Partnership. 2018. "Nurse–Family Partnership national snapshot." Denver, CO: Nurse–Family Partnership.

Olds, D. L., H. Kitzman, M. D. Knudtson, E. Anson, J. A. Smith, and R. Cole. 2014. "Effect of home visiting by nurses on maternal and child mortality: Results of a 2-decade follow-up of a randomized clinical trial." *JAMA Pediatr* 168(9): 800–806. doi:10.1001/jamapediatrics.2014.472.

Organisation for Economic Co-operation and Development. 2019. "OECD Family Database: CO2.2: Child Poverty." https://www.oecd.org/els/family/database.htm

Oshri, A., E. Hallowell, S. Liu, J. MacKillop, A. Galvan, S. M. Kogan, and L. H. Sweet. 2019. "Socioeconomic hardship and delayed reward discounting: Associations with working memory and emotional reactivity." *Dev Cogn Neurosci* 37: 100642. https://doi.org/10.1016/j.dcn.2019.100642.

Patrick, H., and T. A. Nicklas. 2005. "A review of family and social determinants of children's eating patterns and diet quality." *J Am Coll Nutr* 24(2): 83–92. doi:10.1080/07315724.2005.10719448.

Peacock-Chambers, E., K. Ivy, and M. Bair-Merritt. 2017. "Primary care interventions for early childhood development: A systematic review." *Pediatrics* 140(6): e20171661. doi:10.1542/peds.2017-1661.

Petts, R. J. 2017. "Time off after childbirth and mothers' risk of depression, parenting stress, and parenting practices." *J Fam Issues* 39(7): 1827–1854. doi:10.1177/0192513X17728984.

Puma, M., S. Bell, R. Cook, C. Heid, P. Broene, F. Jenkins, A. J. Mashburn, and J. T. Downer. 2012. "Third grade follow-up to the Head Start Impact Study: Final report." U.S. Department of Health & Human Services. https://www.acf.hhs.gov/opre/report/third-grade-follow-head-start-impact-study-final-report.

Puma, M., S. Bell, R. Cook, C. Heid, G. Shapiro, P. Broene, F. Jenkins, et al. 2010. "Head Start Impact Study. Final report." U.S. Department of Health & Human Services. https://www.acf.hhs.gov/sites/default/files/documents/opre/head_start_report_0.pdf

Raub, A., A. Nandi, A. Earle, N. De Guzman Chorny, E. Wong, P. Chung, P. Batra, et al. 2018. "Paid parental leave: A detailed look at approaches across OECD countries." Los Angeles, CA: World Policy Analysis Center, UCLA Fielding School of Public Health.

Reach Out and Read. 2014. "About Reach Out and Read: Giving young children a foundation for success." http://www.reachoutandread.org/about-us.

Reach Out and Read. 2019. "Reach Out and Read: Our story." http://reachoutandread.org/our-story/30th.

Resnicow, K., F. McMaster, A. Bocian, D. Harris, Y. Zhou, L. Snetselaar, R. Schwartz, et al. 2015. "Motivational interviewing and dietary counseling for obesity in primary care: An RCT." *Pediatrics* 135(4): 649–657. doi:10.1542/peds.2014-1880.

Reynolds, A. J., S. R. Ou, C. F. Mondi, and M. Hayakawa. 2017. "Processes of early childhood interventions to adult well-being." *Child Dev* 88(2): 378–387. doi:10.1111/cdev.12733.

Reynolds, A. J., J. A. Temple, S. R. Ou, D. L. Robertson, J. P. Mersky, J. W. Topitzes, and M. D. Niles. 2007. "Effects of a school-based, early childhood intervention on adult health and well-being: A 19-year follow-up of low-income families." *Arch Pediatr Adolesc Med* 161(8): 730–739. doi:10.1001/archpedi.161.8.730.

Robin Dion, M., H. Zaveri, and P. Holcomb. 2015. "Responsible fatherhood programs in the Parents and Children Together (PACT) evaluation." *Family Court Rev* 53(2): 292–303. https://doi.org/10.1111/fcre.12140.

Romeo, R. R., J. A. Leonard, S. T. Robinson, M. R. West, A. P. Mackey, M. L. Rowe, and J. D. E. Gabrieli. 2018. "Beyond the 30-million-word gap: Children's conversational exposure is associated WITH language-related brain function." *Psychol Sci* 29(5): 700–710. doi:10.1177/0956797617742725.

Rowe, M. L. 2012. "A longitudinal investigation of the role of quantity and quality of child-directed speech in vocabulary development." *Child Dev* 83(5): 1762–1774. doi:10.1111/j.1467-8624.2012.01805.x.

Ruhm, C. J. 2000. "Parental leave and child health." *J Health Econ* 19(6): 931–960. doi:10.1016/s0167-6296(00)00047-3.

Schweinhart, L. J. 2004. "The High/Scope Perry Preschool Study through age 40: Summary, conclusions, and frequently asked questions." https://nieer.org/wp-content/uploads/2014/09/specialsummary_rev2011_02_2.pdf

Shah, R., D. DeFrino, Y. Kim, and M. Atkins. 2017. "Sit Down and Play: A preventive primary care-based program to enhance parenting practices." *J Child Fam Stud* 26(2): 540–547. doi:10.1007/s10826-016-0583-6.

Shonkoff, J. P. 2016. "Capitalizing on advances in science to reduce the health consequences of early childhood adversity." *JAMA Pediatr* 170(10): 1003–1007. doi:10.1001/jamapediatrics.2016.1559.

Shonkoff, J. P., and P. A. Fisher. 2013. "Rethinking evidence-based practice and two-generation programs to create the future of early childhood policy." *Dev Psychopathol* 25(4 Pt 2): 1635–1653. doi:10.1017/s0954579413000813.

Shonkoff, J. P., and A. S. Garner. 2012. "The life-long effects of early childhood adversity and toxic stress." *Pediatrics* 129(1): e232–246. doi:10.1542/peds.2011-2663.

Shonkoff, J. P., N. Slopen, and D. R. Williams. 2021. "Early childhood adversity, toxic stress, and the impacts of racism on the foundations of health." *Annu Rev Public Health* 42(1): 115–134. doi:10.1146/annurev-publhealth-090419-101940.

Takeuchi, H., Y. Taki, H. Hashizume, K. Asano, M. Asano, Y. Sassa, S. Yokota, et al. 2015. "The impact of parent–child interaction on brain structures: Cross-sectional and longitudinal analyses." *J Neurosci* 35(5): 2233–2245. doi:10.1523/jneurosci.0598-14.2015.

The Center for High Impact Philanthropy. 2017. "Invest in a strong start for children: A toolkit for donors on early childhood." University of Pennsylvania. https://www.impact.upenn.edu/toolkits/early-childhood-toolkit.

The Children's Defense Fund. 2018. "The state of America's children 2017 report." https://www.childrensdefense.org/reports/2017/the-state-of-americas-children-2017-report.

The PNC Financial Services Group. 2017. "Grow up Great." https://www.pnc.com/en/about-pnc/corporate-responsibility/grow-up-great.html.

Thévenon, O., T. Manfredi, Y. Govind, and I. Klauzner. 2018. "Child poverty in the OECD: Trends, determinants and policies to tackle it." OECD Social, Employment and Migration Working Papers No. 218. Paris, France: Organisation for Economic Co-operation and Development.

Thorland, W., and D. W. Currie. 2017. "Status of birth outcomes in clients of the Nurse–Family Partnership." *Matern Child Health J* 21(5): 995–1001. doi:10.1007/s10995-017-2267-2.

Thorland, W., D. Currie, E. R. Wiegand, J. Walsh, and N. Mader. 2017. "Status of breastfeeding and child immunization outcomes in clients of the Nurse–Family Partnership." *Matern Child Health J* 21(3): 439–445. doi:10.1007/s10995-016-2231-6.

U.S. Bureau of Labor Statistics. 2018. "National Compensation Survey: Employee benefits in the United States." Washington, DC: U.S. Department of Labor.

U.S. Census Bureau. 2018. "Annual Social and Economic Supplement. Age and Sex of All People, Family Members and Unrelated Individuals Iterated by Income-to-Poverty Ratio and Race." Washington, DC: U.S. Census Bureau.

U.S. Department of Agriculture Food and Nutrition Service. 2017. "WIC frequently asked questions (FAQs)." https://www.fns.usda.gov/wic/frequently-asked-questions-about-wic.

U.S. Department of Health and Human Services. 2018. "Implementing Healthy Families America." https://homvee.acf.hhs.gov/Implementation/3/Healthy-Families-America-HFA-Model-Overview/10.

Vargas, C. M., E. M. Stines, and H. S. Granado. 2017. "Health-equity issues related to childhood obesity: A scoping review." *J Public Health Dent* 77(Suppl 1): S32–S42. doi:10.1111/jphd.12233.

Vasquez, E. A., and J. Howard-Field. 2016. "Too (mentally) busy to chill: Cognitive load and inhibitory cues interact to moderate triggered displaced aggression." *Aggress Behav* 42(6): 598–604. doi:10.1002/ab.21654.

Williams, D. R. 1999. "Race, socioeconomic status, and health. The added effects of racism and discrimination." *Ann N Y Acad Sci* 896: 173–188. doi:10.1111/j.1749-6632.1999.tb08114.x.

Woolf, S. H., and L. Y. Aron. 2013. "The US health disadvantage relative to other high-income countries: Findings from a National Research Council/Institute of Medicine report." *JAMA* 309(8): 771–772. doi:10.1001/jama.2013.91.

Yazejian, N., and D. M Bryant. 2012. "Educare implementation study findings—August 2012." Chapel Hill, NC: The University of North Carolina, Frank Porter Graham Child Development Institute.

Yazejian, N., D. M. Bryant, S. Hans, D. Horm, L. St. Clair, N. File, and M. Burchinal. 2017. "Child and parenting outcomes after 1 year of Educare." *Child Dev* 88(5): 1671–1688. doi:10.1111/cdev.12688.

Yoshikawa, H., C. Weiland, J. Brooks-Gunn, M. R. Burchinal, L. M. Espinoza, W. T. Gormley, J. Ludwig, K. A. Magnuson, D. Phillips, and M. J. Zaslow. 2013. *Investing in Our Future: The Evidence Base on Preschool Education*. New York, NY: Foundation for Child Development.

CHAPTER 7

Healthy and Unhealthy Places

Neighborhoods, Health, and Health Disparities

7.1. HEALTH VARIES DRAMATICALLY BY NEIGHBORHOOD

An infant born in one neighborhood in Philadelphia can be expected to live 20 fewer years than an infant born in another neighborhood just a few miles away. Figure 7.1 displays the average life expectancy at birth in several areas within Philadelphia—68 years in poverty-stricken North Philadelphia West and 88 years in the gentrified neighborhoods near the center of the city. Philadelphia is not unique in this respect. Figures 7.2 and 7.3 show additional examples of how people living in adjacent or nearby neighborhoods within the same U.S. cities can experience vastly different burdens of disease. For example, Figure 7.2 reveals that rates of diabetes in Columbus, Ohio, are as much as four or more times higher in some census tracts compared with other census tracts that are adjacent or nearby. Figure 7.3 shows even larger differences in rates of coronary heart disease across different census tracts in Mesa, Arizona (Centers for Disease Control and Prevention [CDC] 2018). Throughout the United States, large and growing disparities in life expectancy have been documented repeatedly when comparing populations in different counties and/or census tracts (Arias et al. 2018; Dwyer-Lindgren et al. 2017). Large geographic disparities also have been observed throughout the United States in many of the most common diseases and health-related behaviors and conditions that drive poor health and early death. These include disparities across different census tracts in diabetes (CDC 2018), cardiovascular disease (CDC 2018), smoking (Fitzpatrick et al. 2018), and obesity (Leas et al. 2019) and disparities across different counties in cardiovascular disease (Roth et al. 2017).

Large variations in health across populations living in close proximity to each other raise questions about whether differences in the personal characteristics of an area's inhabitants, distinguished from characteristics of the areas where they live, might play a role. Dramatic differences in health across different geographic areas have often been observed, however, even after taking individual characteristics—such as household income or educational attainment—into account. This suggests that the observed geographic differences in health could be explained not only by people's characteristics but also by features of the places where they spend their time. Even after controlling for

The Social Determinants of Health and Health Disparities. Paula Braveman, Oxford University Press. © Oxford University Press 2023.
DOI: 10.1093/oso/9780190624118.003.0007

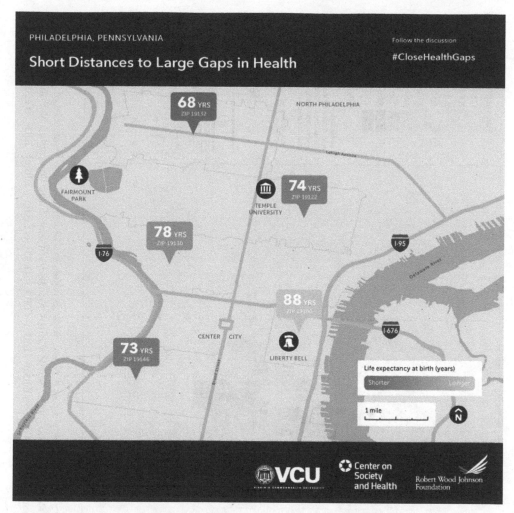

FIGURE 7.1 Twenty-year difference in life expectancy in different Philadelphia neighborhoods. Average life expectancy at birth, Philadelphia, Pennsylvania. *Source*: Reproduced with permission from the Virginia Commonwealth University's Center on Society and Health. Life expectancy at birth was calculated using U.S. Census Bureau data from 2000 and 2010 and mortality data for 2003–2012 from the National Vital Statistics System of the U.S. Centers for Disease Control and Prevention.

individuals' characteristics, many studies have linked a range of physical, economic, and social characteristics of neighborhoods (defined in different ways; see Box 7.1) with diverse health indicators, including mortality, general health status, birth outcomes (e.g., low birthweight and preterm birth), early childhood health, chronic conditions, health-related behaviors and other risk factors for chronic disease, and mental health (Arcaya et al. 2016; Diez Roux and Mair 2010; Oakes et al. 2015). The importance for health of characteristics of places versus of the people in them is explored further later in this chapter.

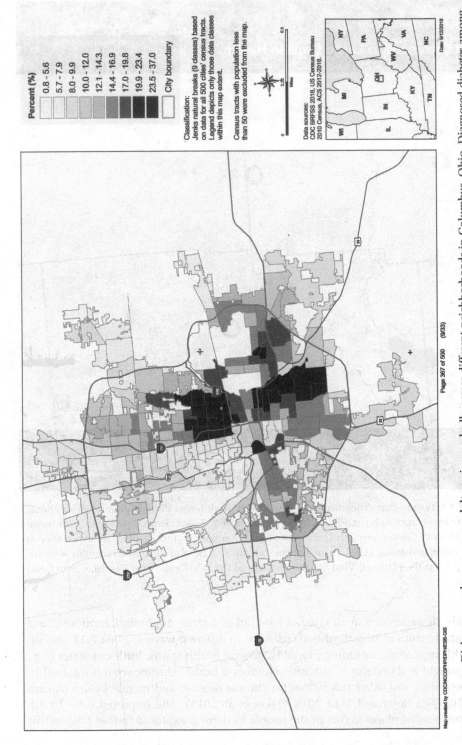

Percent (%)

- 0.8 - 5.6
- 5.7 - 7.9
- 8.0 - 9.9
- 10.0 - 12.0
- 12.1 - 14.3
- 14.4 - 16.9
- 17.0 - 19.8
- 19.9 - 23.4
- 23.5 - 37.0
- City boundary

Classification:
Jenks natural breaks (9 classes) based on data for all 500 cities' census tracts. Legend depicts only those data classes within this map extent.

Census tracts with population less than 50 were excluded from the map.

Data sources:
CDC BRFSS 2016, US Census Bureau
2010 Census, ACS 2012-2016.

Date: 9/12/2018

Map created by CDCNCCDPHPDPHESB GIS

Page 367 of 500   (9/33)

FIGURE 7.2 Diabetes prevalence among adults varies markedly across different neighborhoods in Columbus, Ohio. Diagnosed diabetes among adults aged 18 years or older by census tract, Columbus, Ohio, 2016. *Source:* Centers for Disease Control and Prevention, National Center for Chronic Disease Prevention and Health Promotion, Division of Population Health. 500 Cities Project data [online]. 2018[accessed November 8, 2019]. https://www.cdc.gov/500cities.

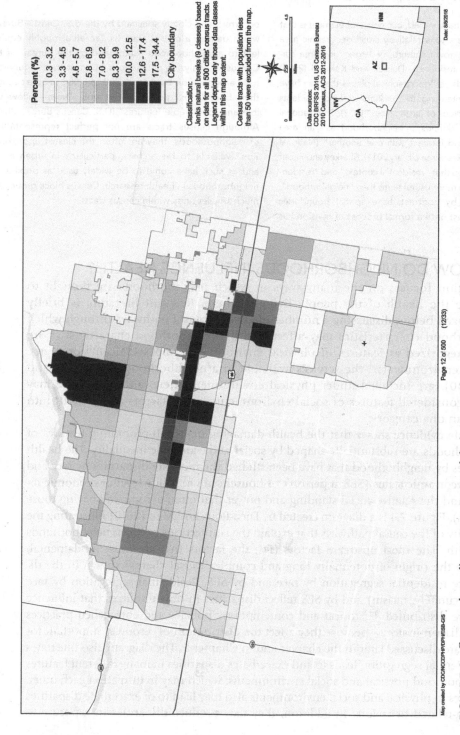

Percent (%)

- 0.3 - 3.2
- 3.3 - 4.5
- 4.6 - 5.7
- 5.8 - 6.9
- 7.0 - 8.2
- 8.3 - 9.9
- 10.0 - 12.5
- 12.6 - 17.4
- 17.5 - 34.4
- City boundary

Classification:
Jenks natural breaks (9 classes) based on data for all 500 cities' census tracts. Legend depicts only those data classes within this map extent.

Census tracts with population less than 50 were excluded from the map.

Data sources:
CDC BRFSS 2016, US Census Bureau
2010 Census, ACS 2012-2016

Date: 8/6/2018

Map created by CDC/NCCDPHP/DPH/ESB-GIS   Page 12 of 500   (12/33)

FIGURE 7.3 Coronary heart disease rates among adults in Mesa, Arizona, vary markedly by census tract. Coronary heart disease among adults aged 18 years or older by census tract, Mesa, Arizona, 2016. *Source:* Centers for Disease Control and Prevention, National Center for Chronic Disease Prevention and Health Promotion, Division of Population Health. 500 Cities Project data [online]. 2018 [accessed November 26, 2019]. https://www.cdc.gov/500cities.

| BOX 7.1 | What Is a Neighborhood? |

Although definitions have varied, one constant element is that a *neighborhood* refers to a relatively small geographic area within a county, city, town, suburb, or larger rural area surrounding a person's residence. Duncan and Kawachi (2018) define neighborhoods as "geographical places that can have social and cultural meaning to residents and nonresidents alike and are subdivisions of large places" (p. 2). The National Geographic Society defines a neighborhood as "an area where people live and interact with one another" (National Geographic Society Resource Library 2011). Sharkey and Faber (2014) have suggested that "residential context" and "residential environment" are more useful terms than "neighborhood".

Census tracts, by contrast, have spatial boundaries that are fixed (at least until a formal process of revision has occurred) and clearly specified by the U.S. Census Bureau, which defines a census tract as "an area roughly equivalent to a neighborhood established by the Bureau of the Census for analyzing populations." Census tracts "generally have a population between 1,200 to 8,000 people . . . and their boundaries generally—but not always—follow visible and identifiable features" (U.S. Census Bureau 2019). Although census tracts are not perfect representations of neighborhoods, they are often the closest approximation available to researchers, particularly in urban areas, and as such have come to be widely used as proxies for neighborhoods in health research. Census block groups are much smaller units within census tracts.

7.2. HOW DO NEIGHBORHOODS INFLUENCE HEALTH?

This section focuses on the many ways in which neighborhoods are thought to influence the health of the people living in them. Relevant literature is briefly summarized below, discussing a number of general causal pathways through which neighborhood characteristics may affect health. Neighborhood characteristics are often categorized as features of physical environments and social environments. "Service environments," the services available in a neighborhood (Diez Roux and Mair 2010), are included under physical environments here, although some may also be considered features of social environments; other factors also may fit into more than one category.

Ample evidence shows that the health-damaging or health-promoting features of neighborhoods are substantially shaped by social and economic inequality. The health disparities by neighborhood that have been studied the most are disparities by race and by socioeconomic status (SES; a person's or household's absolute level of economic resources and the relative social standing and power that often accompany having those resources). Figure 7.4 is a diagram created by Diez-Roux and Mair (2010) illustrating the complexity of the causal pathways that explain the connections between neighborhoods and health. The most upstream factors (i.e., the factors that are most fundamental, closest to the origin of potentially long and complex causal chains) shown in the diagram are residential segregation by race and by SES. Residential segregation by race (more accurately, racism) and by SES reflect disparities in how resources that influence health are distributed. Historical and contemporary policies and entrenched practices that are discriminatory—because they affect the distribution of resources important for health—are discussed later in the chapter and in Chapter 5. The diagram also illustrates that residential segregation leads to and exacerbates disparities in many different features of neighborhood physical and social environments, which may in turn affect each other. Disparities in physical and social environments also may lead to or exacerbate disparities in health-related behaviors. In addition, they may produce disparities in exposure to

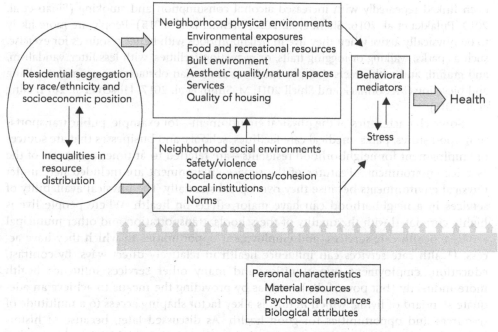

FIGURE 7.4 Schematic representation of the contributions of neighborhood environments to health inequalities. Many aspects of the social and physical environments of neighborhoods, interacting with characteristics of the people living in them, influence health, in often complex ways. *Source*: Diez Roux and Mair (2010).

stress, which in turn can affect health, both directly and through effects on health-related behaviors. These associations are discussed below.

Neighborhood Physical Environments and Health

Perhaps the most obvious and direct way in which neighborhoods can influence health is through their physical characteristics. For example, health can be adversely affected by poor air and water quality or proximity to facilities that produce or store hazardous substances (Brender, Maantay, and Chakraborty 2011). Health also can be affected by: substandard housing conditions that expose residents to lead paint, mold, dust, or pest infestation; lack of access to nutritious foods and safe places to exercise, especially when accompanied by heavy exposure to fast-food outlets and liquor stores; and adverse traffic conditions. Research has examined how the physical characteristics of buildings, streets, and other constructed features of neighborhoods—often referred to as the "built environment"— can affect smoking, drinking, exercise, and obesity (Grasser et al. 2013; Hirsch et al. 2014; Golden et al. 2019; Sherk et al. 2018). Whereas some studies have found relationships between the availability of sources of healthy food (e.g., from full-service supermarkets) or unhealthy food (e.g., from a high concentration of fast-food outlets and convenience stores) and residents' diets or obesity, other studies have not (Cobb et al. 2015; Block, Seward, and James 2018). Living in or in close proximity to an area with a high density of tobacco and alcohol retailers—disproportionately found in low-income neighborhoods—has been linked repeatedly with increased alcohol consumption and smoking (Finan et al. 2019; Pulakka et al. 2016; Sherk et al. 2018; Brenner et al. 2015). People are more likely to be physically active when they live in neighborhoods with better resources for exercise, such as parks, walking or jogging trails, or recreation facilities; with less litter, vandalism, and graffiti; and with streets that present fewer pedestrian obstacles or promote walking and bicycling (McCormack and Shiell 2011; M. Smith et al. 2017; Hirsch et al. 2014; Ding et al. 2011).

Some characteristics of the physical environment—for example, public transportation, food stores, parks, medical care facilities, schools, and businesses that are sources of employment for neighborhood residents—are referred to at times as aspects of the "service environment." Features of the service environment are included here under physical environments because they overlap substantially. The physical availability of services in a neighborhood can have major effects on health. Where people live is highly correlated with the quality of the schools, transportation and other municipal services, health care services, and employment opportunities to which they have access. Health care services can influence health in relatively direct ways. By contrast, education, employment opportunities, and many other services influence health more indirectly (but powerfully), such as by providing the means to achieve an adequate standard of living, which in turn is a key factor shaping access to a multitude of resources and opportunities for good health. As discussed later, because of historical and ongoing discrimination, physical characteristics of neighborhoods vary dramatically according to the race and SES of their residents. Racial and socioeconomic differences across neighborhoods in education and employment opportunities, for example, can create and exacerbate large disparities in health (Phelan and Link 2015; Williams and Collins 2001; Andersson et al. 2018).

Neighborhood Social Environments and Health

Health can also be shaped by the social environments of neighborhoods—that is, by the nature and strength of the social relationships among neighborhood residents, including the degree of mutual trust and feelings of connectedness among neighbors. Residents of "close-knit" neighborhoods may be more likely to work together to achieve common goals that can directly or indirectly influence health, such as improved schools or cleaner and safer public spaces. Neighbors who feel connected with each other may be more likely to exchange information regarding child care, job opportunities, and other resources that affect health; and chances are greater that they will work together to maintain informal social controls that discourage crime or other health-damaging behaviors, such as smoking or alcohol use among youths, littering, or graffiti (Putnam 1993; Kawachi, Subramanian, and Kim 2008; Carpiano 2008). Children in more close-knit neighborhoods may be more likely to receive guidance from multiple adults and less likely to engage in health-damaging behaviors such as smoking, drinking, drug use, or gang involvement (Erickson et al. 2012; Leventhal and Dupéré 2019). Neighborhoods in which residents express mutual trust and share a willingness to intervene for the public good have had lower rates of homicide and other violent crimes (Sampson, Raudenbush, and Earls 1997; Pratt and Cullen 2005). Conversely, less closely knit neighborhoods and more social disorder in a neighborhood have been related to anxiety, depression, and poorer subjective well-being (Almedom and Glandon 2008; Ehsan and De Silva 2015; Baranyi et al. 2020; Ludwig et al. 2012).

Some researchers have suggested that the observed inverse relationship between neighborhood social ties and violent crime rates may be explained by underlying links of both social ties and violent crime with other aspects of a neighborhood's social and economic advantages or disadvantages (Hipp and Wickes 2017). For example, in neighborhoods that face severe economic deprivation, residents' ability to maintain informal social controls and work together for the collective good may be undermined, even when residents do maintain close social ties (Sampson et al. 1997; Sampson, Morenoff, and Gannon-Rowley 2002). Profoundly disadvantaged neighborhoods may have fewer role models of healthy behavior, which could influence the health-related behaviors of neighborhood residents, particularly children.

Neighborhood Effects on Health May Vary for Different Population Groups

Some groups of people may be more affected by neighborhood conditions than others. Children may be particularly vulnerable to unhealthy and unsafe conditions in neighborhoods, with consequences for health, development, and achievement both in childhood and later in life (Chetty, Hendren, and Katz 2016; Sharkey 2010; Jutte, Miller, and Erickson 2015). Findings from Moving to Opportunity, a large experimental study of housing vouchers that enabled families to move from high-poverty to lower poverty neighborhoods, initially showed that the program had beneficial health effects for girls but no beneficial, or sometimes even harmful, health effects for boys (Kling, Liebman, and Katz 2007; Orr et al. 2003; Osypuk, Tchetgen, et al. 2012; Osypuk, Schmidt, et al. 2012; Sanbonmatsu et al. 2011). A follow-up study, however, found beneficial effects on health-related social outcomes (higher rates of college attendance, higher earnings, and reduced likelihood of single parenthood) for both boys and girls, although only among those who were younger than age 13 years when they moved (Chetty et al. 2016). That finding suggests that the timing and duration of older children's exposures to the more socially advantaged neighborhoods were insufficient to improve their economic trajectories, which may have been determined to a large degree in earlier childhood, by the time they moved. This and other studies highlight the potential importance of cumulative exposure over time to neighborhood social and economic advantage or disadvantage for health, development, and opportunity (Wodtke, Harding, and Elwert 2011; Sharkey and Faber 2014). On the other hand, as indicated by the earlier findings from Moving to Opportunity about boys' health and other research, some lower-income individuals who move to more advantaged neighborhoods may paradoxically fare worse than their counterparts living in disadvantaged neighborhoods. This may reflect additional stressors, including higher costs or increased awareness, anticipation, and/or, for persons of color, experiences of discrimination (because of more

> Children—especially younger children—may be particularly vulnerable to unhealthy conditions in neighborhoods, with consequences for health not only in childhood but also later in life.

contact with White people and/or the presence of fewer neighbors of color), with possible differences by gender; or the negative psychological effects of feeling inferior to more socioeconomically advantaged neighbors (DeLuca et al. 2012; H. Smith et al. 2012).

7.3. WHAT IS MORE IMPORTANT FOR HEALTH— PEOPLE OR PLACES?

The weight of the evidence indicates that many neighborhood characteristics are associated with health. But could the observed links between neighborhood conditions and health be largely a function of the characteristics of the individuals living in particular neighborhoods rather than features of those neighborhoods themselves? In other words, do neighborhood conditions really matter once the individual characteristics of their residents are taken into account? Are people who live in poor neighborhoods less healthy only because they themselves as individuals experience the health disadvantages of poverty, or do features of the neighborhoods they live in add something extra to the mix beyond individual circumstances? Do the health effects related to being poor differ depending on whether a poor person lives in a more or less advantaged neighborhood? These and similar questions have been the focus of many studies (Arcaya et al. 2016; Oakes et al. 2015).

Some researchers have hypothesized that the widely observed associations between characteristics of neighborhoods and many health outcomes in fact reflect unmeasured characteristics of the individuals living in the neighborhoods. Extensive literature certainly shows that individual characteristics—for example, one's income, wealth, educational attainment, or experiences of discrimination—can be important determinants of health. Many studies, however, have found relationships between neighborhood disadvantage and health even after considering individual characteristics—that is, the links between neighborhood characteristics and health do not appear to be due only to characteristics of the individuals. For example, a widely cited study that compared heart disease among people living in different neighborhoods found that individuals who lived in the most socioeconomically disadvantaged neighborhoods were more likely to develop heart disease than socioeconomically similar individuals who lived in the most advantaged neighborhoods, even after considering individual characteristics (Diez Roux et al. 2001). Evidence from the Moving to Opportunity experiment showed that randomly selected household heads who were given housing vouchers to move out of high-poverty neighborhoods to lower poverty neighborhoods had improved physical and mental health—including reductions in diabetes, obesity, and major depression—compared with otherwise similar household heads in the control group who did not move (Ludwig et al. 2011, 2012; Sanbonmatsu et al. 2012). As discussed above, improvements in health-related social and economic outcomes were seen for children in the Moving to Opportunity study who moved when they were young, although not necessarily for children who moved after age 13 years. The researchers interpreted the age differences to suggest the importance of duration of exposures in early childhood. Because it randomly assigned households to the experimental and control groups to ensure that their individual characteristics—including unmeasured characteristics—were similar, this study generated important evidence indicating independent neighborhood effects on health (Chetty et al. 2016).

Many other studies, however, have not found such effects (Schootman et al. 2007; Jokela 2014; Cummins, Flint, and Matthews 2014), and some experts argue that the scientific evidence regarding the relative importance of neighborhood and individual effects on health is inconclusive (Oakes 2004; Oakes et al. 2015). Teasing out the independent effects of neighborhood characteristics remains challenging, in part because controlling for individual effects may be inappropriate. For example, because a neighborhood feature (e.g., inferior schools) may affect health by shaping individual characteristics (e.g., low educational attainment), controlling for the individual characteristics will obscure the pathway by which the neighborhood feature affects health and lead to erroneous null findings. There has been increasing recognition among researchers that features of *both* people and places influence health and that people and places may influence each other in complex ways (Oakes et al. 2015; Sharkey and Faber 2014; Duncan and Kawachi 2018). Recent work has called for less focus on disentangling individual and neighborhood effects and more emphasis on better identifying: the specific neighborhood factors that lead to better or worse health; the relative importance of the timing and duration of exposures to these factors; and the populations who are most vulnerable to neighborhood effects (Oakes et al. 2015; Sharkey and Faber 2014).

There has been considerable discussion among researchers about the most appropriate geographic level—county, census tract, or census block group—at which to examine neighborhood effects on health. The most appropriate geographic level will vary with both the outcome being studied and the causal pathways involved (Sharkey and Faber 2014). It will also depend on the size and distribution of the population being examined and whether each neighborhood unit includes enough residents for statistically significant comparisons. Neighborhoods can also be operationalized in research using boundaries based on social rather than administrative patterns—for example, by using residents' own perceptions of neighborhood boundaries; constructing buffer zones around individual homes based on characteristics described in geographic information system databases; or using GPS technology to more thoroughly assess individuals' daily activity patterns and exposures to different environments (Duncan, Regan, and Chaix 2018).

Despite the methodologic controversies, most experts agree that where one lives can shape one's health in many important ways. The physical features, social relationships, services, and opportunities available in people's neighborhoods can either enhance or constrain their exposures and options, with potentially lasting consequences for health and well-being. The overwhelming weight of evidence indicates that both features of neighborhoods and characteristics of their individual residents influence health. Both places and people matter.

7.4. SOME GROUPS OF PEOPLE FACE GREATER OBSTACLES TO LIVING IN A HEALTHY NEIGHBORHOOD: THE ROLE OF RACISM

As of 2010, more than one-fourth of all Americans—approximately 77 million people—lived in poor neighborhoods (Bishaw 2014). Defined as census tracts in which at least 20% of residents are poor, these neighborhoods are also referred to as neighborhoods with concentrated poverty, high-poverty areas, or sometimes simply "poverty areas." The percentage of people who live in poor neighborhoods varies considerably across states, from a low of 6.8% in New Hampshire to a high of 48.5% in Mississippi, in 2010 (Bishaw 2014). Nationally, the number of Americans living in neighborhoods with concentrated poverty has been increasing over time: Between 2000 and 2010, the number of Americans living in poor neighborhoods grew by approximately 56% (Bishaw 2011, 2014).

There Are Large and Persistent Racial and Socioeconomic Disparities in Neighborhood Disadvantage

Some groups of people are more likely than others to live in neighborhoods that do not promote health or that damage health. It may not be surprising to learn that individuals or households with incomes at or below the federal poverty guidelines are more likely than their non-poor counterparts to live in disadvantaged neighborhoods (Bishaw 2014). It may be particularly discouraging, however, to learn that between 1970 and 2009, poor U.S. families became more likely to live in neighborhoods with concentrated poverty, whereas high-income families became more likely to live in neighborhoods with concentrated affluence (Bischoff and Reardon 2014). This increasing inequality is of concern in part because it means increasing separation of the affluent and the poor. Wilkinson and Pickett have articulated the idea that the increasing separation of rich and poor is a threat to society as a whole. They have attributed this to the rich becoming increasingly removed from the reality of the struggles of the poor, and hence increasingly unlikely to support policies that would benefit society as a whole (Wilkinson and Pickett 2009, 2020).

The relationship between low household income and residing in a high-poverty area tells only part of the story, however, and can obscure the role of powerful and enduring societal forces that have created and sustained not only socioeconomic but also racial/ethnic disparities in where people live. These forces are explored below. African Americans, American Indians/Alaska Natives, and Latinos/Hispanics are far more likely than Whites to live in poor neighborhoods; for example, between 2006 and 2010, nearly half of all Blacks lived in poor neighborhoods compared with less than one in five Whites (Bishaw 2011) (Figure 7.5). This uneven pattern of neighborhood disadvantage across racial or ethnic groups is not fully explained by differences in family income. Even among families with similar incomes, Blacks and Latinos/Hispanics live in neighborhoods with higher concentrations of poverty than Whites (Reardon, Fox, and Townsend 2015; Sharkey 2014).

Systemic or Structural Racism Has Produced Disparities in Who Lives in Healthy Neighborhoods

Striking and long-standing racial/ethnic disparities in residence in poor neighborhoods reflect what is widely called "systemic" or "structural" (or sometimes "institutional") racism. This refers to systems, laws, policies, and entrenched practices and beliefs that produce and perpetuate racial discrimination (unfair treatment based on race/ethnic group). The powerful structures, deeply rooted in historical

> Reflecting systemic or structural racism, at almost any level of household income, Black people and Latinos are more likely to live in economically disadvantaged neighborhoods than White people of similar income.

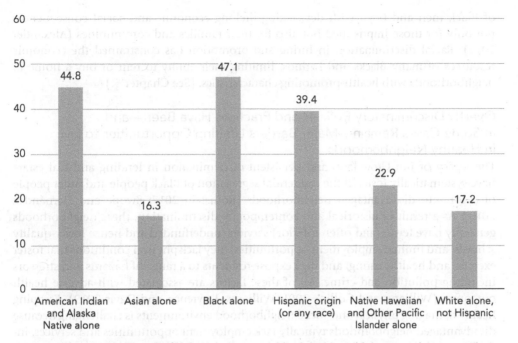

FIGURE 7.5 The likelihood of living in a poor neighborhood varies by a person's race or ethnic group. Percentage of people in different racial or ethnic groups living in poor neighborhoods, 2006–2010. A poor neighborhood is one in which at least 20% of residents have incomes at or below the federal poverty guidelines. *Source*: Bishaw, A. 2011. "Areas with concentrated poverty: 2006–2010." Publication of the U.S. Census Bureau.

injustices, persist and have their discriminatory effects regardless of whether any particular individual now consciously intends to discriminate. For African Americans, the systems and structures began with 250 years of slavery, which denied enslaved people all rights and, to justify that, developed an ideology according to which Africans and African Americans were considered inferior to Whites. Outright slavery was followed by nearly 100 years of "Jim Crow" laws enacted in formerly Confederate states deliberately and systematically to constrain the rights and opportunities of Black people following the end of legal slavery. Based on the racist ideology used to justify slavery and enforced by vigilante terrorism typified by the Ku Klux Klan, Jim Crow laws reinforced racial segregation in all aspects of life, including residential location, schools, transportation, and other public services. Although Jim Crow and other discriminatory laws officially ended with passage of the Civil Rights Act of 1964, enforcement has been an ongoing struggle. For example, despite the Voting Rights Act of 1965, persistent voter suppression systematically targeting people of color has been well documented; laws disproportionately disenfranchising low-income people and people of color proliferated with a 2013 Supreme Court ruling allowing key changes to the Voting Rights Act (Bentele and O'Brien 2013; American Civil Liberties Union 2019), and laws that differentially make it more difficult for people of color to vote have passed or are under consideration in many states. Racial discrimination in policing and sentencing has led to mass incarceration of Black men and boys, with devastating lifelong economic and social consequences not only for those imprisoned but also for their families and communities (Alexander 2012). Racial discrimination in hiring and promotion has constrained the economic resources of many Blacks and Latinos, limiting their ability to rent or buy a home in neighborhoods with health-promoting characteristics. (See Chapter 5.)

Overtly Discriminatory Policies and Practices Have Been—and in Some Cases Remain—Major Barriers Limiting Opportunities to Live in Healthy Neighborhoods

The legacy of Jim Crow laws and persistent discrimination in lending and real estate have systematically fostered the residential segregation of Black people and other people of color into disadvantaged neighborhoods (Rothstein 2017; Swope and Hernández 2019). As a result of historical and contemporary discrimination, these neighborhoods generally have fewer (and often inferior) services, underfunded and hence lower-quality schools, and limited employment opportunities; they lack physical conditions that foster exercise and healthy eating; and they expose residents to a range of hazards and stressors including pollution and crime. All of these factors are associated with adverse health outcomes (Williams and Collins 2001; Williams, Lawrence, and Davis 2019). Escaping health-damaging physical and social neighborhood environments is challenging because disadvantaged neighborhoods typically lack employment opportunities and services, including well-resourced schools, that foster upward social and economic mobility. As a result of racial segregation, Blacks and Latinos are also more likely than Whites to live in poor-quality housing with detrimental effects (Jacobs 2011), posing a greater risk of exposure to conditions that can contribute to poor health, such as lead poisoning of children (Muller, Sampson, and Winter 2018) and indoor allergens that can exacerbate asthma (Hughes et al. 2017; Kanchongkittiphon et al. 2014). (See Chapter 8.)

Discriminatory lending practices also have played a major role. Guidelines established by the federal Home Owners' Loan Corporation (HOLC) beginning in the 1930s, and later adopted by private banks, explicitly considered the racial/ethnic composition and income level of neighborhoods in determining and ranking the riskiness of mortgage lending in those areas. "Redlining" derives its name from the red shading of areas on HOLC maps representing the neighborhoods assigned the poorest ranking of "hazardous" for giving out loans. For decades, areas with high concentrations of residents of color were disproportionately red-lined, severely limiting opportunities to escape poverty and accumulate wealth in communities of color. Economic and racial segregation, as well as lower homeownership rates, home values, and credit scores in these areas, persist to the present day (Aaronson, Hartley, and Mazumder 2017; Mitchell and Franco 2018). Red-lining has played a major role in constraining access, particularly among Black people, to opportunities for improving housing and neighborhoods, limiting the ability to accumulate and pass on wealth to the next generation, and limiting other general economic opportunities, with major implications for health.

During the U.S. housing bubble of the late 2000s, studies found that non-White borrowers were more likely to receive high-cost, subprime mortgage loans even when controlling for standard indicators of creditworthiness and risk (Bayer, Ferreira, and Ross 2014). This in turn led to much higher foreclosure rates within predominantly

Black, Latino, or racially integrated neighborhoods relative to predominately White neighborhoods (Bocian et al. 2011; Hall, Crowder, and Spring 2015b). This foreclosure crisis may have set back progress in narrowing racial inequities in wealth, homeowner-ship, and residential segregation (Hall, Crowder, and Spring 2015a; Goodman, McCargo, and Zhu 2018). Furthermore, research has linked foreclosure to poor mental and physical health outcomes and declines in health care services utilization, both among individuals who experience foreclosure and among people residing in areas with high foreclosure rates (Downing 2016; Arcaya 2018).

Other historical and contemporary policies and practices contribute to inequitable residential patterns. Land-use zoning—either for exclusively single-family or for more commercial or industrial use—is strongly linked with the socioeconomic and racial/ethnic makeup of neighborhoods, contributing to racial and economic segregation and affecting property values, wealth accumulation, and health-relevant environmental exposures (Swope and Hernández 2019). The greater likelihood of environmental hazards (e.g., hazardous waste disposal sites contaminating the soil, freeways and industries polluting the air, and polluted water) within or near neighborhoods with high concentrations of poor people—particularly poor people of color—has also been documented repeatedly (Cushing, Morello-Frosch, et al. 2015; Morello-Frosch and Lopez 2006; Cushing, Faust, et al. 2015).

Gentrification, or the movement of capital and higher-income people into neighborhoods that have historically experienced poverty and disinvestment (N. Smith 1979; Izenberg, Mujahid, and Yen 2018), may displace residents in segregated and poor neighborhoods due to rising housing costs. Gentrification may change neighborhood conditions in both positive and negative ways with differential health effects for different groups, often exacerbating racial health disparities (Izenberg et al. 2018).

7.5. STRATEGIES FOR MAKING NEIGHBORHOODS HEALTHIER

Evidence indicates that physical and social characteristics of neighborhoods can influence people's health in important ways, including through direct exposures to health-harming or health-promoting conditions and indirectly by shaping people's choices and behaviors. Often in medicine and public health, the focus is exclusively on people's choices and behaviors or harm-reducing treatments such as medications. This is, however, unlikely to be adequate for improving health and certainly will not diminish health disparities, unless attention is also paid to enhancing the health-related opportunities and reducing the barriers in the places where people live. A wide range of public and private sector policies have been proposed to make neighborhoods healthier places for everyone, and particularly for those who both experience the most health-damaging environments and face the greatest obstacles to changing their environments. For example, interventions have been proposed, and in some cases implemented, with the overlapping goals of improving the physical quality of neighborhoods, including housing, public spaces, and transportation (Diez Roux 2016); reducing racial and economic segregation; and investing in the economic development of disadvantaged communities. Because chil-dren are likely to be particularly vulnerable to unhealthy conditions in neighborhoods, with consequences for health both in childhood and later in life, proposals focusing on healthier neighborhoods for families with children deserve special consideration (Jutte et al. 2015).

Because neighborhood contexts are likely to affect health through multiple, complex, and interrelated pathways, interventions that produce changes in multiple neighborhood characteristics may be most likely to have an impact (Diez Roux 2016; Williams and Cooper 2019). It is beyond the scope of this chapter to assess which specific policies appear most promising, particularly because rigorous research on the effectiveness of different interventions is limited. However, enough is known to indicate that economic development must be central to any strategy to make neighborhoods healthier. Noted below are a range of interventions that appear to deserve consideration, based on the best available knowledge. Given current gaps in knowledge and the importance of filling those gaps to inform policies for improving health, high priority should be given to well-conceived research assessing the health impacts of these and other approaches to improving neighborhoods in ways likely to improve health and reduce social disparities in health.

> The weight of evidence indicates that physical, social, and service characteristics of neighborhoods can influence health in important ways, including by shaping choices and behaviors. Interventions need to target multiple conditions.

In addition to the examples noted in this chapter, Box 7.2 describes a range—by no means exhaustive—of diverse and sometimes overlapping strategies that warrant consideration as potential approaches to increasing opportunities for good health for all, particularly for those who live in conditions presenting the greatest threats to health. Although the current evidence is limited, we have enough foundational knowledge to identify promising approaches and carefully evaluate them, with the goal of informing future policies.

7.6. KEY POINTS

- Considerable evidence shows that physical and social features of the places where people live can directly or indirectly affect the health of the people living in them. For example, levels of air pollution vary across different neighborhoods, as do the quality of schools and the presence of employment opportunities, all of which influence health; and walkability and the density of stores selling tobacco and alcohol can influence behaviors that strongly influence health.

- Racism, particularly systemic or structural racism, has been and continues to be a major factor determining who has the opportunity to live in health-promoting places. Because the obstacles are systemic and structural, it will take more than making people more aware of racism to dismantle the obstacles.

- Hazardous waste disposal sites and other environmental

> Despite gaps in knowledge about what works best to make neighborhoods healthier, we know enough now based on existing evidence to design, implement, and carefully evaluate a range of promising approaches.

BOX 7.2   Neighborhood-Level Interventions

Following are several examples—selected to illustrate a range of approaches—of neighborhood-level interventions that merit consideration based on the best available knowledge:

- Several multipronged *community development and revitalization initiatives* designed to promote neighborhood economic development and improve physical and social environments in neighborhoods have been recognized as important approaches for improving community health (Sharkey 2016). The U.S. Public Health Service Task Force on Community Preventive Services and a team of experts have recognized the large potential health impact of such initiatives (Anderson et al. 2003).

- An important aspect of revitalization and other relevant neighborhood improvement initiatives is *community organizing* to strengthen capacity for leadership and collective action within communities. It aims to motivate action and bring people together to work collectively and feel empowered to improve their neighborhoods. Without ongoing advocacy from within communities, improvements may not be initiated, adequate, or sustained. Pogo Park in Richmond, California—which builds green spaces for children—is an example of efforts that are both community-based and community-led (https://pogopark.org).

- *"Environmental justice" initiatives* seek to reduce toxic exposures in the physical environment within communities with large concentrations of low-income residents, particularly low-income Black and Hispanic residents. Although eliminating health hazards in all communities is important, it is well documented that hazardous waste, pollution, and other toxic substances are differentially concentrated in such communities (Cushing, Faust, et al. 2015; Cushing, Morello-Frosch, et al. 2015; Morello-Frosch and Lopez 2006)—hence the widely used term "environmental justice." WeACT, a grassroots initiative in Harlem, New York, seeks to build community capacity as it challenges environmental injustice (https://www.weact.org).

- Other promising approaches with potential health implications include strategies to *reduce residential segregation* along socioeconomic and racial/ethnic lines through a range of initiatives, such as zoning measures (Tuller 2018; Pastor and Turner 2010); expanding the supply of affordable housing in neighborhoods that offer opportunities for employment and quality schools (Pastor and Turner 2010); and enforcement of fair housing laws, including the Federal Fair Housing Act (National Fair Housing Alliance 2018). As noted in this chapter, there is debate about the advisability of approaches that enable to move out of disadvantaged neighborhoods versus improving conditions within those neighborhoods.

- Although findings from research on health outcomes have been mixed, *bringing healthy retail food markets into disadvantaged communities* has received attention for its theoretical ability to increase the availability of affordable, healthful food choices in neighborhoods where current options are most limited (Flournay 2010; Bell et al. 2013). There has also been interest in promoting community gardens to improve health and well-being (Kunpeuk et al. 2020; Malberg Dyg, Christensen, and Peterson 2020; Genter et al. 2015; Garcia et al. 2018). Such approaches may be useful adjuncts to efforts that focus on economic development.

Because the evidence indicates that both people and places matter for health, many interventions focused on individuals also can be expected to contribute to improving the quality of neighborhoods from a health perspective. The following are examples:

- *Housing mobility programs* that provide recipients of public housing assistance greater choices about where they live can enable people to move into healthier neighborhoods with lower exposures to crime and social disorder (Sharkey 2016; Gale 2018; Chetty, Hendren, and Katz 2016). This chapter discusses potential strengths and limitations of such programs.

- Studies have shown that the Earned Income Tax Credit, a federal *poverty reduction* policy directly benefiting low-income working households, significantly concentrates financial resources in poor neighborhoods while also leading to improvements in health (Spencer 2007; Muennig et al. 2016).

- *Homeownership assistance* to families could contribute to neighborhood stability and development, as individual assets become investments in neighborhoods (Rohe and Lindblad 2013).

hazards (e.g., sources of air and water pollution) have disproportionately been located in or near low-income communities of color.

7.7. QUESTIONS FOR DISCUSSION

1. How can racial residential segregation damage health?
2. What historical policies and ongoing practices have led to and sustained racial residential segregation?
3. Discuss potential health consequences of racial residential segregation
4. How could being poor (i.e., being part of a household living in poverty) in an affluent neighborhood have different health effects than being poor in a neighborhood with a high percentage of households living in poverty?
5. Why is it so difficult to disentangle the health effects associated with a neighborhood's overall characteristics from those associated with the characteristics of its residents?
6. Are there other ways that neighborhoods can affect health that were not mentioned in this chapter?

ACKNOWLEDGMENT

This chapter builds on material from the following source:

Braveman P., C. Cubbin, S. Egerter, and V. Pedregon. 2011. *Neighborhoods and Health*. Princeton, NJ: Robert Wood Johnson Foundation.

REFERENCES

Aaronson, D., D. Hartley, and B. Mazumder. 2017. "The effects of the 1930s HOLC 'redlining' maps." Working Paper No. 2017–12. Chicago, IL: Federal Reserve Bank of Chicago.

Alexander, M. 2012. *The New Jim Crow: Mass Incarceration in the Age of Color-Blindness*. New York: New Press.

Almedom, A. M., and D. Glandon. 2008. "Social capital and mental health." In *Social Capital and Health*, edited by I. Kawachi, S. V. Subramanian, and D. Kim, 191–214. New York, NY: Springer.

American Civil Liberties Union. 2019. "The case for restoring and updating the Voting Rights Act." Report to the U.S. House Committee on the Judiciary.

Anderson, L. M., S. C. Scrimshaw, M. T. Fullilove, and J. E. Fielding. 2003. "The Community Guide's model for linking the social environment to health." *Am J Prev Med* 24(3, Suppl): 12–20. https://doi.org/10.1016/S0749-3797(02)00652-9.

Andersson, F., J. C. Haltiwanger, M. J. Kutzbach, H. O. Pollakowski, and D. H. Weinberg. 2018. "Job displacement and the duration of joblessness: The role of spatial mismatch." *Rev Econ Stat* 100(2): 203–218. doi:10.1162/REST_a_00707.

Arcaya, M. 2018. "Neighborhood foreclosure and health." In *Neighborhoods and Health*, edited by D. T. Duncan and I. Kawachi, 2nd ed., 293–319. New York, NY: Oxford University Press.

Arcaya, M. C., R. D. Tucker-Seeley, R. Kim, A. Schnake-Mahl, M. So, and S. V. Subramanian. 2016. "Research on neighborhood effects on health in the United States: A systematic review of study characteristics." *Soc Sci Med* 168: 16–29. https://doi.org/10.1016/j.socscimed.2016.08.047.

Arias, E., L. A. Escobedo, J. Kennedy, C. Fu, and J. Cisewki. 2018. "U.S. Small-Area Life Expectancy Estimates Project: Methodology and results summary." *Vital Health Stat* 2(181): 1–40.

Baranyi, G., S. Sieber, S. Cullati, J. Pearce, C. Dibben, and D. S. Courvoisier. 2020. "The longitudinal association of perceived neighborhood disorder and lack of social cohesion with depression among adults aged 50 and over: An individual participant data meta-analysis from 16 high-income countries." *Am J Epidemiol* 189(4): 343–353. doi:10.1093/aje/kwz209.

Bayer, P., F. Ferreira, and S. L. Ross. 2014. "Race, ethnicity and high-cost mortgage lending." Working Paper No. 20762. Cambridge, MA: National Bureau of Economic Research.

Bell, J., G. Mora, E. Hagan, V. Rubin, and A. Karpyn. 2013. "Access to healthy food and why it matters: A review of the research." Philadelphia, PA: Policy Link and The Food Trust. https://www.policylink.org/resources-tools/access-to-healthy-food-and-why-it-matters

Bentele, K. G., and E. E. O'Brien. 2013. "Jim Crow 2.0? Why states consider and adopt restrictive voter access policies." *Perspect Politics* 11(4): 1088–1116. doi:10.1017/S1537592713002843.

Bischoff, K., and S. F. Reardon. 2014. "Residential segregation by income, 1970–2009." In Diversity and *Disparities*: America Enters a *New Century*, edited by J. Logan, 208–233. New York, NY: Russell Sage Foundation.

Bishaw, A. 2011. "Areas with concentrated poverty: 2006–2010." Vol. 9. Washington, DC: U.S. Census Bureau.

Bishaw, A. 2014. "Changes in areas with concentrated poverty: 2000 to 2010." Washington, DC: U.S. Department of Commerce, Economics and Statistics Administration.

Block, J., M. Seward, and P. James. 2018. "Food environment and health." *Neighborhoods Health* 247–277.

Bocian, D. G., W. Li, C. Reid, and R. G. Quercia. 2011. "Lost ground, 2011: Disparities in mortgage lending and foreclosures." Durham, NC: Center for Responsible Lending.

Brender, J. D., J. A. Maantay, and J. Chakraborty. 2011. "Residential proximity to environmental hazards and adverse health outcomes." *Am J Public Health* 101(Suppl 1): S37–S52. doi:10.2105/ajph.2011.300183.

Brenner, A. B., L. N. Borrell, T. Barrientos-Gutierrez, and A. V. Diez Roux. 2015. "Longitudinal associations of neighborhood socioeconomic characteristics and alcohol availability on drinking: Results from the Multi-Ethnic Study of Atherosclerosis (MESA)." *Soc Sci Med* 145: 17–25. doi:10.1016/j.socscimed.2015.09.030.

Carpiano, R. M. 2008. "Actual or potential neighborhood resources for health." In *Social Capital and Health*, edited by I. Kawachi, S. V. Subramanian, and D. Kim, 83–93. New York, NY: Springer.

Centers for Disease Control and Prevention. 2018. "500 Cities Project data." Accessed November 8, 2019. https://www.cdc.gov/places/about/500-cities-2016-2019/index.html

Chetty, R., N. Hendren, and L. F. Katz. 2016. "The effects of exposure to better neighborhoods on children: New evidence from the Moving to Opportunity Experiment." *Am Econ Rev* 106(4): 855–902.

Cobb, L. K., L. J. Appel, M. Franco, J. C. Jones-Smith, A. Nur, and C. A. M. Anderson. 2015. "The relationship of the local food environment with obesity: A systematic review of methods, study quality, and results." *Obesity* 23(7): 1331–1344.

Cummins, S., E. Flint, and S. A. Matthews. 2014. "New neighborhood grocery store increased awareness of food access but did not alter dietary habits or obesity." *Health Affairs* 33(2): 283–291.

Cushing, L., J. Faust, L. M. August, R. Cendak, W. Wieland, and G. Alexeeff. 2015. "Racial/ethnic disparities in cumulative environmental health impacts in California: Evidence from a statewide environmental justice screening tool (CalEnviroScreen 1.1)." *Am J Public Health* 105(11): 2341–2348. doi:10.2105/AJPH.2015.302643.

Cushing, L., R. Morello-Frosch, M. Wander, and M. Pastor. 2015. "The haves, the have-nots, and the health of everyone: The relationship between social inequality and environmental quality." *Annu Rev Public Health* 36(1): 193–209. doi:10.1146/annurev-publhealth-031914-122646.

DeLuca, S., G. J. Duncan, M. Keels, and R. Mendenhall. 2012. "The notable and the null: Using mixed methods to understand the diverse impacts of residential mobility programs." In *Neighbourhood Effects Research: New Perspectives*, edited by M. van Ham, D. Manley, N. Bailey, L. Simpson, and D. Maclennan, 195–223. Dordrecht, the Netherlands: Springer.

Diez Roux, A. V. 2016. "Neighborhoods and health: What do we know? What should we do?" *Am J Public Health* 106(3): 430–431. doi:10.2105/ajph.2016.303064.

Diez Roux, A. V., and C. Mair. 2010. "Neighborhoods and health." *Ann N Y Acad Sci* 1186(1): 125–145. doi:10.1111/j.1749-6632.2009.05333.x.

Diez Roux, A. V., S. S. Merkin, D. Arnett, L. Chambless, M. Massing, F. J. Nieto, P. Sorlie, M. Szklo, H. A. Tyroler, and R. L. Watson. 2001. "Neighborhood of residence and incidence of coronary heart disease." *N Engl J Med* 345(2): 99–106. doi:10.1056/Nejm200107123450205.

Ding, D., J. F. Sallis, J. Kerr, S. Lee, and D. E. Rosenberg. 2011. "Neighborhood environment and physical activity among youth: A review." *Am J Prev Med* 41(4): 442–455. https://doi.org/10.1016/j.amepre.2011.06.036.

Downing, J. 2016. "The health effects of the foreclosure crisis and unaffordable housing: A systematic review and explanation of evidence." *Soc Sci Med* 162: 88–96.

Duncan, D., and I. Kawachi. 2018. "Neighborhoods and health: A progress report." In *Neighborhoods and Health*, edited by D. T. Duncan and I. Kawachi, 2nd ed., 1–16. New York, NY: Oxford University Press.

Duncan, D., S. D. Regan, and B. Chaix. 2018. "Operationalizing neighborhood definitions in health research: Spatial misclassification and other issues." In *Neighborhoods and Health*, edited by D. T. Duncan and I. Kawachi, 2nd ed., 19–56. New York, NY: Oxford University Press.

Dwyer-Lindgren, L., A. Bertozzi-Villa, R. W. Stubbs, C. Morozoff, J. P. Mackenbach, F. J. van Lenthe, A. H. Mokdad, and C. J. L. Murray. 2017. "Inequalities in life expectancy among US counties, 1980 to 2014: Temporal trends and key drivers." *JAMA Intern Med* 177(7): 1003–1011. doi:10.1001/jamainternmed.2017.0918.

Ehsan, A. M., and M. J. De Silva. 2015. "Social capital and common mental disorder: A systematic review." *J Epidemiol Community Health* 69(10): 1021–8. doi:10.1136/jech-2015-205868.

Erickson, P. G., L. Harrison, S. Cook, M.-M. Cousineau, and E. M. Adlaf. 2012. "A comparative study of the influence of collective efficacy on substance use among adolescent students in Philadelphia, Toronto, and Montreal." *Addict Res Theory* 20(1): 11–20. doi:10.3109/16066359.2010.530710.

Finan, L. J., S. Lipperman-Kreda, M. Abadi, J. W. Grube, E. Kaner, A. Balassone, and A. Gaidus. 2019. "Tobacco outlet density and adolescents' cigarette smoking: A meta-analysis." *Tob Control* 28(1): 27–33. doi:10.1136/tobaccocontrol-2017-054065.

Fitzpatrick, K. M., X. Shi, D. Willis, and J. Niemeier. 2018. "Obesity and place: Chronic disease in the 500 largest U.S. cities." *Obes Res Clin Pract* 12(5): 421–425. doi:10.1016/j.orcp.2018.02.005.

Flournay, R. 2010. "Healthy food, healthy communities: Promising strategies to improve access to fresh, healthy food and transform communities 5." PolicyLink. https://www.healthyfoodaccess.org/resources-tools-library-promising-strategies-to-improve-access.

Gale, R. 2018. "Housing mobility programs and health outcomes." Health Affairs. https://www.healthaffairs.org/do/10.1377/hpb20180313.616232.

Garcia, M. T., S. M. Ribeiro, A. C. C. G. Germani, and C. M. Bógus. 2018. "The impact of urban gardens on adequate and healthy food: A systematic review." *Public Health Nutr* 21(2): 416–425. doi:10.1017/S1368980017002944.

Genter, C., A. Roberts, J. Richardson, and M. Sheaff. 2015. "The contribution of allotment gardening to health and wellbeing: A systematic review of the literature." *Br J Occup Ther* 78(10): 593–605.

Golden, S. D., T.-M. Kuo, A. Y. Kong, C. D. Baggett, L. Henriksen, and K. M. Ribisl. 2019. "County-level associations between tobacco retailer density and smoking prevalence in the USA, 2012." *Prev Med Rep* 17: 101005. https://doi.org/10.1016/j.pmedr.2019.101005.

Goodman, L., A. McCargo, and J. Zhu. 2018. "A closer look at the fifteen-year drop in Black homeownership. Technical report. Washington, DC: Urban Institute.

Grasser, G., D. Van Dyck, S. Titze, and W. Stronegger. 2013. "Objectively measured walkability and active transport and weight-related outcomes in adults: A systematic review." *Int J Public Health* 58(4): 615–625. doi:10.1007/s00038-012-0435-0.

Hall, M., K. Crowder, and A. Spring. 2015a. "Neighborhood foreclosures, racial/ethnic transitions, and residential segregation." *Am Soc Rev* 80(3): 526–549. doi:10.1177/0003122415581334.

Hall, M., K. Crowder, and A. Spring. 2015b. "Variations in housing foreclosures by race and place, 2005–2012." *Annal Am Acad Polit Soc Sci* 660(1): 217–237. doi:10.1177/0002716215576907.

Hipp, J. R., and R. Wickes. 2017. "Violence in urban neighborhoods: A longitudinal study of collective efficacy and violent crime." *J Quant Criminol* 33(4): 783–808. doi:10.1007/s10940-016-9311-z.

Hirsch, J. A., K. A. Moore, P. J. Clarke, D. A. Rodriguez, K. R. Evenson, S. J. Brines, M. A. Zagorski, and A. V. Diez Roux. 2014. "Changes in the built environment and changes in the amount of walking over time: Longitudinal results from the Multi-Ethnic Study of Atherosclerosis." *Am J Epidemiol* 180(8): 799–809. doi:10.1093/aje/kwu218.

Hughes, H. K., E. C. Matsui, M. M. Tschudy, C. E. Pollack, and C. A. Keet. 2017. "Pediatric asthma health disparities: Race, hardship, housing, and asthma in a national survey." *Acad Pediatr* 17(2): 127–134. https://doi.org/10.1016/j.acap.2016.11.011.

Izenberg, J. M., M. S. Mujahid, and I. H. Yen. 2018. "Health in changing neighborhoods: A study of the relationship between gentrification and self-rated health in the state of California." *Health Place* 52: 188–195. https://doi.org/10.1016/j.healthplace.2018.06.002.

Jacobs, D. E. 2011. "Environmental health disparities in housing." *Am J Public Health* 101(Suppl 1): S115–S122. doi:10.2105/AJPH.2010.300058.

Jokela, M. 2014. "Are neighborhood health associations causal? A 10-year prospective cohort study with repeated measurements." *Am J Epidemiol* 180(8): 776–784. doi:10.1093/aje/kwu233.

Jutte, D. P., J. L. Miller, and D. J. Erickson. 2015. "Neighborhood adversity, child health, and the role for community development." *Pediatrics* 135(Suppl 2): S48. doi:10.1542/peds.2014-3549F.

Kanchongkittiphon, W., M. J. Mendell, J. M. Gaffin, G. Wang, and W. Phipatanakul. 2014. "Indoor environmental exposures and exacerbation of asthma: An update to the 2000 review by the Institute of Medicine." *Environ Health Perspect* 123(1): 6–20.

Kawachi, I., S. V. Subramanian, and D. Kim. 2008. "Social capital and health." In *Social Capital and Health: A Decade of Progress and Beyond*, edited by I. Kawachi, S. V. Subramanian, and D. Kim, 1–26. New York, NY: Springer.

Kling, J. R., J. B. Liebman, and L. F. Katz. 2007. "Experimental analysis of neighborhood effects." *Econometrica* 75(1): 83–119.

Kunpeuk, W., W. Spence, S. Phulkerd, R. Suphanchaimat, and S. Pitayarangsarit. 2020. "The impact of gardening on nutrition and physical health outcomes: A systematic review and meta-analysis." *Health Promot Int* 35(2): 397–408.

Leas, E. C., N. C. Schleicher, J. J. Prochaska, and L. Henriksen. 2019. "Place-based inequity in smoking PREVALENCE in the largest cities in the United States." *JAMA Intern Med* 179(3): 442–444. doi:10.1001/jamainternmed.2018.5990.

Leventhal, T., and V. Dupéré. 2019. "Neighborhood effects on children's development in experimental and nonexperimental research." *Annu Rev Dev Psychol* 1: 149–176. doi:10.1146/annurev-devpsych-121318-085221.

Ludwig, J., G. J. Duncan, L. A. Gennetian, L. F. Katz, R. C. Kessler, J. R. Kling, and L. Sanbonmatsu. 2012. "Neighborhood effects on the long-term well-being of low-income adults." *Science* 337(6101): 1505–1510. doi:10.1126/science.1224648.

Ludwig, J., L. Sanbonmatsu, L. Gennetian, E. Adam, G. J. Duncan, L. F. Katz, R. C. Kessler, et al. 2011. "Neighborhoods, obesity, and diabetes—A randomized social experiment." *N Engl J Med* 365(16): 1509–1519. doi:10.1056/NEJMsa1103216.

Malberg Dyg, P., S. Christensen, and C. J. Peterson. 2020. "Community gardens and wellbeing amongst vulnerable populations: A thematic review." *Health Promot Int* 35(4): 790–803.

McCormack, G. R., and A. Shiell. 2011. "In search of causality: A systematic review of the relationship between the built environment and physical activity among adults." *Int J Behav Nutr Phys Activity* 8(1): 125. doi:Artn12510.1186/1479-5868-8-125.

Mitchell, B., and J. Franco. 2018. "HOLC 'redlining' maps: The persistent structure of segregation and economic inequality." National Community Reinvestment Coalition. https://ncrc.org/holc.

Morello-Frosch, R., and R. Lopez. 2006. "The riskscape and the color line: Examining the role of segregation in environmental health disparities." *Environ Res* 102(2): 181–196. https://doi.org/10.1016/j.envres.2006.05.007.

Muennig, P. A., B. Mohit, J. Wu, H. Jia, and Z. Rosen. 2016. "Cost effectiveness of the Earned Income Tax Credit as a health policy investment." *Am J Prev Med* 51(6): 874–881. https://doi.org/10.1016/j.amepre.2016.07.001.

Muller, C., R. J. Sampson, and A. S. Winter. 2018. "Environmental inequality: The social causes and consequences of lead exposure." *Annu Rev Sociol* 44(1): 263–282. doi:10.1146/annurev-soc-073117-041222.

National Fair Housing Alliance. 2018. "Making every neighborhood a place of opportunity: 2018 fair housing trends report." Washington, DC: National Fair Housing Alliance.

National Geographic Society Resource Library. 2011. "Neighborhood.". https://www.nationalgeographic.org/encyclopedia/neighborhood.

Oakes, J. M. 2004. "The (mis)estimation of neighborhood effects: Causal inference for a practicable social epidemiology." *Soc Sci Med* 58(10): 1929–1952. doi:10.1016/j.socscimed.2003.08.004.

Oakes, J. M., K. E. Andrade, I. M. Biyoow, and L. T. Cowan. 2015. "Twenty years of neighborhood effect research: an assessment." *Curr Epidemiol Rep* 2(1): 80–87.

Orr, L., J. Feins, R. Jacob, E. Beecroft, L. Sanbonmatsu, L. F. Katz, J. B. Liebman, and J. R. Kling. 2003. "Moving to opportunity: Interim impacts evaluation." Washington, DC: U.S. Department of Housing and Urban Development.

Osypuk, T. L., N. M. Schmidt, L. M. Bates, E. J. Tchetgen-Tchetgen, F. J. Earls, and M. M. Glymour. 2012. "Gender and crime victimization modify neighborhood effects on adolescent mental health." *Pediatrics* 130(3): 472–481.

Osypuk, T. L., E. J. Tchetgen, D. Acevedo-Garcia, F. J. Earls, A. Lincoln, N. M. Schmidt, and M. M. Glymour. 2012. "Differential mental health effects of neighborhood relocation among youth in vulnerable families: Results from a randomized trial." *Arch Gen Psychiatry* 69(12): 1284–1294.

Pastor, M., and M. A. Turner. 2010. "Reducing poverty and economic distress after ARRA: Potential roles for place-conscious strategies." Washington, DC: Urban Institute.

Phelan, J. C., and B. G. Link. 2015. "Is racism a fundamental cause of inequalities in health?" *Annu Rev Sociol* 41(1): 311–330. doi:10.1146/annurev-soc-073014-112305.

Pratt, T. C., and F. T. Cullen. 2005. "Assessing macro-level predictors and theories of crime: A meta-analysis." *Crime Justice* 32: 373–450. doi:10.1086/655357.

Pulakka, A., J. I. Halonen, I. Kawachi, J. Pentti, S. Stenholm, M. Jokela, I. Kaate, M. Koskenvuo, J. Vahtera, and M. Kivimaki. 2016. "Association between distance from home to tobacco outlet and smoking cessation and relapse." *JAMA Intern Med* 176(10): 1512–1519. doi:10.1001/jamainternmed.2016.4535.

Putnam, R. D. 1993. "The prosperous community: Social capital and public life." *The American Prospect* (13): 35–42.

Reardon, S. F., L. Fox, and J. Townsend. 2015. "Neighborhood income composition by household race and income, 1990–2009." *Annals Am Acad Polit Soc Sci* 660(1): 78–97.

Rohe, W. M., and M. Lindblad. 2013. "Reexamining the social benefits of homeownership after the housing crisis." Cambridge, MA: Joint Center for Housing Studies of Harvard University.

Roth, G. A., L. Dwyer-Lindgren, A. Bertozzi-Villa, R. W. Stubbs, C. Morozoff, M. Naghavi, A. H. Mokdad, and C. J. L. Murray. 2017. "Trends and patterns of geographic variation in cardiovascular mortality among US counties, 1980–2014." *JAMA* 317(19): 1976–1992. doi:10.1001/jama.2017.4150.

Rothstein, R. 2017. *The color of law: A forgotten history of how our government segregated America.* New York: Liveright.

Sampson, R. J., J. D. Morenoff, and T. Gannon-Rowley. 2002. "Assessing 'neighborhood effects': Social processes and new DIRECTIONS in research." *Annu Rev Sociol* 28(1): 443–478. doi:10.1146/annurev.soc.28.110601.141114.

Sampson, R. J., S. W. Raudenbush, and F. Earls. 1997. "Neighborhoods and violent crime: A multilevel study of collective efficacy." *Science* 277(5328): 918–924. doi:10.1126/science.277.5328.918.

Sanbonmatsu, L., L. F. Katz, J. Ludwig, L. A. Gennetian, G. J. Duncan, R. C. Kessler, E. K. Adam, T. McDade, and S. T. Lindau. 2011. "Moving to opportunity for fair housing demonstration program: Final impacts evaluation." Washington, DC: U.S. Department of Housing and Urban Development.

Sanbonmatsu, L., N. A. Potter, E. Adam, G. J. Duncan, L. F. Katz, R. C. Kessler, J. Ludwig, et al. 2012. "The long-term effects of moving to opportunity on adult health and economic self-sufficiency." *Cityscape* 14(2): 109–136.

Schootman, M., E. M. Andresen, F. D. Wolinsky, T. K. Malmstrom, J. P. Miller, and D. K. Miller. 2007. "Neighbourhood environment and the incidence of depressive symptoms among middle-aged African Americans." *J Epidemiol Community Health* 61(6): 527. doi:10.1136/jech.2006.050088.

Sharkey, P. 2010. "The acute effect of local homicides on children's cognitive performance." *Proc Natl Acad Sci USA* 107(26): 11733–11738. doi:10.1073/pnas.1000690107.

Sharkey, P. 2014. "Spatial segmentation and the Black middle class." *Am J Sociol* 119(4): 903–954.

Sharkey, P. 2016. "Neighborhoods, cities, and economic mobility." *RSF* 2(2): 159. doi:10.7758/RSF.2016.2.2.07.

Sharkey, P., and J. W. Faber. 2014. "Where, when, why, and for whom do residential contexts matter? Moving away from the dichotomous understanding of neighborhood effects." *Annu Rev Sociol* 40: 559–579.

Sherk, A., T. Stockwell, T. Chikritzhs, S. Andréasson, C. Angus, J. Gripenberg, H. Holder, et al. 2018. "Alcohol consumption and the physical availability of take-away alcohol: Systematic reviews and meta-analyses of the days and hours of sale and outlet density." *J Stud Alcohol Drugs* 79(1): 58–67. doi:10.15288/jsad.2018.79.58.

Smith, H. J., T. F. Pettigrew, G. M. Pippin, and S. Bialosiewicz. 2012. "Relative deprivation: A theoretical and meta-analytic review." *Pers Soc Psychol Rev* 16(3): 203–232. doi:10.1177/1088868311430825.

Smith, M., J. Hosking, A. Woodward, K. Witten, A. MacMillan, A. Field, P. Baas, and H. Mackie. 2017. "Systematic literature review of built environment effects on physical activity and active transport—An update and new findings on health equity." *Int J Behav Nutr Phys Act* 14(1): 158. doi:10.1186/s12966-017-0613-9.

Smith, N. 1979. "Toward a theory of gentrification a back to the city movement by capital, not people." *J Am Planning Assoc* 45(4): 538–548.

Spencer, J. H. 2007. "Neighborhood economic development effects of the Earned Income Tax Credit in Los Angeles: Poor places and policies for the working poor." *Urban Affairs Rev* 42(6): 851–873. doi:10.1177/1078087407300515.

Swope, C. B., and D. Hernández. 2019. "Housing as a determinant of health equity: A conceptual model." *Soc Sci Med* 243: 112571. https://doi.org/10.1016/j.socscimed.2019.112571.

Tuller, D. 2018. "Housing and health: The role of inclusionary zoning." HealthAffairs. https://www.healthaffairs.org/do/10.1377/hpb20180313.668759.

U.S. Census Bureau. 2019. "Census tract." https://www.census.gov/programs-surveys/geography/about/glossary.html#par_textimage_13.

Wilkinson, R. D., and K. Pickett. 2009. *The Spirit Level: Why More Equal Societies Almost Always Do Better.* New York, NY: Bloomsbury.

Wilkinson, R. G., and K. Pickett. 2020. *How More Equal Societies Reduce Stress, Restore Sanity and Improve Everyone's Well-Being*. New York, NY: Penguin.

Williams, D. R., and C. Collins. 2001. "Racial residential segregation: A fundamental cause of racial disparities in health." *Public Health Rep* 116(5): 404–416. doi:10.1093/phr/116.5.404.

Williams, D. R., and A. L. Cooper. 2019. "Reducing racial inequities in health: Using what we already know to take action."

Int J Environ Res Public Health 16(4), 606. doi:10.3390/ijerph16040606.

Williams, D. R., J. A. Lawrence, and B. A. Davis. 2019. "Racism and health: Evidence and needed research." *Annu Rev Public Health* 40(1): 105–125. doi:10.1146/annurev-publhealth-040218-043750.

Wodtke, G. T., D. J. Harding, and F. Elwert. 2011. "Neighborhood effects in temporal perspective." *Am Sociol Rev* 76(5): 713–736. doi:10.1177/0003122411420816.

CHAPTER 8

Housing, Health, and Health Disparities

8.1. INTRODUCTION

Where we live is at the core of our daily lives. A home is a place of shelter, safety, security, and, for many people, being with family. Housing generally represents a family's greatest single expenditure, and for homeowners, it is often their major source of wealth. Given the centrality of home in people's lives, it is not surprising that factors related to housing have the potential to promote—or harm—health in major ways. This chapter examines the many ways in which housing can influence health and health disparities, focusing on four important and interrelated aspects of residential housing: physical conditions within homes; housing affordability; housing insecurity and homelessness; and, briefly, conditions in the neighborhoods surrounding homes. Housing and neighborhood conditions are strongly linked; discussion of neighborhoods is limited here, however, because Chapter 7 focuses on the role of neighborhoods in health and health disparities. This chapter also notes examples of general strategies for improving housing that appear worth considering in order to improve health and reduce health disparities.

8.2. HOW THE PHYSICAL CONDITIONS OF HOUSING AFFECT HEALTH

Most Americans spend approximately 90% of their time indoors, with an estimated two-thirds of that time spent in the home (Klepeis et al. 2001). Very young children spend even more time at home (Klepeis, Tsang, and Behar 1996) and are especially vulnerable to household hazards. Given the amount of time people generally spend at home, homes have a potentially strong influence on the health of their residents. When adequate housing protects individuals and families from harmful exposures and provides them with a sense of privacy, security, stability, and control, it can set a strong foundation for good health. In contrast, inadequate housing contributes to health problems throughout life, including infectious and chronic diseases, mental health problems, injuries, overall poor health, and diminished cognitive and developmental outcomes among children (Swope and Hernández 2019; Krieger and Higgins 2002; Dunn 2020; Singh et al. 2019;

The Social Determinants of Health and Health Disparities. Paula Braveman, Oxford University Press. © Oxford University Press 2023. DOI: 10.1093/oso/9780190624118.003.0008

Coley et al. 2013). Households with fewer financial resources are most likely to experience unhealthy and unsafe housing conditions; they also are least likely to have the resources needed to remedy these conditions, further contributing to disparities in health across socioeconomic groups (Swope and Hernández 2019). This section discusses several physical hazards in housing:

- *Lead poisoning.* Lead poisoning irreversibly affects brain and nervous system development and leads to lower intelligence, reading disabilities, and behavioral problems. It provides a good example of how housing-related disparities can affect health. In the United States, an estimated 535,000 children aged 1–5 years have elevated blood lead levels (Centers for Disease Control and Prevention 2013). Most lead exposures occur in the home, particularly in homes built before 1978 that often contain lead-based paint and lead in plumbing systems. Deteriorating paint in older homes is the primary source of lead exposure among children, who ingest paint chips and inhale lead-contaminated dust. A 2005–2006 survey of American homes estimated that 23 million homes—nearly one-fourth of the nation's housing—had one or more lead-based paint hazards; those hazards were found in 29% of low-income households compared with 18% of higher income households (U.S. Department of Housing and Urban Development 2011). Higher blood lead levels have been found among children in low-income households and neighborhoods; they are also more prevalent among children of color, whose families face constrained housing choices—across virtually all income levels—due to racial segregation and housing discrimination (Muller, Sampson, and Winter 2018; White, Bonilha, and Ellis 2016; Sampson and Winter 2016). In 2014, dangerous lead levels were discovered in the water supply of Flint, Michigan, attributed to cost-saving measures by city officials. Many believe that both the contamination and officials' inadequate initial response reflected systemic disregard for the welfare of Flint's largely Black population (Michigan Civil Rights Commission 2017; Mohai 2018). In the 18 months before the city took action, the incidence of elevated blood lead levels in young children doubled, with likely serious implications for affected children's long-term health and life trajectories (Hanna-Attisha et al. 2015).

- *Asthma and substandard housing.* Substandard housing conditions such as water leaks, poor ventilation, dirty carpets, and pest infestation can lead to increases in mold, mites, and other allergens; these conditions are concentrated in low-income households. Indoor allergens and damp housing conditions play an important role in the development and exacerbation of respiratory problems, including asthma (Kanchongkittiphon et al. 2014), which currently affects nearly 25 million Americans (Centers for Disease Control and Prevention 2019) and is the most common chronic disease among children. In 2010, the estimated cost of preventable hospitalizations for asthma was $1.9 billion (Torio, Elixhauser, and Andrews 2013). Approximately 40% of diagnosed asthma among children is believed to be attributable to residential exposures (Lanphear, Aligne, et al. 2001; Lanphear, Kahn, et al. 2001). Children in low-income families and Black and Puerto Rican children have higher rates of asthma compared with both higher income children and children in other racial groups (Zahran et al. 2018);

differential exposure to poor-quality housing is thought to be an important contributor to those racial disparities (Hughes et al. 2017).

- *Injuries at home.* Each year on average, in the United States, injuries occurring at home result in more than 30,000 deaths (Mack et al. 2013). In 2013, 3.5 million children were seen in emergency rooms for injuries commonly occurring in the home (Safe Kids Worldwide 2015). Housing-related contributing factors include structural features, such as steep staircases and balconies, and a lack of safety devices, such as window guards and smoke detectors (Gielen, McDonald, and Shields 2015).

- *Residential crowding.* Residential crowding has been linked both with physical illness, including infectious diseases such as tuberculosis and respiratory infections, and with psychological distress and other mental health problems (Shannon et al. 2018). Children who live in crowded housing may have poorer cognitive development and educational achievement; they may also experience greater social withdrawal, psychological distress, or aggression (Evans 2006; Solari and Mare 2012). Residential crowding is closely tied to housing affordability. Low-income families may need to "double-up" with other family members or friends to cope with high housing and other costs. A nationally representative study of families with young children in large U.S. cities found that nearly half of all children had lived in a doubled-up household at some point before age 9 years (Pilkauskas, Garfinkel, and McLanahan 2014). Residential crowding, which greatly increases the risks of viral transmission, is thought to be a major factor in the elevated rates of COVID-19 infection observed among Latino/Hispanic immigrants and incarcerated people (Chen and Krieger 2021).

- *Poor indoor air quality.* Residents can be exposed to carcinogenic air pollutants in their homes. Radon—a natural, radioactive gas released from the ground that has been linked with lung cancer—is found at elevated levels in an estimated 1 in 15 U.S. homes (U.S. Environmental Protection Agency 2018). Residential exposures to environmental tobacco smoke, volatile organic compounds, and asbestos have been linked with respiratory irritation or illness and some types of cancer (World Health Organization 2018; Jones 1999). Both racial and socioeconomic disparities in exposure to poor indoor air quality have been observed (Homa et al. 2015; Adamkiewicz et al. 2013).

- *Extremes in indoor temperatures.* Extremes in indoor temperatures can also be detrimental to health. Cold indoor conditions have been associated with poorer health, including an increased risk of cardiovascular and respiratory disease and mental health conditions (Marmot et al. 2011). Both extremely low

Multiple coexisting substandard housing conditions are common. Poor indoor air quality, lead paint, lack of home safety devices, and other housing hazards often coexist in homes, placing children and families at greater risk of multiple health problems. Families with fewer financial resources are generally likely to experience the most unhealthy and unsafe housing conditions, and financially least able to remedy them, contributing to disparities in health across socioeconomic groups (Swope and Hernández 2019).

and extremely high temperatures have been associated with increased mortality, especially among vulnerable populations such as the elderly (Institute of Medicine 2011). Exposure to both excessive heat and cold during pregnancy has been associated with preterm birth, with stronger evidence for heat (Zhang, Yu, and Wang 2017). Black people are less likely to have air conditioning at home and/or convenient access to air-conditioned public spaces than White people (Klein Rosenthal, Kinney, and Metzger 2014; Voelkel et al. 2018; O'Neill, Zanobetti, and Schwartz 2005). Low-income people are more likely to experience difficulty paying energy bills, with resulting shut-offs. (U.S. Energy Information Administration 2018). Residents of low-income and racially segregated neighborhoods are less likely to live in energy-efficient homes, which also contributes to disparities in exposure to unhealthy indoor temperatures (Hernández 2016; Reames 2016).

8.3. HOW HOUSING AFFORDABILITY CAN AFFECT HEALTH

The affordability of housing influences people's options for where they and their families live, with major implications for health. A shortage of affordable housing can relegate lower-income families to inadequate housing in poorer and resource-scarce neighborhoods. It also can increase the risks that they and their children will, at some point, experience housing insecurity or homelessness.

Housing is commonly considered to be "affordable" when a family spends 30% or less of its income to rent or buy a residence; a family that spends more than 30% of its income on housing is considered "housing-cost-burdened." In 2017, an estimated 37.8 million households in the United States spent more than 30% of their incomes on housing; 18.2 million of these households spent more than 50% of their incomes on housing, making them "severely housing-cost-burdened" (Joint Center for Housing Studies of Harvard University 2019). It is important to note that a given percentage of income can reflect very different burdens depending on a family's overall level of financial resources; for example, having 50% of a $200,000 annual income left to spend after paying for housing costs presents dramatically different options than having 50% of a $19,000 annual income. Not surprisingly, lower-income families are more likely to lack affordable housing (Figure 8.1).

Lack of access to affordable housing places many families under tremendous and constant financial strain, with potential health consequences; for example, the financial pressure of indebtedness has been associated with suicidal ideation, depression, poor subjective health, and adverse health-related behaviors (Turunen and Hiilamo 2014).

"A family with one full-time worker earning the minimum wage cannot afford the local fair-market rent for a two-bedroom apartment anywhere in the United States" (National Low Income Housing Coalition 2019, p. 2).

Spending more than 30% of one's income on housing has been associated with a number of poor health outcomes, including poor self-rated health (Pollack, Griffin, and Lynch 2010), hypertension (Pollack et al. 2010; Leung and Lau 2017), arthritis (Pollack et al. 2010),

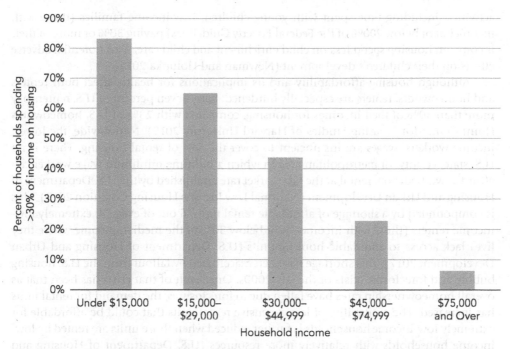

FIGURE 8.1 The percentage of American families of different income levels who spend more than 30% of their income on housing decreases dramatically as income increases. *Source:* 2017 American Community Survey tabulations from *The State of the Nation's Housing: 2019* (Joint Center for Housing Studies of Harvard University 2019).

and poor mental health (Bentley et al. 2011; Mason et al. 2013; Leung and Lau 2017; Singh et al. 2019).

The financial burden of unaffordable housing can prevent families, particularly low-income families, from meeting other basic needs. High housing-related costs often force low-income families to make trade-offs between shelter and food, heating, medical care, medicine, and other basic needs (Knowles et al. 2016; Hernández 2016). Compared with low-income families with affordable housing, low-income families experiencing severe housing-cost-burden spent 35% less on food and 74% less on health care in 2017 (Joint Center for Housing Studies of Harvard University 2019). High housing-cost-burden (Meltzer and Schwartz 2016) and frequent worry about (Stahre et al. 2015) or difficulty making housing payments (Kushel et al. 2006; Pollack et al. 2010; Sandel et al. 2018) have each been associated with postponing needed health care or failing to take prescribed medications. In a study of more than 20,000 low-income caregivers with children younger than age 3 years, household crowding and more than two moves in the past year—both indicators of lack of affordable housing—were associated with not being able to afford balanced and nutritious food and with skipping or reducing the size of meals due to cost (Cutts et al. 2011). People also make other kinds of trade-offs related to housing costs. To obtain affordable housing, many people live far away from their work, requiring them to spend more time and money commuting and less time engaging in health-promoting activities, including time spent with young children. Low-income families (those with incomes at or below 200% of the Federal Poverty Guidelines) paying 30% or more of their income on housing spend less on child enrichment and child care, with potential adverse effects on their children's development (Newman and Holupka 2014).

Although housing affordability and its implications for health affect both renters and homeowners, renters are especially burdened. Forty-seven percent of U.S. renters pay more than 30% of their incomes for housing, compared with 23% of U.S. homeowners (Joint Center for Housing Studies of Harvard University 2019). Nationwide, the lowest income workers' wages are insufficient to cover the cost of rental housing. There is no U.S. state, county, or metropolitan area in which a full-time minimum wage worker can afford a two-bedroom rental at the fair market rate established by the U.S. Department of Housing and Urban Development (National Low Income Housing Coalition 2019). This is compounded by a shortage of affordable rental units; 6 out of every 10 extremely low-income renters (those with incomes at or below 30% of the median income where they live) lack access to affordable housing units (U.S. Department of Housing and Urban Development 2017). This shortage has been exacerbated by fallout from the U.S. housing bubble and foreclosure crisis of the late 2000s. One result of that crisis has been that as overall homeownership rates have fallen due to foreclosures, the demand for rental units has increased. The availability of less expensive rental units that could be affordable for extremely low-income households is further reduced when those units are rented by low-income households with relatively more resources (U.S. Department of Housing and Urban Development 2017).

Homeownership is a major source of household wealth and stability that is out of reach for families at greater social and economic disadvantage, who are less likely to own their own homes. The Black–White gap in homeownership has persisted for decades, reflecting discriminatory policies and practices, described later in this chapter and in Chapter 5, that have led to gaps in household and intergenerational wealth, income, and marital status (Choi et al. 2019). The racial gap in homeownership has widened since the 2010 U.S. foreclosure crisis (Choi et al. 2019); even before then, homeowners of color were particularly likely to receive subprime loans and end up in foreclosure—even after controlling for creditworthiness and risk (Bayer, Ferreira, and Ross 2014; Bocian et al. 2011; Hall, Crowder, and Spring 2015). The experience of foreclosure alone has been linked with poor physical and mental health outcomes and declines in health care utilization (Downing 2016; Arcaya 2018). A decade later, the number of U.S. homeowners has begun to increase again, with home prices reaching near pre-crisis levels and increases in mortgage interest rates (Joint Center for Housing Studies of Harvard University 2019). These pressures may be pushing homeownership further out of reach for many, particularly in high-priced metro areas (Joint Center for Housing Studies of Harvard University 2019).

8.4. THE HEALTH IMPACTS OF HOUSING INSECURITY AND HOMELESSNESS

Housing insecurity is a multidimensional concept that reflects threats to an individual's or a family's secure, stable, and adequate housing (Frederick et al. 2014; Cox et al. 2019).

There is no one uniform definition of housing insecurity. When measuring housing security, researchers sometimes take into account both housing affordability, as measured by difficulty making housing payments or by extreme housing costs relative to income, and the physical adequacy and safety of housing and the surrounding neighborhoods. Housing instability—including frequent moves, doubling up with other families, and overcrowding—is a dimension of housing insecurity that has been associated with poor health outcomes (Frederick et al. 2014; Cox et al. 2019). Children may be especially vulnerable to the effects of family housing instability. Aspects of housing instability have been associated with caregiver reports of poorer child health (Cutts et al. 2011; Sandel et al. 2018; Busacker and Kasehagen 2012), concerns about child development (Sandel et al. 2018; Cutts et al. 2011), lower child weight-for-age (Cutts et al. 2011), and child food insecurity and foregone medical care (Sandel et al. 2018). Housing instability has also been linked with emotional, behavioral, and academic problems during childhood and with increased risk of teen pregnancy, early drug use, and depression during adolescence (Jelleyman and Spencer 2008; Cutuli et al. 2013; Ziol-Guest and McKenna 2014). Although many children experiencing housing instability display resilience in the face of this stressor, many do not (Cutuli et al. 2013), and the impacts of these health, developmental, and academic disadvantages in childhood can have longer term adverse consequences for health and well-being.

According to widely used definitions, if a family or individual loses their home and ends up in a shelter, on the street, or without a regular place to stay and is moving between the homes of friends/family, they are considered to be experiencing homelessness. The causes of homelessness can be complex and multidimensional. Unaffordable housing, low wages, and lack of employment opportunities are major drivers of homelessness. Other causes include lack of adequate safety nets for people facing acute financial crises and inadequate services and supports for people experiencing mental health or substance use problems, disability, family violence or abuse, or other childhood and adult trauma (Batterham 2019; Fazel, Geddes, and Kushel 2014). Communities throughout the United States conduct an annual single-night count of people staying in shelters, on the street, or in other places not suitable for human habitation; this "point-in-time" count is reported to Congress as one way to monitor U.S. homelessness. On a single night in 2019, nearly 568,000 people were experiencing homelessness in the United States, including 103,000 children younger than age 18 years living with family and approximately 35,000 unaccompanied youth younger than age 25 years (U.S. Department of Housing and Urban Development 2020). Approximately 96,000 people were chronically homeless, meaning they had either been homeless for at least 1 year or experienced at least four episodes of homelessness during the prior 3 years that, when combined, represented at least 1 year of homelessness. Nearly two-thirds of the people experiencing chronic homelessness were unsheltered, meaning they were staying outdoors or in other places such as vehicles or abandoned buildings not suitable for human habitation (U.S. Department of Housing and Urban Development 2020). African Americans have been considerably overrepresented in these point-in-time counts, accounting for 40% of all people experiencing homelessness and 52% of homeless families with children (U.S. Department of Housing and Urban Development 2020), despite being only approximately 13% of the population (U.S. Census Bureau 2020).

Although annual point-in-time counts offer a meaningful snapshot of American homelessness, they underestimate the extent of the problem because they do not include the millions of individuals and families who experience shorter episodes of homelessness at any other time during a year. Point-in-time counts may especially undercount homeless children, who are less likely to be living in shelters or on the streets and are more likely to be moving between the homes of family members and friends or staying in hotels or motels. One report using an expanded definition of homelessness (that included these kinds of unstable housing situations) estimated that 2.5 million American children younger than age 18 years—or 1 in every 30—had experienced homelessness at some time during 2013 (The National Center on Family Homelessness 2014).

Homelessness, especially when chronic, can have significantly detrimental impacts on health. The risk of death among homeless individuals is commonly reported to be two to five times the rate among same-aged housed individuals in the general population (Fazel et al. 2014). Homeless individuals are more likely to suffer from mental health and substance use disorders (Fazel et al. 2008), both of which are not only risk factors for but also exacerbated by homelessness (Fazel, Geddes, and Kushel 2014). Experiencing homelessness can also increase a person's exposure to other health-damaging conditions, including poor nutrition, infectious diseases, harsh living conditions, and victimization and unintentional injuries (Fazel et al. 2014). Among older homeless adults, these risks appear to accelerate by an estimated 10–15 years the onset of chronic diseases and age-related conditions that are typical in the general population (Fazel et al. 2014). Among children, homelessness has been linked with increased risks of infections, respiratory diseases, injuries, malnutrition, stunting, obesity, abuse, trauma, emotional distress, and developmental delays (American Academy of Pediatrics 2013). Homelessness in an infant's first year is associated with subsequent caregiver reports of fair or poor health and concerns about development (Cutts et al. 2018).

8.5. HOMES AND NEIGHBORHOODS AFFECT HEALTH

In addition to conditions in the home, conditions in the neighborhoods where homes are located may also have powerful effects on health (Duncan and Kawachi 2018). Although the connection between neighborhoods and health is examined in more depth in Chapter 7, neighborhood conditions are mentioned briefly here because they are so closely linked with housing conditions and are therefore an important aspect of how housing can affect health. Many—but not all—studies have observed that the social, physical, and economic characteristics of neighborhoods are associated with short- and long-term health quality and longevity, even after taking into account the characteristics of the individuals who live in them. From a methodologic perspective, fully disentangling individual and neighborhood effects on health is challenging. Despite these challenges, however, there is wide consensus that neighborhood characteristics can—but may not always—influence residents' health; for example, the health implications of living in a poor household may depend at least in part on whether that household is located in a more or less economically advantaged neighborhood.

> Residing in a disadvantaged neighborhood can limit opportunities to be healthy, regardless of a family's own level of resources.

A neighborhood's physical characteristics may promote health by providing places for children to play and for adults to exercise that are free from crime, violence, and pollution. Walkable neighborhoods with bike paths, green spaces, and convenient public transportation can promote physical activity (M. Smith et al. 2017; Ding et al. 2011). Social and economic conditions in neighborhoods may also influence residents' health through access to employment opportunities and public resources, including good schools and transportation. Neighborhoods with strong ties (social cohesion) and high levels of trust among residents may also promote health through a range of mechanisms (Kim, Subramanian, and Kawachi 2008; Almedom and Glandon 2008). All of these factors provide potential opportunities and resources for health.

Housing discrimination, a product of systemic racism, however, has limited the ability of many low-income and minority families to move to health-promoting neighborhoods. The concentration of substandard housing in less advantaged neighborhoods further compounds racial and ethnic as well as socioeconomic disparities in health. Neighborhood conditions can pose risks to health through exposures to air, ground, or water pollution; excessive noise; or violence, including violence by police. Research on the health effects of living in "food deserts"—that is, places without nearby full-service grocery stores—has yielded inconsistent results (Block, Seward, and James 2018; Cobb et al. 2015). Similarly, higher concentrations of fast-food outlets or liquor and convenience stores ("food swamps") have been associated with higher risks of obesity in some, but not all, studies (Block et al. 2018; Cobb et al. 2015). (The lack of consistent findings on the effects of food deserts and food swamps may reflect how causal relationships can be altered in different contexts and populations.) Higher density of liquor stores and convenience stores has been linked with smoking cigarettes and alcohol use (Finan et al. 2019; Pulakka et al. 2016; Brenner et al. 2015). Largely minority neighborhoods have been deliberately and systematically targeted by liquor and tobacco companies with more intensive billboard advertising and promoting, with content designed deliberately and specifically to appeal to young people of color (Lee et al. 2015; Martino et al. 2018).

8.6. HOUSING DISCRIMINATION AS A DETERMINANT OF HEALTH DISPARITIES

Historical and contemporary discriminatory policies and practices have, for a long time, constrained housing choices for people of color and low-income people in the United States, with implications for housing quality, affordability, security/stability, and home ownership—all of which influence health, as noted above. Swope and Hernández (2019) highlight these policies and practices in their diagram illustrating discrimination in housing as a determinant of health inequity (Figure 8.2). Some of these policies and practices are discussed below.

Many federal and local policies in the United States have contributed to persistent economic and racial residential segregation, with consequences for health disparities.

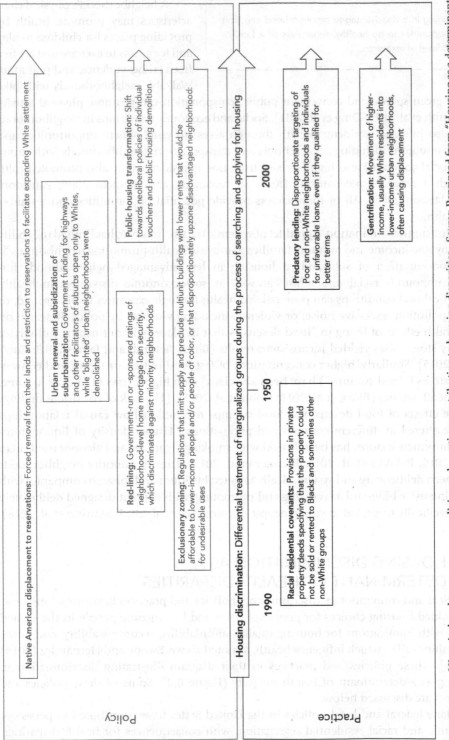

FIGURE 8.2 Historical and contemporary policies and practices contributing to housing disparities. *Source:* Reprinted from "Housing as a determinant of health equity: A conceptual model," Swope and Hermandez (2019), with permission from Elsevier.

The figure contains the following elements:

Policy

Native American displacement to reservations: Forced removal from their lands and restriction to reservations to facilitate expanding White settlement

Urban renewal and subsidization of suburbanization: Government funding for highways and other facilitators of suburbs open only to Whites, while 'blighted' urban neighborhoods were demolished

Red-lining: Government-run or -sponsored ratings of neighborhood-level home mortgage loan security, which discriminated against minority neighborhoods

Public housing transformation: Shift towards neoliberal policies of individual vouchers and public housing demolition

Exclusionary zoning: Regulations that limit supply and preclude multiunit buildings with lower rents that would be affordable to lower-income people and/or people of color, or that disproportionately upzone disadvantaged neighborhood.

Racial residential covenants: Provisions in private property deeds specifying that the property could not be sold or rented to Blacks and sometimes other non-White groups

Practice

Housing discrimination: Differential treatment of marginalized groups during the process of searching and applying for housing

Predatory lending: Disproportionate targeting of Poor and non-White neighborhoods and individuals for unfavorable loans, even if they qualified for better terms

Gentrification: Movement of higher-income, usually White residents into lower-income urban neighborhoods, often causing displacement

1990   1950   2000

In the 19th and early 20th centuries, American Indians were forcibly removed from their lands and restricted to living on reservations in poor-quality housing, on generally undesirable land, with severely limited economic opportunities. Beginning in the 1930s, guidelines established by the federal Home Owners' Loan Corporation (HOLC) and later adopted by private banks explicitly used neighborhood racial/ethnic composition and income level in determining the riskiness of mortgage lending (Swope and Hernández 2019). During decades when federal loan programs expanded homeownership among White people, particularly in the growing suburbs, non-White and low-income areas were disproportionately "red-lined." Red-lining refers to the red shading on HOLC maps of neighborhoods deemed "hazardous" for lending. Differences in homeownership, home values, and credit scores due to red-lining persist to the present day (Aaronson, Hartley, and Mazumder 2017; Mitchell and Franco 2018). In the 1950s, Black migration into cities increased, and White people increasingly moved to the suburbs. Federal funding for highways increased greatly to serve the suburban communities and often had destructive effects on urban Black communities. Black residents, concentrated in cities, were effectively locked out of suburban communities and prevented from accumulating wealth (see Chapter 2s). Other widespread discriminatory practices have also constrained housing choices for low-income people and people of color. In addition to discriminatory lending programs and policies, racial residential covenants, or agreements not to sell or rent property to people of color, were legally enforceable until the mid-20th century.(Boustan 2013)

In the late 1940s and 1950s, federally subsidized urban renewal programs in cities throughout the country cleared "blighted" neighborhoods, displacing low-income residents of color and turning these areas over for development by private investors or, later, for highway construction (Avila and Rose 2009). Conditions in public housing projects in cities began to deteriorate in the 1950s and 1960s due to stigmatization of poor tenants, declining political support, poor construction and management, and inadequate funding for maintenance (Hunt 2018). Cities that had built public housing saw White tenants leave as civil rights legislation banning segregation was enforced. Public housing projects in many cities thus predominantly housed Black families, who had fewer choices due to discrimination in both housing and employment (Hunt 2018). In the 1970s, some cities began to demolish public housing projects, often further stigmatizing and displacing residents. In both the 1970s and the 1980s, U.S. public housing policy shifted away from government-funded public housing projects toward housing voucher programs providing subsidies for families to rent in the private market or privately developed public housing (Vale and Freemark 2012) (Box 8.1).

Existing public housing and voucher programs fall far short of meeting the need for affordable public housing today. At the same time, families with subsidized housing vouchers face widespread discrimination in the private rental market (Cunningham et al. 2018). Some of that discrimination is structural rather than interpersonal. For example, some local land-use zoning practices, including limits on density, have tended to exclude low-income or minority households from wealthier and predominantly White areas (Lens and Monkkonen 2016). Conversely, zoning for commercial or industrial enterprises that would be unwanted in affluent White neighborhoods has often been concentrated in largely low-income or minority neighborhoods (Banzhaf, Ma, and

BOX 8.1   Seeking Healthier Alternatives to Traditional Public Housing

Two alternatives to high-density housing projects have been rigorously evaluated, with results showing that the issues are complex. Evidence from these initiatives indicates that simply moving low-income families to higher income neighborhoods may not improve health, without broader strategies.

Housing Subsidies to Low-Income Families Enabling Them to Rent in the Private Sector

Housing vouchers help individuals rent privately owned houses that meet certain criteria for quality standards and rent guidelines. Moving to Opportunity for Fair Housing Demonstration Program, a large, randomized controlled experiment in five cities, was designed to test long-term effects on well-being and health associated with moving from public housing in high-poverty areas to private-market housing in lower poverty neighborhoods. Although early findings suggested favorable outcomes for families, effects varied by the age and gender of participants; teenage boys experienced adverse outcomes, including more delinquent and risky behaviors (Kling, Liebman, and Katz 2007; Orr et al. 2003; Osypuk, Schmidt, et al. 2012; Osypuk, Tchetgen, et al. 2012; Sanbonmatsu et al. 2011), which could be due to the stresses of moving and specifically of moving to areas where most peers were better off. Results of longer term follow-up were more reassuring, with favorable results among adults and among boys as well as girls, particularly those who had moved before age 13 years (Chetty, Hendren, and Katz 2016).

Replacing Traditional Public Housing with More Health-Promoting Designs

Since its creation in 1992, the HOPE VI program has invested $6.3 billion to demolish, reconfigure, or replace the nation's worst housing projects. As of June 2006, more than 78,000 units had been demolished and another 10,400 were slated for redevelopment. The health evaluations of this program did not include randomization or control groups, as Moving to Opportunity had done. However, housing development residents who relocated generally moved to lower poverty and safer neighborhoods and reported less fear and anxiety for their own and their children's safety. Following their moves, children in relocated families had fewer reported behavior problems, and this effect was strongest among girls. Despite evidence of improved living conditions among program participants who relocated, there have been no conclusive findings of corresponding improvements in health; rates of mortality appeared higher among some relocated participants relative to other vulnerable populations (Manjarrez, Popkin, and Guernsey 2007; Lindberg et al. 2010; Popkin, Levy, and Buron 2009). Many initiatives have focused on developing mixed-income housing, and some may assist eligible households in buying homes; however, the potential health effects have not been adequately evaluated.

Timmins 2019). Factors such as these have contributed to and reinforced racial and economic segregation in housing, with adverse impacts on property values and wealth accumulation, and health-harming environmental exposures for many low-income people, particularly people of color (Swope and Hernández 2019).

Although illegal since the Fair Housing Act of 1968, housing discrimination on an individual level remains a common practice (Oh and Yinger 2015; Cunningham et al. 2018). To test for the presence and sources of housing discrimination, paired housing audits have been conducted throughout the United States. Findings from these experiments, in which trained auditors with different racial backgrounds present nearly identical qualifications (e.g., education, income, and employment) to landlords and real estate agents, have consistently documented discriminatory treatment of Black people and other people of color seeking housing (Oh and Yinger 2015). Despite declines over recent decades in some of the most blatant racially discriminatory practices—such as refusing to meet with a home-seeker or to provide information about available housing—landlords and real estate agents recommend and show fewer available apartments and homes to Black, Latino/Hispanic, and Asian people compared with White people with equal qualifications (Turner et al. 2013; Oh and Yinger 2015). Discriminatory practices such as these make it more difficult and time-consuming for people of color to secure housing.

Predatory mortgage lending continues to disadvantage homebuyers of color. As noted previously, during the U.S. housing bubble of the late 2000s, borrowers of color were more likely to receive high-cost, subprime mortgage loans even when controlling for common indicators of creditworthiness and risk (Bayer et al. 2014). This resulted in much higher foreclosure rates in predominantly Black, Latino, or racially integrated neighborhoods (Bocian et al. 2011; Hall et al. 2015); it may have contributed to a slowing of prior progress in narrowing racial inequities in wealth, homeownership, and residential segregation (Hall et al. 2015; Goodman and Mayer 2018). Gentrification, or the movement of capital and higher income people into neighborhoods that have historically experienced poverty and disinvestment (N. Smith 1979; Izenberg, Mujahid, and Yen 2018), often displaces residents in segregated and poor neighborhoods as housing costs rise. The resulting changes in neighborhood conditions—and their differential impacts on residents' health—further reinforce socioeconomic and health inequalities along racial lines (Izenberg et al. 2018).

8.7. EXAMPLES OF INITIATIVES WORTH CONSIDERING TO IMPROVE HEALTH AND REDUCE HEALTH DISPARITIES BY IMPROVING HOUSING

The research reviewed in this chapter indicates that health and health equity could be improved in important ways through actions that target housing-related issues, particularly for low-income people. History has demonstrated the importance of addressing issues such as fire hazards, lead, sanitation, ventilation, mold, and crowding to reduce injuries and certain infectious diseases. Now, in light of the growing body of evidence about the many additional ways that housing can affect health, it is clear that strategies must be multifaceted. Increasing affordable housing is crucial. Strategies also must focus not only on improving the physical quality of housing but also on strengthening health-promoting social as well as physical conditions in neighborhoods. Experience has shown that for some homeless people, housing is needed that is "supportive"—that is, accompanied by a range of mental health and other social services; for many homeless people, however, affordability is the crucial issue (Elder and King 2019).

It is beyond the scope of this chapter to assess which strategies merit highest priority, particularly given a widespread lack of sufficient information from rigorous studies of health impact. Although we lack definitive information on the health impact of many housing interventions, we know enough now to develop and test a range of promising approaches. The non-exhaustive list below includes a number of general approaches that have received serious consideration by experts and public agencies and/or that appear worth considering based on current knowledge. Many of the strategies are relevant to more than one category.

Improving physical conditions in homes:

- Programs providing low-income households with free environmental health assessments, tenant and landlord education, and assistance in correcting hazards (e.g., lead, injury prevention, fire hazards, excess moisture/mold, dust and other allergens, ventilation, and toxins). Because housing hazards often coexist, it may be more efficient for programs to address all the major home hazards together rather than the typical approach targeting one hazard at a time through separate programs.

- Improving and enforcing federal, state, and local housing codes and guidelines to reflect current knowledge regarding hazards within the home environment (World Health Organization 2018; Krieger and Higgins 2002).
- National, state, and local public campaigns and programs to inform and motivate private- and public-sector housing tenants, managers/providers, and owners about the dangers of unsafe and unhealthy housing and about their rights and responsibilities.
- Increasing resources and expanding the role of public health agencies in housing education, inspections, and enforcements at the local, state, and national levels (Krieger and Higgins 2002).
- Public and private initiatives to encourage viable "green" building in residential construction and federal affordable housing programs by setting standards; providing resources to help with costs of implementation; providing incentives to private developers and builders to help meet sustainable goals; and developing supportive financing mechanisms such as "on-bill utility financing," in which the cost of "green" upgrades is absorbed by the utility (and may be later repaid in installments on the utility bill) (Howell, Mueller, and Wilson 2019).

Efforts to improve housing affordability:

- Constructing and adequately maintaining affordable housing for low-income households (below 200% of the Federal Poverty Guidelines) and for lower-middle-income households (200–300% of Federal Poverty Guidelines)
- Rent control, particularly in high-cost areas
- Targeted rent subsidies for low- and lower-middle-income households in high-cost areas
- Raising the minimum wage to a level that would enable households to afford rental housing in the same city/town where they work
- Changing zoning ordinances to permit new construction or conversion of existing structures into affordable multi-unit housing in a wider range of locations
- Expansion of the Earned Income Tax Credit, which would make more low- and middle-income households able to afford housing

Critical elements for eliminating homelessness:

- Because lack of affordable housing is the crucial issue for many homeless people, see above examples of improving affordability, including adequate minimum wage/income support.
- Mental health services (Stergiopoulos et al. 2019).
- "Supportive housing," including on-site mental health and other social services, often funded by Medicaid; social services should include employment assistance.
- The Housing First model provides homeless people with housing without requiring sobriety as a precondition; once housed, participants are provided a

range of mental health and social services, including services focused on lessening substance abuse. Outcomes have been favorable (Woodhall-Melnik and Dunn 2016; Elder and King 2019).

Making neighborhoods healthier includes the following:

- Developing healthier alternatives to traditional public housing, which historically has tended to create pockets of concentrated poverty with its associated disadvantages, including substandard schools and low opportunity for employment or starting a business. Alternatives include vouchers (subsidies) to move to less disadvantaged neighborhoods. Studies of the effectiveness of vouchers permitting public housing residents to move to private housing have observed mixed results; however, the longest term comprehensive assessment of outcomes of this approach for children produced generally favorable results (Chetty et al. 2016). Another option is to redesign existing public housing and its surroundings to make it more health-promoting; this would have the advantage of not leaving many people (those who did not receive vouchers enabling them to move) behind in unhealthy neighborhood contexts.

Directly addressing racial discrimination in housing:

- Strengthening monitoring and enforcement of fair housing laws, including the Federal Fair Housing Act of 1968 and other state and local regulations prohibiting racial discrimination in housing markets (National Fair Housing Alliance 2018)
- Strengthening monitoring and enforcement of laws prohibiting racial discrimination in bank lending for mortgages
- Continuing federal involvement in setting lending and fairness standards for banking and loan institutions
- Improving banking and lending procedures of the private sector to create equal opportunities for credit

General considerations in strategies to improve health and reduce health disparities through housing interventions:

- Increasing collaboration across government agencies at all levels and between stakeholders from community groups, public health agencies, and private groups (e.g., employers) to ensure a coordinated approach to housing as a determinant of health and health disparities (Elder and King 2019; Krieger and Higgins 2002).
- Rigorous research evaluating health outcomes of housing interventions. Because many relevant outcomes manifest only after decades of exposure, the health outcomes evaluated will often be intermediate outcomes (e.g., physiologic markers of risk for adverse outcomes later in life or health behaviors).

8.8. KEY POINTS

- Housing can influence health in many ways, including exposure to toxins, other physical hazards, and crowding; and effects of lack of affordability and consequent instability (e.g., stress and inability to pay for food, housing, medical care, heat, or other necessities).

- Differential exposure to substandard housing is a major cause of racial disparities in asthma, the most common chronic disease in children.
- Housing is considered unaffordable when its cost represents 30% or more of household income. High housing costs can lead families to make potentially health-harming trade-offs, such as being unable to purchase adequate food, heat, or needed medical care and medications.
- Unaffordable housing is a major cause of homelessness. Lack of adequate social, economic, and mental health safety nets feature prominently as well.
- In addition to homelessness, lack of housing security (also called residential instability) is associated with emotional, behavioral, and school problems in children and with teen pregnancy, early drug use, and depression in adolescence.
- Racial discrimination in mortgage lending has excluded many people of color from homeownership and therefore the opportunity to accumulate wealth. Although racial discrimination in housing has been illegal since 1964, evidence indicates this bias persists, although to a lesser degree than before 1964.

8.9. QUESTIONS FOR DISCUSSION

1. How can physical conditions in homes and housing affordability affect health? Give specific examples.
2. How has housing discrimination—both legal and illegal—contributed to large racial disparities in home ownership and home values, which represent the major source of wealth for most U.S. households? Give examples of recent/contemporary as well as historical discrimination.
3. What are potential solutions for homelessness?
4. What are some advantages and disadvantages of providing housing subsidies or vouchers enabling low-income households to seek private or public housing elsewhere versus building more (and improving) public housing in disadvantaged communities?

ACKNOWLEDGMENTS

This chapter builds on material from the following source:
Braveman, P., M. Dekker, S. Egerter, T. Sadegh-Nobari, and C. Pollack. 2011. *Housing and Health*. Princeton, NJ: Robert Wood Johnson Foundation.
Miranda Brillante also made substantive contributions to this chapter.

REFERENCES

Aaronson, D., D. Hartley, and B. Mazumder. 2017. "The effects of the 1930s HOLC 'redlining' maps." Working Paper No. 2017-12. Chicago, IL: Federal Reserve Bank of Chicago.

Adamkiewicz, G., J. D. Spengler, A. E. Harley, A. Stoddard, M. Yang, M. Alvarez-Reeves, and G. Sorensen. 2013. "Environmental conditions in low-income urban housing: Clustering and associations with self-reported health." *Am J Public Health* 104(9): 1650–1656. doi:10.2105/AJPH.2013.301253.

Almedom, A. M., and D. Glandon. 2008. "Social capital and mental health." In *Social Capital and Health*, edited by I. Kawachi, S. V. Subramanian, and D. Kim, 191–214. New York, NY: Springer.

American Academy of Pediatrics. 2013. "Providing care for children and adolescents facing homelessness and housing insecurity." *Pediatrics* 131(6): 1206. doi:10.1542/peds.2013-0645.

Arcaya, M. 2018. "Neighborhood foreclosure and health." In *Neighborhoods and health*, edited by D. T. Duncan and I. Kawachi, 293–319. New York, NY: Oxford University Press.

Avila, E., and M. H. Rose. 2009. "Race, culture, politics, and urban renewal: An introduction." *Journal of Urban History* 35(3): 335–347. doi:10.1177/0096144208330393.

Banzhaf, H. S., L. Ma, and C. Timmins. 2019. "Environmental justice: Establishing causal relationships." *Annu Rev Resour Econ* 11(1): 377–398. doi:10.1146/annurev-resource-100518-094131.

Batterham, D. 2019. "Defining 'at-risk of homelessness': Re-connecting causes, mechanisms and risk." *Housing, Theory Society* 36(1): 1–24.

Bayer, P., F. Ferreira, and S. L. Ross. 2014. "Race, ethnicity and high-cost mortgage lending." National Bureau of Economic Research. https://www.nber.org/system/files/working_papers/w20762/w20762.pdf

Bentley, R., E. Baker, K. Mason, S. V. Subramanian, and A. M. Kavanagh. 2011. "Association between housing affordability and mental health: A longitudinal analysis of a nationally representative household survey in Australia." *Am J Epidemiol* 174(7): 753–760. doi:10.1093/aje/kwr161.

Block, J., M. Seward, and P. James. 2018. "Food environment and health." In *Neighborhoods and health*, edited by D. T. Duncan and I. Kawachi, 247–277. New York, NY: Oxford University Press.

Bocian, D. G., W. Li, C. Reid, and R. G. Quercia. 2011. "Lost ground, 2011: Disparities in mortgage lending and foreclosures." Center for Responsible Lending. https://www.respons iblelending.org/mortgage-lending/research-analysis/Lost-Ground-2011.pdf

Boustan, L. P. 2013. "Racial residential segregation in American cities." National Bureau of Economic Research. https://www.nber.org/system/files/working_papers/w19045/w19045.pdf

Brenner, A. B., L. N. Borrell, T. Barrientos-Gutierrez, and A. V. Diez Roux. 2015. "Longitudinal associations of neighborhood socioeconomic characteristics and alcohol availability on drinking: Results from the Multi-Ethnic Study of Atherosclerosis (MESA)." *Soc Sci Med* 145: 17–25. doi:10.1016/j.socscimed.2015.09.030.

Busacker, A., and L. Kasehagen. 2012. "Association of residential mobility with child health: An analysis of the 2007 National Survey of Children's Health." *Matern Child Health J* 16(1): 78–87. doi:10.1007/s10995-012-0997-8.

Centers for Disease Control and Prevention. 2013. "Blood lead levels in children aged 1–5 years—United States, 1999–2010." *MMWR Morb Mortal Wkly Rep* 62(13): 245–248.

Centers for Disease Control and Prevention. 2019. "Current asthma population estimates—in thousands by age, United States: National Health Interview Survey, 2018." https://www.cdc.gov/asthma/nhis/2018/table3-1.htm.

Chen, J. T., and N. Krieger. 2021. "Revealing the unequal burden of COVID-19 by income, race/ethnicity, and household crowding: US county versus zip code analyses." *J Public Health Manag Pract* 27(Suppl 1): S43–S56. doi:10.1097/phh.0000000000001263.

Chetty, R., N. Hendren, and L. F. Katz. 2016. "The effects of exposure to better neighborhoods on children: New evidence from the Moving to Opportunity experiment." *Am Econ Rev* 106(4): 855–902.

Choi, J. H., A. McCargo, M. Neal, L. Goodman, and C. Young. 2019. *Explaining the Black–White homeownership gap*. Washington, DC: Urban Institute.

Cobb, L. K., L. J. Appel, M. Franco, J. C. Jones-Smith, A. Nur, and C. A. M. Anderson. 2015. "The relationship of the local food environment with obesity: A systematic review of methods, study quality, and results." *Obesity* 23(7): 1331–1344.

Coley, R. L., T. Leventhal, A. D. Lynch, and M. Kull. 2013. "Relations between housing characteristics and the well-being of low-income children and adolescents." *Dev Psychol* 49(9): 1775.

Cox, R., B. Henwood, S. Rodnyansky, E. Rice, and S. Wenzel. 2019. "Road map to a unified measure of housing insecurity." *Cityscape* 21(2): 93–128.

Cunningham, M., M. M. Galvez, C. L. Aranda, R. Santos, D. A. Wissoker, A. D. Oneto, R. Pitingolo, and J. Crawford. 2018. *A pilot study of landlord acceptance of Housing Choice Vouchers.* Washington, DC: Urban Institute.

Cutts, D. B., A. Bovell-Ammon, S. Ettinger de Cuba, R. Sheward, M. Shaefer, C. Huang, M. M. Black, et al. 2018. "Homelessness during infancy: Associations with infant and maternal health and hardship outcomes." *Cityscape* 20(2): 119–132.

Cutts, D. B., A. F. Meyers, M. M. Black, P. H. Casey, M. Chilton, J. T. Cook, J. Geppert, et al. 2011. "US housing insecurity and the health of very young children." *Am J Public Health* 101(8): 1508–1514. doi:10.2105/AJPH.2011.300139.

Cutuli, J. J., C. D. Desjardins, J. E. Herbers, J. D. Long, D. Heistad, C.-K. Chan, E. Hinz, and A. S. Masten. 2013. "Academic achievement trajectories of homeless and highly mobile students: Resilience in the context of chronic and acute risk." *Child Dev* 84(3): 841–857. doi:10.1111/cdev.12013.

Ding, D., J. F. Sallis, J. Kerr, S. Lee, and D. E. Rosenberg. 2011. "Neighborhood environment and physical activity among youth: A review." *Am J Prev Med* 41(4): 442–455. https://doi.org/10.1016/j.amepre.2011.06.036.

Downing, J. 2016. "The health effects of the foreclosure crisis and unaffordable housing: A systematic review and explanation of evidence." *Soc Sci Med* 162: 88–96.

Duncan, D. T., and I. Kawachi (Eds.). 2018. *Neighborhoods and Health.* Oxford University Press Oxford, UK.

Dunn, J. R. 2020. "Housing and healthy child development: Known and potential impacts of interventions." *Annu Rev Public Health* 41: 381–396. doi:10.1146/annurev-publhealth-040119-094050.

Elder, J., and B. King. 2019. "Housing and homelessness as a public health issue: Executive summary of policy adopted by the American Public Health Association." *Med Care* 57(6): 401–405. doi:10.1097/mlr.0000000000001115.

Evans, G. W. 2006. "Child development and the physical environment." *Annu Rev Psychol* 57: 423–451.

Fazel, S., J. R. Geddes, and M. Kushel. 2014. "The health of homeless people in high-income countries: Descriptive epidemiology, health consequences, and clinical and policy recommendations." *Lancet* 384(9953): 1529–1540.

Fazel, S., V. Khosla, H. Doll, and J. Geddes. 2008. "The prevalence of mental disorders among the homeless in Western countries: Systematic review and meta-regression analysis." *PLoS Med* 5(12): e225–e225. doi:10.1371/journal.pmed.0050225.

Finan, L. J., S. Lipperman-Kreda, M. Abadi, J. W. Grube, E. Kaner, A. Balassone, and A. Gaidus. 2019. "Tobacco outlet density and adolescents' cigarette smoking: a meta-analysis." *Tob Control* 28(1): 27–33. doi:10.1136/tobaccocontrol-2017-054065.

Frederick, T. J., M. Chwalek, J. Hughes, J. Karabanow, and S. Kidd. 2014. "How stable is stable? Defining and measuring housing stability." *J Community Psychol* 42(8): 964–979. doi:10.1002/jcop.21665.

Gielen, A. C., E. M. McDonald, and W. Shields. 2015. "Unintentional home injuries across the life span: Problems and solutions." *Annu Rev Public Health* 36(1): 231–253. doi:10.1146/annurev-publhealth-031914-122722.

Goodman, L. S., and C. Mayer. 2018. "Homeownership and the American dream." *J Econ Perspect* 32(1): 31–58.

Hall, M., K. Crowder, and A. Spring. 2015. "Neighborhood foreclosures, racial/ethnic transitions, and residential segregation." *Am Sociol Rev* 80(3): 526–549. doi:10.1177/0003122415581334.

Hanna-Attisha, M., J. LaChance, R. C. Sadler, and A. C. Schnepp. 2015. "Elevated blood lead levels in children associated with the Flint drinking water crisis: A spatial analysis of risk and public health response." *Am J Public Health* 106(2): 283–290. doi:10.2105/AJPH.2015.303003.

Hernández, D. 2016. "Understanding 'energy insecurity' and why it matters to health." *Soc Sci Med* 167: 1–10.

Homa, D. M., L. J. Neff, B. A. King, R. S. Caraballo, R. E. Bunnell, S. D. Babb, B. E. Garrett, C. S. Sosnoff, and L. Wang. 2015. "Vital signs: Disparities in nonsmokers' exposure to secondhand smoke—United States, 1999–2012." *MMWR Morb Mortal Wkly Rep* 64(4): 103.

Howell, K. L., E. J. Mueller, and B. Brown Wilson. 2019. "One size fits none: Local context and planning for the preservation of affordable housing." *Housing Policy Debate* 29(1): 148–165. doi:10.1080/10511482.2018.1476896.

Hughes, H. K., E. C. Matsui, M. M. Tschudy, C. E. Pollack, and C. A. Keet. 2017. "Pediatric asthma health disparities: Race, hardship, housing, and asthma in a national survey." *Acad Pediatr* 17(2): 127–134. https://doi.org/10.1016/j.acap.2016.11.011.

Hunt, D. B. 2018. "Public housing in urban America." In Oxford Research Encyclopedia of American History. New York, NY: Oxford University Press. https://oxfordre.com/americanhistory/view/10.1093/acrefore/9780199329175.001.0001/acrefore-9780199329175-e-61.

Institute of Medicine. 2011. *Climate Change, the Indoor Environment, and Health*. Washington, DC: Institute of Medicine.

Izenberg, J. M., M. S. Mujahid, and I. H. Yen. 2018. "Health in changing neighborhoods: A study of the relationship between gentrification and self-rated health in the state of California." *Health Place* 52: 188–195. https://doi.org/10.1016/j.healthplace.2018.06.002.

Jelleyman, T., and N. Spencer. 2008. "Residential mobility in childhood and health outcomes: A systematic review." *J Epidemiol Community Health* 62(7): 584. doi:10.1136/jech.2007.060103.

Joint Center for Housing Studies of Harvard University. 2019. *The State of the Nation's Housing: 2019*. Cambridge, MA: Joint Center for Housing Studies of Harvard University.

Jones, A. P. 1999. "Indoor air quality and health." *Atmospheric Environ* 33(28): 4535–4564. https://doi.org/10.1016/S1352-2310(99)00272-1.

Kanchongkittiphon, W., M. J. Mendell, J. M. Gaffin, G. Wang, and W. Phipatanakul. 2014. "Indoor environmental exposures and exacerbation of asthma: An update to the 2000 review by the Institute of Medicine." *Environ Health Perspect* 123(1): 6–20.

Kim, D., S. V. Subramanian, and I. Kawachi. 2008. "Social capital and physical health." In *Social Capital and Health*, edited by I. Kawachi, S. V. Subramanian, and D. Kim, 139–190. New York, NY: Springer.

Klein Rosenthal, J., P. L. Kinney, and K. B. Metzger. 2014. "Intra-urban vulnerability to heat-related mortality in New York City, 1997–2006." *Health Place* 30: 45–60. https://doi.org/10.1016/j.healthplace.2014.07.014.

Klepeis, N. E., W. C. Nelson, W. R. Ott, J. P. Robinson, A. M. Tsang, P. Switzer, J. V. Behar, S. C. Hern, and W. H. Engelmann. 2001. "The National Human Activity Pattern Survey (NHAPS): A resource for assessing exposure to environmental pollutants." *J Exposure Sci Environ Epidemiol* 11(3): 231–252.

Klepeis, N. E., A. M. Tsang, and J. V. Behar. 1996. "Analysis of the National Human Activity Pattern Survey (NHAPS) respondents from a standpoint of exposure assessment." Washington, DC: U.S. Environmental Protection Agency.

Kling, J. R., J. B. Liebman, and L. F. Katz. 2007. "Experimental analysis of neighborhood effects." *Econometrica* 75(1): 83–119.

Knowles, M., J. Rabinowich, S. Ettinger de Cuba, D. B. Cutts, and M. Chilton. 2016. "'Do you wanna breathe or eat?' Parent perspectives on child health consequences of food insecurity, trade-offs, and toxic stress." *Matern Child Health J* 20(1): 25–32. doi:10.1007/s10995-015-1797-8.

Krieger, J., and D. L Higgins. 2002. "Housing and health: Time again for public health action." *Am J Public Health* 92(5): 758–768.

Kushel, M. B., R. Gupta, L. Gee, and J. S. Haas. 2006. "Housing instability and food insecurity as barriers to health care among low-income Americans." *J Gen Intern Med* 21(1): 71–77. doi:10.1111/j.1525-1497.2005.00278.x.

Lanphear, B. P., C. A. Aligne, P. Auinger, M. Weitzman, and R. S. Byrd. 2001. "Residential exposures associated with asthma in US children." *Pediatrics* 107(3): 505–511.

Lanphear, B. P., R. S. Kahn, O. Berger, P. Auinger, S. M. Bortnick, and R. W. Nahhas. 2001. "Contribution of residential exposures to asthma in US children and adolescents." *Pediatrics* 107(6): e98.

Lee, J. G., L. Henriksen, S. W. Rose, S. Moreland-Russell, and K. M. Ribisl. 2015. "A systematic review of neighborhood disparities in point-of-sale tobacco marketing." *Am J Public Health* 105(9): e8–e18. doi:10.2105/AJPH.2015.302777.

Lens, M. C., and P. Monkkonen. 2016. "Do strict land use regulations make metropolitan areas more segregated by income?" *J Am Planning Assoc* 82(1): 6–21. doi:10.1080/01944363.2015.1111163.

Leung, L. A., and C. Lau. 2017. "Effect of mortgage indebtedness on health of U.S. homeowners." *Rev Econ Household* 15(1): 239–264. doi:10.1007/s11150-014-9250-0.

Lindberg, R. A., E. D. Shenassa, D. Acevedo-Garcia, S. J. Popkin, A. Villaveces, and R. L. Morley. 2010. "Housing interventions at the neighborhood level and health: A review of the evidence." *J Public Health Manag Pract* 16(5): S44–S52.

Mack, K. A., R. A. Rudd, A. D. Mickalide, and M. F. Ballesteros. 2013. "Fatal unintentional injuries in the home in the U.S., 2000–2008." *Am J Prev Med* 44(3): 239–246. doi:10.1016/j.amepre.2012.10.022.

Manjarrez, C. A., S. J. Popkin, and E. Guernsey. 2007. *Poor Health: Adding Insult to Injury for HOPE VI Families*. Washington, DC: Urban Institute.

Marmot, M., I. Geddes, E. Bloomer, J. Allen, and P. Goldblatt. 2011. "The health impacts of cold homes and fuel poverty." London, UK: Friends of the Earth & the Marmot Review Team.

Martino, S., R. L. Collins, S. A. Kovalchik, C. M. Setodji, E. J. D'Amico, K. Becker, W. G. Shadel, and A. A. Tolpadi. 2018. "Drinking it in: The impact of youth exposure to alcohol advertising." RAND Corporation. https://www.rand.org/pubs/research_briefs/RB10015.html

Mason, K. E., E. Baker, T. Blakely, and R. J. Bentley. 2013. "Housing affordability and mental health: Does the relationship differ for renters and home purchasers?" *Soc Sci Med* 94: 91–97. https://doi.org/10.1016/j.socscimed.2013.06.023.

Meltzer, R., and A. Schwartz. 2016. "Housing affordability and health: Evidence from New York City." *Housing Policy Debate* 26(1): 80–104. doi:10.1080/10511482.2015.1020321.

Michigan Civil Rights Commission. 2017. *The Flint Water Crisis: Systemic Racism Through the Lens of Flint*. Lansing, MI: Michigan Civil Rights Commission.

Mitchell, B., and J. Franco. 2018. "HOLC 'redlining' maps: The persistent structure of segregation and economic inequality." National Community Reinvestment Coalition. https://ncrc.org/holc.

Mohai, P. 2018. "Environmental justice and the Flint water crisis." *Michigan Sociol Rev* 32: 1–41.

Muller, C., R. J. Sampson, and A. S. Winter. 2018. "Environmental inequality: The social causes and consequences of lead exposure." *Annu Rev Sociol* 44(1): 263–282. doi:10.1146/annurev-soc-073117-041222.

National Fair Housing Alliance. 2018. *Making Every Neighborhood a Place of Opportunity: 2018 Fair Housing Trends Report*. Washington, DC: National Fair Housing Alliance.

National Low Income Housing Coalition. 2019. "Out of reach report." Washington, DC: National Low Income Housing Coalition.

Newman, S. J., and C. Scott Holupka. 2014. "Housing affordability and investments in children." *J Housing Econ* 24: 89–100. https://doi.org/10.1016/j.jhe.2013.11.006.

Oh, S. J., and J. Yinger. 2015. "What have we learned from paired testing in housing markets?" *Cityscape* 17(3): 15–60.

O'Neill, M. S., A. Zanobetti, and J. Schwartz. 2005. "Disparities by race in heat-related mortality in four US cities: The role of air conditioning prevalence." *J Urban Health* 82(2): 191–197. doi:10.1093/jurban/jti043.

Orr, L., J. Feins, R. Jacob, E. Beecroft, L. Sanbonmatsu, L. F. Katz, J. B. Liebman, and J. R. Kling. 2003. "Moving to opportunity: Interim impacts evaluation." Washington, DC: U.S. Department of Housing and Urban Development.

Osypuk, T. L., N. M. Schmidt, L. M. Bates, E. J. Tchetgen-Tchetgen, F. J. Earls, and M. M.

Glymour. 2012. "Gender and crime victimization modify neighborhood effects on adolescent mental health." *Pediatrics* 130(3): 472–481.

Osypuk, T. L., E. J. Tchetgen Tchetgen, D. Acevedo-Garcia, F. J. Earls, A. Lincoln, N. M. Schmidt, and M. M. Glymour. 2012. "Differential mental health effects of neighborhood relocation among youth in vulnerable families: Results from a randomized trial." *Arch Gen Psychiatry* 69(12): 1284–1294.

Pilkauskas, N. V., I. Garfinkel, and S. S. McLanahan. 2014. "The prevalence and economic value of doubling up." *Demography* 51(5): 1667–1676. doi:10.1007/s13524-014-0327-4.

Pollack, C. E., B. A. Griffin, and J. Lynch. 2010. "Housing affordability and health among homeowners and renters." *Am J Prev Med* 39(6): 515–521. https://doi.org/10.1016/j.amepre.2010.08.002.

Popkin, S. J., D. K. Levy, and L. Buron. 2009. "Has Hope VI transformed residents' lives? New evidence from the Hope VI Panel Study." *Housing Stud* 24(4): 477–502. doi:10.1080/02673030902938371.

Pulakka, A., J. I. Halonen, I. Kawachi, J. Pentti, S. Stenholm, M. Jokela, I. Kaate, M. Koskenvuo, J. Vahtera, and M. Kivimaki. 2016. "Association between distance from home to tobacco outlet and smoking cessation and relapse." *JAMA Intern Med* 176(10): 1512–1519. doi:10.1001/jamainternmed.2016.4535.

Reames, T. G. 2016. "Targeting energy justice: Exploring spatial, racial/ethnic and socioeconomic disparities in urban residential heating energy efficiency." *Energy Policy* 97: 549–558. https://doi.org/10.1016/j.enpol.2016.07.048.

Safe Kids Worldwide. 2015. *Report to the Nation: Protecting Children in Your Home.* Washington, DC: Safe Kids Worldwide.

Sampson, R. J., and A. S. Winter. 2016. "The racial ecology of lead poisoning: Toxic inequality in Chicago neighborhoods, 1995–2013." *Du Bois Rev* 13(2): 261–283. doi:10.1017/S1742058X16000151.

Sanbonmatsu, L., J. Ludwig, L. F. Katz, L. A. Gennetian, G. J. Duncan, R. C. Kessler, E. Adam, T. W. McDade, and S. T. Lindau. 2011. "Moving to Opportunity for Fair Housing Demonstration Program—Final impacts evaluation." Washington, DC: U.S. Department of Housing & Urban Development.

Sandel, M., R. Sheward, S. Ettinger de Cuba, S. M. Coleman, D. A. Frank, M. Chilton, M. Black, et al. 2018. "Unstable housing and caregiver and child health in renter families." *Pediatrics* 141(2): e20172199. doi:10.1542/peds.2017-2199.

Shannon, H., C. Allen, M. Clarke, D. Davila, L. Fletcher-Wood, S. Gupta, K. Keck, S. Lang, R. Ludolph, and D. A. Kahangire. 2018. "Web Annex A: Report of the systematic review on the effect of household crowding on health." WHO Housing and Health Guidelines. Geneva, Switzerland: World Health Organization.

Singh, A., L. Daniel, E. Baker, and R. Bentley. 2019. "Housing disadvantage and poor mental health: A systematic review." *Am J Prev Med* 57(2): 262–272.

Smith, M., J. Hosking, A. Woodward, K. Witten, A. MacMillan, A. Field, P. Baas, and H. Mackie. 2017. "Systematic literature review of built environment effects on physical activity and active transport—An update and new findings on health equity." *Int J Behav Nutr Phys Act* 14(1): 158. doi:10.1186/s12966-017-0613-9.

Smith, N. 1979. "Toward a theory of gentrification a back to the city movement by capital, not people." *J Am Planning Assoc* 45(4): 538–548.

Solari, C. D., and R. D. Mare. 2012. "Housing crowding effects on children's wellbeing." *Soc Sci Res* 41(2): 464–476. https://doi.org/10.1016/j.ssresearch.2011.09.012.

Stahre, M., J. VanEenwyk, P. Siegel, and R. Njai. 2015. "Housing insecurity and the association with health outcomes and unhealthy behaviors, Washington State, 2011." *Prev Chronic Dis* 12: E109–E109. doi:10.5888/pcd12.140511.

Stergiopoulos, V., C. Mejia-Lancheros, R. Nisenbaum, R. Wang, J. Lachaud, P. O'Campo, and S. W. Hwang. 2019. "Long-term effects of rent supplements and mental health support services on housing and health outcomes of homeless adults with mental illness: Extension study of the At Home/Chez Soi randomised controlled trial." *Lancet Psychiatry* 6(11): 915–925. https://doi.org/10.1016/S2215-0366(19)30371-2.

Swope, C. B., and D. Hernández. 2019. "Housing as a determinant of health equity: A conceptual model." *Soc Sci Med* 243: 112571. https://doi.org/10.1016/j.socscimed.2019.112571.

The National Center on Family Homelessness. 2014. "America's youngest outcasts: A report card on child homelessness." Waltham, MA: American Institutes for Research.

Torio, C. M., A. Elixhauser, and R. M. Andrews. 2013. "Trends in potentially preventable hospital admissions among adults and children, 2005–2010: Statistical Brief No. 151." Rockville, MD: Agency for Healthcare Research and Quality.

Turner, M. A., R. Santos, D. K. Levy, D. Wissoker, C. L. Aranda, R. Pitingolo, and the Urban Institute. 2013. "Housing discrimination against racial and ethnic minorities 2012: Full report." Washington, DC: U.S. Department of Housing and Urban Development.

Turunen, E., and H. Hiilamo. 2014. "Health effects of indebtedness: A systematic review." *BMC Public Health* 14(1): 489. doi:10.1186/1471-2458-14-489.

U.S. Census Bureau. 2020. https://www.census.gov/census.gov.

U.S. Department of Housing and Urban Development. 2011. "American Healthy Homes Survey: Lead and arsenic findings." Washington, DC: US Department of Housing and Urban Development.

U.S. Department of Housing and Urban Development. 2017. "Worst case housing needs, 2017 report to Congress. Washington, DC: US Department of Housing and Urban Development.

U.S. Department of Housing and Urban Development. 2020. "The 2019 annual homeless assessment report (AHAR) to Congress. Part 1: Point-in-time estimates of homelessness." Washington, DC: U.S. Department of Housing and Urban Development, Office of Community Planning and Development.

U.S. Energy Information Administration. 2018. "One in three U.S. households faces a challenge in meeting energy needs." https://www.eia.gov/todayinenergy/detail.php?id=37072#.

U.S. Environmental Protection Agency. 2018. "Home buyer's and seller's guide to radon." https://www.epa.gov/sites/default/files/2015-05/documents/hmbuygud.pdf.

Vale, L. J., and Y. Freemark. 2012. "From public housing to public–private housing." *J Am Planning Assoc* 78(4): 379–402. doi:10.1080/01944363.2012.737985.

Voelkel, J., D. Hellman, R. Sakuma, and V. Shandas. 2018. "Assessing vulnerability to urban heat: A study of disproportionate heat exposure and access to refuge by sociodemographic status in Portland, Oregon." *Int J Environ Res Public Health* 15(4), 1–14. doi:10.3390/ijerph15040640.

White, B. M., H. S. Bonilha, and C. Ellis. 2016. "Racial/ethnic differences in childhood blood lead levels among children <72 months of age in the United States: A systematic review of the literature." *J Racial Ethnic Health Disparities* 3(1): 145–153. doi:10.1007/s40615-015-0124-9.

Woodhall-Melnik, J. R., and J. R. Dunn. 2016. "A systematic review of outcomes associated with participation in Housing First programs." *Housing Studies* 31(3): 287–304. doi:10.1080/02673037.2015.1080816.

World Health Organization. 2018. *WHO Housing and Health Guidelines*. Geneva, Switzerland: World Health Organization.

Zahran, H. S., C. M. Bailey, S. A. Damon, P. L. Garbe, and P. N. Breysse. 2018. "Vital signs: Asthma in children—United States, 2001–2016." *MMWR Morb Mortal Wkly Rep* 67(5): 149.

Zhang, Y., C. Yu, and L. Wang. 2017. "Temperature exposure during pregnancy and birth outcomes: An updated systematic review of epidemiological evidence." *Environ Pollut* 225: 700–712. https://doi.org/10.1016/j.envpol.2017.02.066.

Ziol-Guest, K. M., and C. C. McKenna. 2014. "Early childhood housing instability and school readiness." *Child Dev* 85(1): 103–113. doi:10.1111/cdev.12105.

CHAPTER 9

Work Can Be Good—or Bad—for Your Health

9.1. INTRODUCTION

Work Affects Health—and Health Affects Work

Without considering unpaid work, on average, American adults spend close to half of their waking hours at work (U.S. Bureau of Labor Statistics 2020a). It is obvious that work can influence health by exposing people to hazardous physical conditions such as toxic materials, dangerous machinery, extreme temperatures, or long hours without breaks, which have recognized health effects. The nature of work and how it is organized also have been shown to affect physical and mental health. Work can, for example, provide a sense of identity, social status and belonging; social support; and purpose in life. Work can influence health by providing a setting in which healthy activities and behaviors can be promoted or undermined. In addition, work affects a worker's life outside of work. For most people, employment is their primary source of income; it determines how much they can spend on food, housing, child care, and educating their children. It affects whether they have the means to live in homes and neighborhoods that promote health, and it influences their ability to pursue health-promoting behaviors. Inadequate pay is a major source of ongoing stress. Most Americans, furthermore, obtain their health care insurance through their jobs.

Not only does work affect health, but health also affects work. Good health is often needed for employment; it may be especially important for low-skilled manual workers who are likely to lack options such as paid sick leave, flexible hours, and the ability to work from home. Lack of employment among those who are unable to work due to illness can lead to adverse economic and social impacts, limiting a person's access to health-promoting resources and opportunities, and thus exacerbating their ill health.

Employment-Related Health Problems Have Significant Human and Economic Costs for Individuals and Society

In 2018, more than 5,250 fatal and 2.8 million nonfatal work-related injuries and illnesses were reported in private industry workplaces in the United States; of the nonfatal injuries,

The Social Determinants of Health and Health Disparities. Paula Braveman, Oxford University Press. © Oxford University Press 2023.
DOI: 10.1093/oso/9780190624118.003.0009

900,380 resulted in time away from work due to recuperation, job transfer, or activity restriction necessitated by the injury (U.S. Bureau of Labor Statistics 2019a, 2019b). Some reports have estimated that the total economic costs of occupational illness and injury in the United States are comparable to those of cancer and nearly comparable to those of heart disease (Leigh 2011). Healthy workers and their families are likely to incur lower medical costs and be more productive, whereas those with chronic health conditions generate higher costs in terms of health care use, absenteeism, disability, and reduced productivity (Asay et al. 2016; Araujo et al. 2020; Fouad et al. 2017). Workplace injuries and work-related illnesses have a major financial impact not only on employers' costs for workers' compensation but also on health care systems, health and disability insurers, and public social safety net programs (Sears, Edmonds, and Coe 2020). In 2017, in the United States, the cost to employers for workers' compensation totaled $97.4 billion, a 9.1% increase since 2013 (Weiss, Murphy, and Boden 2019).

This chapter examines how work (also referred to as occupation) can affect health, exploring the health effects of physical and psychosocial aspects of work and work-related opportunities and resources. It concludes with examples of promising approaches to making work healthier. Unless specified otherwise, in this book, "work" refers to paid work (i.e., employment); however, unpaid work, such as family caregiving, can also have substantial health effects.

9.2. CHANGES IN THE WORKFORCE AND WORK
The profiles of both workers and the nature and structure of work in the United States have evolved considerably over time.

Changes in the Workforce
Compared to decades ago, today's U.S. workforce is older (Toossi and Torpey 2017). From 1970 until the end of the 20th century, workers aged 55 years or older made up the smallest segment of the labor force (Toossi and Torpey 2017). They began to increase their share in the labor force during the 1990s and are projected to further increase their share during the period 2019–2029 (Figure 9.1) (U.S. Bureau of Labor Statistics 2020d).

Although the workforce has become more racially/ethnically diverse compared to decades ago, most U.S. workers are still White. In 2018, White people made up 78% of the labor force, whereas Black and Asian people constituted 13% and 6%, respectively. American Indians and Alaska Natives made up 1% of the workforce, and Native Hawaiians and Other Pacific Islanders accounted for less than 1% (U.S. Bureau of Labor Statistics 2019d). Whereas White people are somewhat overrepresented in the workforce, none of the other groups are markedly underrepresented (U.S. Census Bureau 2018).

The labor force participation rate is calculated as the proportion of a country's working-age population that engages actively in the labor market, either by working or by searching for work. As shown in Figure 9.2, the labor force participation of women aged 16 years or older increased after the 1950s, peaked at 60% in 1999, and has decreased since the peak (to 57.4% in 2017, compared with 69.2% of men) (U.S. Bureau of Labor Statistics 2020c). Not shown in Figure 9.2 are comparable data for 2019, showing a further decline by 2019, when approximately 57.4% of women aged

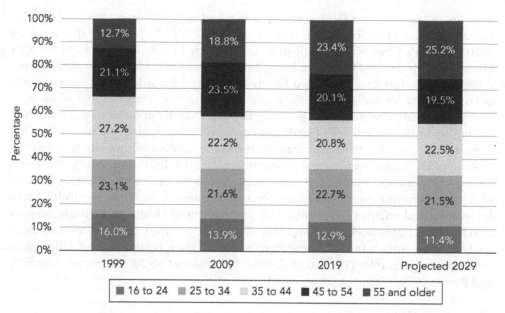

FIGURE 9.1 Percentage distribution of workforce by age group over time, 1999–2019 and projected 2029. Data may not sum to 100.00 due to rounding. *Source*: U.S. Bureau of Labor Statistics (2020d).

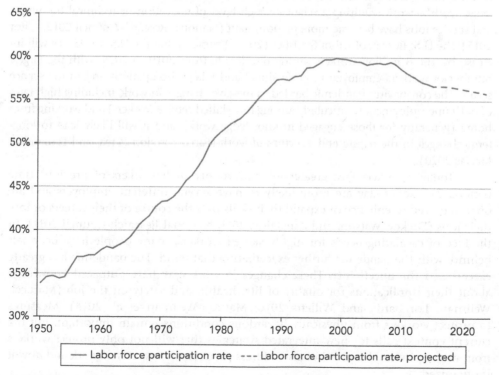

FIGURE 9.2 Women's labor force participation rate, 1950–2015 and projected to 2024. *Source*: Toossi and Morisi (2017).

16 years or older were in the labor force, compared to (a stable) 69.2% of men (U.S. Bureau of Labor Statistics 2020g). Even before the COVID-19 pandemic that began in 2020, women's labor force participation was projected to decline to 55.8% by 2024 (Toossi and Morisi 2017). The pandemic has led to further declines in women's participation in the workforce, attributed largely to the need for at least one parent to stay at home to care for and supervise the education of children (Power 2020; Collins et al. 2021). Child care responsibilities generally fall more heavily upon women. This is only partly due to the persistence of traditional caregiver roles; it also reflects the fact that women often earn less than their male partners, and families cannot afford to lose the income of the higher earner (Pew Research Center 2013; Jolly et al. 2014). The workforce participation of women has major implications for health. For example, the lack of paid maternity leave or provisions for breastfeeding at work are particular issues for women and infants (Rubin 2016; U.S. Department of Health and Human Services 2011). Nonstandard work hours and lack of flexibility in working hours are also more likely to affect women (and their children) adversely, given persistent gender disparities in family caregiver roles (Thomas et al. 2018; Fernandez et al. 2016; Kervezee, Shechter, and Boivin 2018; Champion et al. 2012).

Changes in Work

Along with increased gender diversity, the 21st-century workplace features more multidisciplinary jobs, reliance on technology, and contingent ("gig") jobs and a shift away from manufacturing jobs (Litchfield et al. 2016). As new industries have emerged, both "knowledge work"—work requiring a relatively high level of education or technical training— and service jobs have become more predominant (National Research Council 2012; Autor 2015) The U.S. Bureau of Labor Statistics (2020d) projects that the U.S. workforce will increase by 168.8 million workers during the decade from 2019 to 2029, with the largest number of workers employed in professional and related occupations and in the service sector. The coronavirus pandemic has led to massive changes in work, including high rates of both unemployment (particularly among low-skilled service workers) and working from home (generally for those engaged in knowledge work), and it will likely lead to long-term changes in the nature and structure of work (Fana, Torrejón Pérez, and Fernández-Macías 2020).

• Today's workers face greater job uncertainty than workers of previous time periods. Workers today are more likely to have several different employers and are often required to enhance or expand their skills over the course of their careers or lose their jobs (Dickey, Watson, and Zangelidis 2011; National Research Council 2011). In the face of escalating needs for highly skilled workers, many people have been left behind, with the pandemic further exacerbating that trend. The pandemic has greatly exacerbated the uncertainty. These changes in work may have outpaced knowledge about their implications for quality of life, health, and safety on the job (Marucci-Wellman, Lombardi, and Willetts 2016; Marucci-Wellman et al. 2014). Measures to protect workers from physically hazardous conditions remain important, but the current context calls for new integrated strategies that will not only protect workers from major physical hazards but also address psychosocial aspects of work and how it is organized.

9.3. HOW DOES WORK AFFECT HEALTH AND HEALTH DISPARITIES? AN OVERVIEW

This section discusses both physical and psychosocial aspects of work and evidence of how they affect health (Figure 9.3).

Links Between Health and the Physical Aspects of Work
Physical Working Conditions and Risk of Injury and Illness

There is widespread awareness that both the physical tasks involved in a job and the physical work environment can have important health effects. These concerns have been the traditional domain of occupational health and safety (Burgard and Lin 2013). Workers in particular sectors of the workforce are at increased risk of work-related injuries and illness. Four sectors alone—health care and social assistance, manufacturing, retail trade, and transportation and warehousing—accounted for nearly 56% of nonfatal occupational injuries in 2018 (The National Institute for Occupational Safety and Health 2020b). Incidence rates of severe nonfatal injuries and illnesses vary markedly by occupation. For example, in 2018, the rates of serious nonfatal occupational injury or illness were 127.3 per 10,000 workers in construction and extraction; 120.2 per 10,000 workers in farming, fishing, and forestry; 148.1 per 10,000 workers in installation, maintenance, and repair; and 193.7 per 10,000 workers in transportation and material moving—all heavily blue-collar occupations (The National Institute for Occupational Safety and Health 2020b). By contrast, in the same year, the rates of serious nonfatal occupational injury or illness among workers in the white-collar occupations "management, business, and finance" and "computer, engineering, and science" were far lower: 20.4 per 10,000 workers and 8.2 cases per 10,000 workers, respectively (Figure 9.4) (The National Institute for Occupational Safety and Health 2020b).

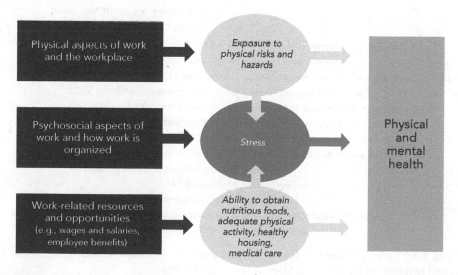

FIGURE 9.3   How does work affect health?

Physically demanding daily tasks and uncomfortable working positions can lead to musculoskeletal strain and injury, increasing the risk of long-term absence (Lallukka et al. 2019; Andersen et al. 2016). Jobs requiring repetitive movements and those with high psychosocial demand and high physical workload, including lifting, pushing, or pulling heavy loads, put workers at higher risk for musculoskeletal injuries and disorders and overextension and repetitive strain injuries such as carpal tunnel syndrome (da Costa and Vieira 2010). Multiple injuries with fractures accounted for the highest median number of days (48 days) away from work among all occupational illness or injuries in 2018 (U.S. Bureau of Labor Statistics 2019c). The ergonomics of equipment and work space are important contributors to occupational health. For example, poorly designed tools, keyboards, and chairs have been linked with persistent arm, back, and shoulder pain, as well as other musculoskeletal disorders (Ranasinghe et al. 2011; Celik et al. 2018). Lack of proper equipment for moving patients can lead to serious musculoskeletal injuries among nursing assistants (S. Choi and Brings 2015). Sedentary jobs adversely affect health by restricting opportunities for movement or exercise, and physical inactivity contributes to risk of obesity and chronic diseases such as diabetes and heart disease (B. Choi et al. 2010).

Workplace conditions such as dampness, inadequate ventilation, and poor temperature control can aggravate health problems such as allergies and asthma (Sundell et al. 2011; Fishwick 2014; Jaakkola, Lajunen, and Jaakkola 2020). The physical environment of a workplace also can expose workers to a variety of potentially hazardous chemicals (Henneberger et al. 2010). Asbestos, lead, pesticides, aerosols, ammonia, and other cleaning products are only a few of the many chemicals commonly found in manufacturing, construction, services, and mining workplaces. Long-term exposure has been associated with poisoning; anemia; cognitive changes; and heart, kidney, and reproductive problems, including problems during pregnancy (Hsieh et al. 2017; Obeng-Gyasi

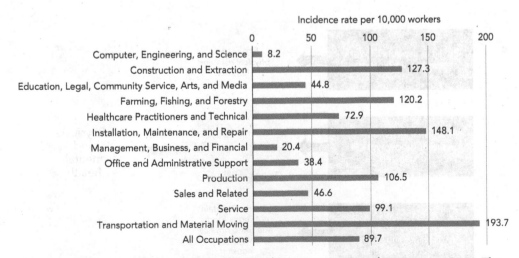

FIGURE 9.4   Count of severe injuries and illnesses by occupation, United States, 2018. *Source*: The National Institute for Occupational Safety and Health (2020b).

2019; Alarcon 2016). Farmworkers are routinely exposed to toxic pesticides (McCauley et al. 2006), extreme heat (Fleischer et al. 2013), and uncomfortable physical positions (Xiao et al. 2013). Noisy work environments are associated with hearing loss, one of the most common occupational injuries worldwide. Workplace noise also raises the risk of accidents (Estill et al. 2017).

Psychosocial Aspects of Work and How Work Is Organized Also Can Affect Health

The experience of work itself—including logistics, psychosocial issues, and the quality of relationships with co-workers and supervisors—can affect workers' physical and mental health. The quality of experiences and relationships at work has been linked repeatedly with health. Work culture (norms and prevailing ways that workers interact with each other and with supervisors), management practices, and office climate affect employee health (Aldana et al. 2012; Cox 1993; Payne et al. 2018). For many people, work is not just a crucial source of income. It also can be a major source of opportunities for personal development and social support. These opportunities appear to be shaped by many characteristics of the work environment, including logistical issues, workplace culture, job demands, and latitude in making decisions about one's work (control at work, "decision latitude"; discussed below).

Work-Related Stress and Health

Working conditions can damage health not only through exposure to physical hazards but also by being stressful. Daily occupational stressors can include constant challenges posed by work environments in which a person may feel disrespected, intimidated, or under constant strain, trying to balance the demands of work and family responsibilities with inadequate resources. The past two decades have seen substantial increases in scientific knowledge about causal pathways and physiologic mechanisms that help explain the links between stress and health (see Chapter 4). One of the most important pathways is that involving physiologic damage to multiple vital organ systems caused by chronic stress acting through neuroendocrine and immune mechanisms (Herman et al. 2016; Ménard et al. 2017; Russell and Lightman 2019). Stressful experiences—such as aspects of working conditions—can trigger the release of cortisol, epinephrine, norepinephrine, inflammatory cytokines, and other substances in the body that, particularly with repeated/prolonged stress over time, can damage immune defenses and vital organs, in part by producing inflammation (Fagundes, Glaser, and Kiecolt-Glaser 2013; McEwen 2017; Wirtz and von Känel 2017). The physiologic chain of events that can accompany chronic stress has been associated with more rapid onset and progression of chronic illnesses including cancer (Powell, Tarr, and Sheridan 2013), cardiovascular disease (Kivimäki and Steptoe 2018; Wirtz and von Känel 2017), chronic kidney disease (Duni et al. 2019), and neurodegenerative diseases (e.g., Alzheimer disease) (Bisht, Sharma, and Tremblay 2018; Mravec, Horvathova, and Padova 2018). The bodily wear and tear due to chronic stress may accelerate aging (Karatsoreos and McEwen 2013; Liguori et al. 2018) and adversely affect cognition and decision-making (McEwen 2017).

Whereas acute stress may temporarily improve immune function and memory, chronic (i.e., repeated over a period of time) stress may lead, over time, to more physiological damage than a single stressful event, even if that event is more dramatic (McEwen 2013). Evidence has also linked chronic stress over the life course with shortening of the length of telomeres, the caps on the ends of chromosomes (Oliveira et al. 2016). Shortening of telomeres appears to be a marker of physiologic aging (Shammas 2011; Prasad, Wu, and Bondy 2017). Many of the working conditions explored in this chapter exert their influence on health by causing stress.

Commuting to Work

The private vehicle is the predominant form of transportation to and from work in the United States. In 2013, approximately 86% of all workers commuted to work by private vehicle, either driving alone or carpooling (U.S. Census Bureau 2013). Longer commutes by both train and automobile have been associated with greater levels of stress (Legrain, Eluru, and El-Geneidy 2015). Long commutes have been linked with health risks including sleep problems, cardiovascular disease, metabolic risk, and increased likelihood of obesity (Hoehner et al. 2012; Halonen et al. 2020; King and Jacobson 2017). Of the 156.9 million people age 16 years or older in the United States who worked outside their homes during 2019, 119.2 million commuted by vehicle alone (i.e., not in carpools), contributing to traffic congestion, air pollution, reduced physical activity, and risk of injury and death due to accidents (U.S. Census Bureau 2019). By contrast, using public transit has been associated with greater physical activity (Lachapelle et al. 2011). The COVID-19 pandemic, however, has undermined the use of public transit due to fears of exposure to COVID-19 (Zheng et al. 2020; Hu et al. 2020).

Work Schedules

Working evening and night shifts, holding multiple jobs, long work hours, and excessive overtime work can be detrimental to health by causing fatigue and disturbances in circadian rhythms. Psychological risks have been shown to be higher among shift workers compared to regular day workers; this may reflect low job control and a lower level of support from managers (Fischer et al. 2019). Shift work and long work hours have been associated with reduced performance on the job, sleep problems, and unhealthy behaviors that lead to increased risk of chronic illness, including type 2 diabetes and coronary artery disease (Vetter et al. 2016; Shan et al. 2018; Caruso 2014). In turn, inadequate sleep leads to decreased concentration and lower cognitive performance, and it can cause mistakes that negatively impact an employee's health, work, or both (Whitney et al. 2017; Lo et al. 2016). Working more than 40 hours per week has been associated with adverse health outcomes such as increased rates of mortality, injury, and illness, including depression, anxiety, and coronary artery disease; effects of long work weeks have been especially pronounced for work shifts longer than 8 hours (Bannai and Tamakoshi 2014; Friedman, Almberg, and Cohen 2019). Because the burden of family caregiving still falls largely on women (Lee and Tang 2015; Revenson et al. 2016), inflexible work schedules and long hours may have particularly adverse health impacts on them.

Flexible work schedules and more worker control over work schedules have been associated with better perceived work–life balance (Brauner et al. 2019), which in turn has been linked with children's perceived family support and life satisfaction (Schnettler et al. 2018). Jobs with long hours, weekend hours, irregular hours, low worker control over work hours, or low supervisor support for workers meeting family obligations can result in workers spending inadequate time with their families and communities (Arlinghaus et al. 2019; Craig and Powell 2011). Parental stress from nonstandard working hours appears to affect children's health and development (Li et al. 2014). Parents' shift work and nonstandard working hours have been associated with an increased likelihood of risky behaviors in adolescence and higher risk of parental separation and divorce (Arlinghaus et al. 2019).

Health Effects of Holding Multiple Jobs

As of June 2020, approximately 4.7% of the U.S. workforce held more than one job, often out of a need to earn more income, although some do so to advance their professional development (U.S. Bureau of Labor Statistics 2020g). Women were more likely to hold multiple jobs than men (U.S. Bureau of Labor Statistics 2020g). Evidence has associated holding multiple jobs with work–family conflict/imbalance, leading to poor work performance and poor mental health, with particular effects on low-income working mothers (Mellor and Decker 2020; Bruns and Pilkauskas 2019). Policies to reduce the number of parents working multiple jobs would likely need to improve minimum wage levels, decrease the costs of child care, and/or increase the availability of affordable housing; lack of affordable housing is a frequent reason for parents working multiple jobs.

Work–Life (Work–Family) Balance

Work–life balance has been measured, for example, using a Likert scale with a question assessing the level of a worker's satisfaction with the balance between their work and their private life (Brauner et al. 2019; Haar et al. 2014). Work–family conflict may be a key mediator of the relationship between nonstandard work schedules (e.g., evening shifts, night shifts, weekend work, and irregular hours) and poor health (Cho 2018; Dettmers 2017). Work–family conflict occurs when pressures from meeting work and family responsibilities are at odds with one another (Greenhaus and Beutell 1985; Leineweber et al. 2012). Work–family imbalance has been associated with psychological distress, sleep deficiency, health risk behaviors (e.g., tobacco use and alcohol abuse), emotional exhaustion, and poorer overall health among workers (Leineweber et al. 2012; Wolff et al. 2013; Jacobsen et al. 2014; Mensah and Adjei 2020).

Notable changes have occurred in family life and family structure in the United States since the 1960s, with two-parent households no longer being the most common family structure (Pew Research Center 2015a). At the height of the post-World War II baby boom, approximately 73% of children were born into two-parent households, whereas by 2014, 4 out of 10 births were occurring to single women or women living with a nonmarital partner (Pew Research Center 2015a). Since 1970, more single mothers have joined the workforce and are working longer hours; in addition, the share of two-parent households in which both parents are employed full-time has increased from 31% in

1970 to 46% in 2019 (Pew Research Center 2015b). Given the extent of women's workforce participation, lack of workplace accommodations for breastfeeding can be an important source of work–life imbalance.

For many families, these changes represent substantial and likely stressful constraints on time for activities such as housework, child care, leisure, and sleep. Compared to married mothers, single mothers have been shown to have greater predicted mortality risk, psychological distress, work–family conflict, and financial hardship, attributed to job strain (discussed later) and family-related stress (Dziak, Janzen, and Muhajarine 2010; Sabbath et al. 2015). In households in which both parents work full-time, mothers do more household chores and child care–related tasks than fathers, including managing children's schedules, activities, and health care (Pew Research Center 2015b). In households in which both parents work at least part-time, approximately half reported that both are equally focused on their careers; when there is an imbalance, however, fathers are three times more likely to focus on their careers (Pew Research Center 2015b).

Policies that promote greater work–family balance may be expected to have positive health impacts for children as well as for workers. Parents' work schedules as well as working conditions (e.g., stressors at work) can affect their ability to care for their children (Li et al. 2014). Socioeconomic resources such as income, wealth, and education are also important for a worker's ability to parent. This should not be surprising; higher income/wealth makes it possible for a working parent to hire assistance with child care and to obtain a range of other services that prevent or reduce stress and free up time to spend with family. Perhaps surprisingly, however, among women of low educational attainment (but not among women of high educational attainment), part-time and full-time working mothers are more likely than unemployed mothers to provide "child learning opportunities" (Augustine 2014; Buehler et al. 2014). This may reflect unmeasured characteristics that differentiate employed from unemployed mothers.

Control at Work, Job Demands, Decision Latitude, and Job Strain

Jobs characterized by high levels of both psychological demands and "decision latitude" (decision-making authority and skill utilization) have been observed to promote a worker's self-esteem and self-efficacy. Conversely, workers whose jobs make high demands yet offer little decision latitude experience "job strain" (Karasek et al. 1981; Slopen et al. 2012). Substantial empirical evidence has shown an association between job strain and several health outcomes, both long- and short-term, including musculoskeletal disorders (Cantley et al. 2016), chronic physical illnesses (e.g., cardiovascular disease) (Kivimäki et al. 2012; Nyberg et al. 2013; Rocco et al. 2017; Landsbergis et al. 2015), poorer mental health (Theorell et al. 2015; Burns, Butterworth, and Anstey 2016), absence from work (M. Wang et al. 2014), and unhealthy behaviors (e.g., smoking, alcohol consumption, and physical inactivity) that contribute to these illnesses (Heikkilä et al. 2013). Control at work has been considered by some scholars to contribute in an important way to socioeconomic differences in coronary heart disease among employed persons (Marmot et al. 1997; Kivimäki et al. 2012; Kristenson et al. 2004).

Jobs characterized by high levels of decision-making authority and skill utilization have been linked to better health and mental well-being, even in the presence of high demands. Conversely, workers whose jobs make high demands of them yet offer little decision latitude are at risk of job strain (Karasek et al. 1981). The job demand–control model, first introduced by sociologist Robert Karasek in 1979 and used in many studies since then (Häusser et al. 2010), is based on the hypothesis that individuals experiencing high-strain jobs (jobs characterized by high demands and low control) are more likely to have work-related stress and emotional exhaustion (Elovainio et al. 2015; Fan et al. 2019).

Although the job demand–control model and variations on it (e.g., the job demands–resources model; Bakker and Demerouti 2014) are still cited and used widely in occupational health studies, a number of conceptual, empiric, and methodologic reservations about the model have been expressed (Bell et al. 2017; Schaufeli and Taris 2014; Alves, Hökerberg, and Faerstein 2013; Van der Doef and Maes 1999; Mausner-Dorsch and Eaton 2000; de Jonge et al. 2000; de Lange et al. 2003). Some scholars, for example, have questioned the direction of causation, noting that worker health and well-being due to an array of factors can influence work performance and work environments, including job strain (Zapf, Dormann, and Frese 1996; de Lange et al. 2005; Tang 2014). Zapf et al. (1996) hypothesized that healthy workers are more likely to enter and remain in favorable work environments, whereas unhealthy workers are more likely to end up in more demanding and less accommodating work environments because their options are more limited. Several reasons have been proposed to explain this phenomenon. One explanation is that for some unhealthy workers, emotional and mental exhaustion may lead to cognitive and behavioral withdrawal, which unfavorably impacts their relationships with supervisors and co-workers (Tang 2014). Strained workers may be less likely to seek and be competitive for new job opportunities in more favorable work environments, given that employers are often reluctant to hire workers perceived to be unhealthy (Tang 2014). All of these factors could result in observing associations between job control and worker health, but the direction of causation would be from worker health to job control rather than vice versa. In fact, the relationships may be bidirectional.

The Balance Between Effort and Rewards

Perceived balance between a worker's efforts and rewards (e.g., in terms of earnings, benefits, recognition, job security, and career opportunities) also has been thought to influence health. The effort–reward imbalance model posits that lack of fairness and lack of reciprocity of efforts create psychological stress in employees, increasing the risk of poor health (Siegrist, Siegrist, and Weber 1986; Siegrist 1996; van Vegchel et al. 2005; Eddy et al. 2018; Siegrist and Li 2016). Involuntary overtime work without commensurate rewards, for example, is associated with high fatigue and low satisfaction (Beckers et al. 2008; Wong, Chan, and Ngan 2019). Psychological reactions to the imbalance between high efforts and low rewards have been associated with a number of adverse health outcomes, including poor physical functioning and increased incidence of coronary heart disease (Dragano et al. 2017), higher blood pressure (Gilbert-Ouimet et al. 2014; Boucher et al. 2017; Trudel et al. 2017), higher risk of being bullied (Notelaers, Törnroos, and Salin 2019), impaired mental and social functioning, and mild psychiatric disorders (de Araújo et al. 2019). The demand–control model and the effort–reward model appear complementary to each other in predicting social inequalities in health, rather than contradictory rivals (Tsutsumi and Kawakami 2004; Ostry et al. 2003).

9.4. HOW DOES WORK AFFECT HEALTH AND HEALTH DISPARITIES? THE ROLE OF ORGANIZATIONAL JUSTICE AND DISCRIMINATION

Organizational Justice

The term *organizational justice* refers to the degree to which employees are treated with justice at work (Colquitt, Greenberg, and Zapata-Phelan 2005; Greenberg 1987). It includes whether decisions are made with input from affected parties and applied consistently and whether bias is systematically avoided. It also includes whether supervisors treat employees with respect, transparency, and fairness. It applies to outcomes, processes, and relationships in the workplace. Theoretical models of organizational justice generally have addressed three major aspects: distributive justice, procedural justice, and interactional justice (Cohen-Charash and Spector 2001; Colquitt et al. 2001; Yean and Yusof 2016). In this literature, distributive justice focuses on perceived fairness in the outcomes of how rewards and recognition—such as pay, promotion, status, and tenure—are given in an organization (Colquitt 2001; Yean and Yusof 2016). Procedural justice focuses on the fairness of the organizational processes themselves (distinguished from the outcomes of the processes) (Yean and Yusof 2016; Colquitt 2001). Interactional justice pertains to aspects of interpersonal treatment and the communication process between management and employees, such as respect, honesty, and whether an employer is providing adequate information and explanations (Colquitt 2001; Yean and Yusof 2016). Organizational injustice may manifest as harassment, abuse, bullying, or discrimination based on various characteristics—for example, racial/ethnic group, class, gender, disability, or sexual orientation or gender identity.

A growing body of literature suggests that organizational injustice may make important contributions to health disparities (Okechukwu et al. 2014). A review by Okechukwu (2014) concluded that workplace injustices have been associated with poor psychological and physical health, health behaviors, and job outcomes (Okechukwu et al. 2014). For example, lower levels of justice at work have been associated with higher self-reported morbidity, increased mental health problems, and stress-related behaviors (e.g., smoking and drinking) among workers (Kobayashi and Kondo 2019). Conversely, organizational justice can contribute to lower sickness absence (Elovainio et al. 2013; Ybema and van den Bos 2010). Although a combination of large effort–reward imbalance and high organizational injustice has been associated with greater health risk than either alone, studies have shown that high organizational injustice was associated with increased health risk independently of adverse effort–reward imbalance and demand–control–support dynamics (Ndjaboué, Brisson, and Vézina 2012).

Health Consequences of Discrimination at Work: Overview

Discrimination—unfair treatment based on characteristics of a person such as racial or ethnic group, skin color, religion, gender, disability, sexual orientation, and gender identity—is an aspect of organizational injustice. Among both women and men and across diverse racial and ethnic groups, perceived discrimination (in general, although not necessarily specifically at work) has been linked with poorer physical and mental health (Lewis, Cogburn, and Williams 2015; Hammond, Gillen, and Yen 2010; Triana,

Jayasinghe, and Pieper 2015). The physical and mental health consequences of discrimination in general have been demonstrated for groups defined by race/ethnicity, gender, disability, immigrant status, gender identity, or sexual orientation (Krieger 2014).

Racial Discrimination in the Workplace

Overwhelming evidence indicates that people of color often face racial discrimination at work. Laws and practices have been put in place to protect employee rights and increase diversity and equity in management practices, notably the enforcement of Title VII of the Civil Rights Act of 1964, which forbids employment discrimination on the basis of race, color, religion, sex, and national origin. A 2020 decision of the U.S. Supreme Court interprets the inclusion of "sex" as a protected characteristic to imply protection against discrimination based on sexual orientation or gender identity (Supreme Court of the United States 2020). Despite the law, however, many people continue to experience racial discrimination in workplaces (Triana et al. 2015). In 2019, the Equal Employment Commission received 72,675 discrimination complaints; of these, racial discrimination was the most prevalent, accounting for one-third of all discrimination claims made during the year (U.S. Equal Employment Opportunity Commission 2020). Black people working in predominantly White environments are especially at risk of experiencing racial discrimination (Assari and Moghani Lankarani 2018).

People of color are more likely to be exposed to physically harmful occupational conditions (Okechukwu et al. 2014; Stanbury and Rosenman 2014; Grineski, Collins, and Morales 2017). Racial discrimination and racial bullying in the workplace have been linked to poor mental and physical health outcomes among people of color (Velez et al. 2018; Attell, Kummerow Brown, and Treiber 2017; McCord et al. 2018; Hammond et al. 2010). The negative health impacts of discrimination in the workplace can be both short term (e.g., greater stress, with elevated blood pressure and other physiological signs associated with stress) and longer term (leading to heart disease, arthritis, other musculoskeletal problems, and other physical illnesses). Racial discrimination in the workplace also is associated with behavioral risk factors such as smoking and alcohol use (Chavez et al. 2015).

Among Americans in every racial or ethnic group, higher levels of education are associated with greater likelihood of being employed and, among those in the workforce, higher earnings (Tamborini, Kim, and Sakamoto 2015). Although Black and Hispanic people increasingly have higher educational attainment and have moved into higher-skilled and higher-paying occupations, they are still underrepresented in management, professional, and related jobs. In 2018, 54% of Asian Americans worked in management and professional occupations compared to 41% of White, 31% of Black, and 22% of Hispanic/Latino workers (U.S. Bureau of Labor Statistics 2019d). Black and Hispanic/Latino workers are overrepresented in the service sector and low-paying jobs. In particular, Hispanic/Latino workers account for only 17% of total employment but are substantially overrepresented in construction and maintenance (55%), agriculture (53%), and housekeeping (49%) (U.S. Bureau of Labor Statistics 2019d). Similarly, Black workers only account for 12% of the workforce but higher proportions of nursing and home health aides (36%), security guards (31%), and licensed vocational nurses (30%) (U.S. Bureau of Labor Statistics 2019d). White Americans continue to dominate chief executive positions, and Asian

Americans are overrepresented in engineering and health care professions (U.S. Bureau of Labor Statistics 2019d).

Reflecting systemic racism (racism that is deeply embedded in systems, laws, and policies), people of color are overrepresented in lower status and lower paying jobs. Workers in these types of jobs are disproportionately exposed to health-impairing working conditions (Burgard and Lin 2013; Landsbergis, Grzywacz, and LaMontagne 2014). Low-paying, blue-collar jobs present more occupational hazards, including environmental and chemical exposures (e.g., pesticides and asbestos), poor working conditions (e.g., shift work with few breaks and potentially harmful tools), and psychosocial stressors (e.g., less control) (Burgard and Lin 2013). For instance, farm workers, the majority of whom are Hispanic/Latino immigrants, are exposed to toxic chemicals in pesticides; their effects have been associated with poor reproductive, maternal, and birth outcomes (James-Todd, Chiu, and Zota 2016), as well as adverse physiological and neurodevelopment in young children (Harley et al. 2013; Eskenazi et al. 2013). Likewise, bus drivers face numerous physical and psychosocial stressors in their jobs, including exposure to chemical fumes and high noise levels; high risk for musculoskeletal strain; pressure to arrive on time; and stress resulting from passenger behavior, traffic, and required paperwork (Crizzle et al. 2017). These workers were also reported to be at higher risk for chronic illnesses such as diabetes and cardiovascular diseases due to poor diet, lack of exercise, and inadequate sleep (Crizzle et al. 2017). Lower wage workers also are less likely to have health-related benefits such as paid sick leave, job flexibility, and access to workplace wellness programs (U.S. Bureau of Labor Statistics 2020c).

Racial Disparities in Earnings

Earnings matter for health. Income has long been associated with health and life expectancy at the population level (World Health Organization 2019; Chetty et al. 2016; Daly et al. 2002) because it plays a fundamental role in shaping one's access to stable and affordable housing, quality education, healthy food, health insurance, a range of services, and more. Conversely, low income is a strong risk factor for behavioral risks to health such as smoking (Casetta et al. 2017), obesity (Ogden et al. 2017), and substance use disorders (Sareen et al. 2011) (See Chapter 2.)

As shown in Figure 9.5, despite an increase in median household income for all racial/ethnic groups since 1967, large racial disparities in income persist, reflecting persistent racism. Black people in general earn less than other racial and ethnic groups. In 2018, the median annual income of Asian, Black, Hispanic or Latino, and White people was $87,194, $41,361, $51,450, and $66,943, respectively (Semega et al. 2019). These figures may, however, somewhat overestimate disparities in earnings from employment, given that White and Asian people are more likely to have part of their income come from accumulated wealth (e.g., dividends from stocks) rather than employment. Multiple sources, however, have documented racial disparities in earnings from employment and have attributed those disparities to discrimination (V. Wilson and Rodgers 2016; Yearby 2019; Brewster and Lynn 2014; Miller 2020). A long history of discriminatory policies and practices—which were legal until the enactment of civil rights legislation in the 1960s—has placed and continues to place particularly large obstacles to

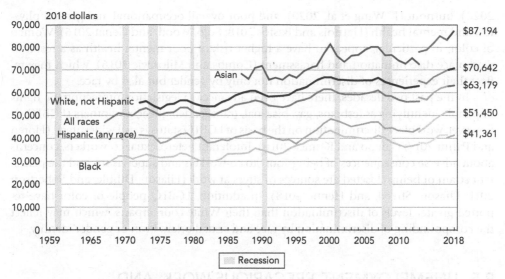

FIGURE 9.5 Real median household income by race and Hispanic origin, 1967–2018. The data for 2017 and beyond are based on an updated processing system. Income questions were redesigned and implemented for data collection in 2013 and beyond. Median household income data are not available prior to 1967. *Source*: Semega et al. (2019).

accumulating wealth for people of color (Herring and Henderson 2016; Rothstein 2017). The disparities noted below, therefore, reflect racial disparities both in earnings from employment and in income from accumulated wealth.

In 2017, the United States had 6.9 million adults who were "working poor"—that is, living in poverty despite being employed at least 27 weeks out of the previous year (U.S. Bureau of Labor Statistics 2019e). Black and Hispanic people were twice as likely to be among the working poor as Whites and Asians, with working-poor rates of 7.9%, 3.9%, and 2.9% among Black, Hispanic, and White people, respectively (U.S. Bureau of Labor Statistics 2019e).

Workplace Discrimination Based on Gender, Gender Identity, or Sexual Orientation

Gender disparities in earnings for comparable work are another manifestation of discrimination in the workplace. Compared with the 1950s, women have markedly increased their workforce participation and their educational attainment (Toossi and Morisi 2017; U.S. Bureau of Labor Statistics 2017). Despite a decline in earning disparities between men and women since the mid-1970s (Mandel and Semyonov 2014), however, a large pay gap by gender persists in today's workforce in almost all occupations. In 2018, females earned 81.6 cents to every dollar earned by males in the United States (U.S. Census Bureau 2022). Not surprisingly given the earnings gap, women are more likely than men to be among the working poor; in 2017, the working poor rate was 5.3% among women and 3.8% among men (U.S. Bureau of Labor Statistics 2019e).

Women continue to experience discrimination and harassment in the workplace, which has been linked to long-term sickness absences (Pietiläinen, Nätti, and Ojala

2020), burnout (L. Wang et al. 2020), and poor overall occupational and general physical and mental health (Harnois and Bastos 2018; Sojo, Wood, and Genat 2016). Women of color, in particular, appear to have a higher risk of poor mental health as a result of workplace discrimination and harassment (Combs and Milosevic 2016), which may reflect their experiences of discrimination not only by gender but also by race.

In the past two decades, there have been advances in legislation protecting the rights of people identifying as lesbians, gay, bisexual, transgender, queer, and others (LGBTQ+); however, workplace discrimination on the basis of LGBTQ status is still widespread (Lloren and Parini 2017; Galupo and Resnick 2016). Intolerant heterosexual co-workers, concerns about adverse consequences of being "out" to co-workers and supervisors, and the persistent strain of being closeted are sources of stress at work (Eliason, Dibble, and Robertson 2011; Eliason, Streed, and Henne 2018). In addition, LGBTQ people of color have reported greater levels of discrimination than their White counterparts, which may reflect the compounding of discrimination by race and sexual orientation or gender identity.

9.5. UNEMPLOYMENT, PRECARIOUS WORK, AND UNPAID WORK

People who are unemployed have a higher prevalence of poor health and excess mortality than their employed counterparts (Matilla-Santander et al. 2021; Norström et al. 2019; Bartley, Ferrie, and Montgomery 2006). Although ill health itself can be a reason for unemployment, findings from longitudinal studies indicate that the health effects of unemployment appear to be independent of preexisting health (Herber et al. 2019; Janlert, Winefield, and Hammarström 2015).

Unemployment may affect physical and mental health in several ways:

- *Lowered income and living standards.* Reductions in income associated with unemployment can lead to deteriorating physical health because of changes in ability to afford nutritious food, healthy housing, and/or appropriate medical care.
- *Psychosocial effects.* Loss of employment is associated with stress-related changes in health, such as increased blood pressure (Khubchandani and Price 2017; Seeman et al. 2018), and can limit access to health-promoting aspects of work, such as physical and mental activity, use of skills, decision latitude, social contact, and social status.
- *Behavioral health risks.* The impact of unemployment on unhealthy coping behaviors such as increased alcohol consumption, smoking, and drug use has been widely studied; however, findings are inconsistent (Perreault et al. 2017; Rosenthal et al. 2012).

Among those who are employed, job insecurity and threat of job loss can contribute to poorer health through similar pathways. Stress associated with the prospect of losing one's job can lead to risky coping behaviors such as smoking, lack of exercise, and forgoing sick or vacation leave, and it may place workers at increased risk of work-related injury and illness (de Wolff 2008).

The number of Americans at risk of the health-damaging effects of job insecurity and unemployment is growing. During the height of the COVID-19 pandemic in 2020, the

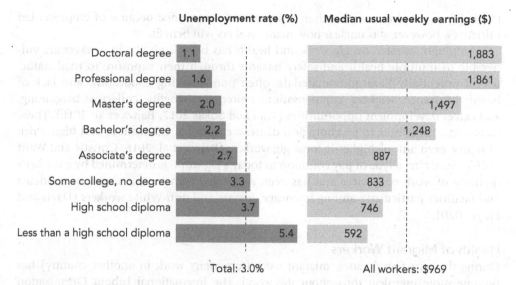

	Unemployment rate (%)	Median usual weekly earnings ($)
Doctoral degree	1.1	1,883
Professional degree	1.6	1,861
Master's degree	2.0	1,497
Bachelor's degree	2.2	1,248
Associate's degree	2.7	887
Some college, no degree	3.3	833
High school diploma	3.7	746
Less than a high school diploma	5.4	592
	Total: 3.0%	All workers: $969

FIGURE 9.6 Unemployment rates and earnings by educational attainment. Data are for persons aged 25 years or older. Earnings are for full-time wage and salary workers. *Source*: U.S. Bureau of Labor Statistics (2020g).

unemployment rate rose to 13% in the United States, up from 3.6% at the end of 2019 (U.S. Bureau of Labor Statistics 2021). And those who were already at greater disadvantage with respect to social factors such as educational attainment and racial or ethnic group were most likely to be unemployed (Figure 9.6).

Gig (Contingent) Work and Health

The U.S. Bureau of Labor Statistics (2020e) defines contingent workers as "people who do not expect their jobs to last or who report that their jobs are temporary"; their work arrangement does not contain an "explicit or implicit contract for long-term employment." In 2017, approximately 3.8% of workers in the United States—nearly 6 million people—were contingent or "gig" workers (U.S. Bureau of Labor Statistics 2018). Since the 2008 economic recession, gig work—a type of contingent work arrangement that requires use of digital platforms—has grown markedly (Tran and Sokas 2017). Digital platforms are used to connect individuals seeking services with those providing services, who generally are not considered employees of those who own and operate the digital platforms. Gig workers—such as truck drivers and contract nurses—do not qualify for minimum wage or overtime pay. Gig businesses such as Uber and meal delivery services, therefore, have not been obligated to treat workers as employees or comply with labor laws; most do not provide benefits such as health insurance, worker's compensation, or paid sick leave (Muntaner 2018; Malos, Lester, and Virick 2018). Unlike typical independent contractors, workers cannot negotiate their rates or work contracts (Tran and Sokas 2017). Approximately 49% of Uber drivers receive employer-sponsored health insurance through a different employer or through their family members (Hall and Krueger 2018). California's AB5, which took effect in 2020, enabled some gig workers in California to qualify as employees rather than independent contractors; because of employer-led initiatives, however, it is unclear how many workers will benefit.

Although research on gig work and health has been limited, gig workers are vulnerable to multiple health and safety hazards through their exposure to road traffic; use of potentially hazardous materials; often poor working conditions; and lack of health insurance, workers' compensation, retirement benefits, collective bargaining, and career development opportunities (Tran and Sokas 2017; Bajwa et al. 2018). These factors can contribute to psychological distress, emotional exhaustion, and higher risk of injury, even among higher-income gig workers (Bajwa et al. 2018; Christie and Ward 2019). Piece rate, a type of pay common to today's gig work, is determined by a worker's quantity of work or services and has been associated with increased risk of accidents and fatalities particularly among low-wage, female and non-White workers (Davis and Hoyt 2020).

Health of Migrant Workers

During the past few decades, migrant work (temporary work in another country) has become more prevalent throughout the world. The International Labour Organization (2018) estimated that 164 million people in the world are migrant workers; 70% of them live in high-income countries, 18.6% in upper middle-income countries, 10.1% in lower middle-income countries, and 3.4% in low-income countries. In 2019, the United States had approximately 28.4 million foreign-born workers, accounting for 17.4% of the U.S. labor force. Workers of Latin American origin accounted for nearly half of the foreign-born labor force, and Asians accounted for one-quarter (U.S. Bureau of Labor Statistics 2020f).

Compared to native-born workers, these workers are more likely to be working in service, construction, maintenance, production, transportation, natural resource, and material moving occupations (U.S. Bureau of Labor Statistics 2020f). Others work as housekeepers, hotel cleaners, and in nail salons, restaurants, and dry-cleaning services. Many of these workers are Mexican immigrants; some are undocumented (Gany et al. 2014). Legal status, educational level, language, and labor skill have been important factors in the overrepresentation of Mexican and other Latino immigrants in these occupations (Gany et al. 2014).

Migrant work is associated with various health risks. Migrant workers typically do not have the power to demand workplace rights and protections; therefore, they often have no other option than to work in hazardous conditions that predispose them to occupational injuries, accidents, and mental health problems. Many migrant workers face language barriers, employer and co-worker prejudice, lack of professional networks, inadequate workplace protections, lack of safety standards, workplace abuse, long work hours, and challenges accessing quality employment opportunities (Yanar, Kosny, and Smith 2018). Migrant workers in agriculture in particular are exposed to environmental risk factors including extreme temperatures, pesticides, chemicals, and hazardous equipment (Moyce and Schenker 2018). Furthermore, hotel cleaners, housekeeping workers, and farm workers are at higher risk of musculoskeletal disorders due to uncomfortable body positions, repetitive movements, need to lift heavy equipment, and the fast pace they must keep (Moyce and Schenker 2018).

Unpaid Work and Health

Women in the United States engage in significantly more unpaid work hours than men (Jung and O'Brien 2019). Unpaid work can take the form of housework, child care, or care of the elderly (Jung and O'Brien 2019). For women, housework has been associated with adverse physical and mental health outcomes and perceived unfairness in the division of household labor (Polachek and Wallace 2015; Adjei and Brand 2018; Tao, Janzen, and Abonyi 2010). Excessive child care responsibilities in relation to employment demands and unequal distribution of child care work among parents have been linked to adverse health outcomes, including distress, depression, and stress related to work–life imbalance (Jung and O'Brien 2019). Caring for the elderly and terminally ill has also been shown to be psychologically challenging for both men and women, as they provide care and bear witness to loss and suffering (Nielsen et al. 2016; Del-Pino-Casado et al. 2019).

9.6. WORK-RELATED RESOURCES ALSO AFFECT HEALTH

In addition to income, many work-related benefits—such as health insurance, paid sick and caregiver leave, workplace wellness programs, child and elder care resources, and retirement benefits—also shape the major health-related options available to individuals and families.

Health Insurance Provided Through Employment

Although most Americans receive their health insurance through their jobs, not all workers have access to this benefit. One of the major building blocks of the Affordable Care Act (ACA) is the employer mandate in which employers may face penalties if they fail to provide their full-time employees and their dependents (e.g., children) affordable coverage. The ACA penalizes employers who either do not provide coverage or who offer coverage that does not meet the minimum value and affordability standards (Jost 2012; Kaiser Family Foundation 2019). As of 2017, most worksites in the United States offered full (39.1%) or partial payment (45.6%) of health insurance premiums for full-time employees, with only 15.4% offering no coverage (Centers for Disease Control and Prevention, National Center for Chronic Disease Prevention and Health Promotion 2017). Nevertheless, the average deductible amounts for covered workers with plans with deductibles have consistently increased during the past 10 years; people employed in smaller firms are more likely to have higher deductibles for their employer-sponsored plans (Kaiser Family Foundation 2020a).

In 2020, 78% of all civilian workers had access to medical care benefits; however, the proportion varies across occupational sectors: 94% of workers in management, business, and financial sectors receive such benefits compared with 50% of service industry workers (U.S. Bureau of Labor Statistics 2020b). Access to employer-based medical care benefits is much lower among part-time workers (23%) compared to full-time workers (87%) (U.S. Bureau of Labor Statistics 2020b). Union workers have a higher rate of medical care benefits (95%) than non-union workers (68%) (U.S. Bureau of Labor Statistics 2020b).

Although more American adults have had access to medical care and the coverage gaps have diminished since the passage of the ACA, the rates of underinsured adults have increased, particularly among those with employer coverage (The Commonwealth Fund 2019). Workers with average wages placing them in the lowest 25% of wage earners have a coverage rate of 45%, whereas those in the highest 25% of wage earners have a coverage rate of 90% (U.S. Bureau of Labor Statistics 2020b). Even if employment-sponsored benefits are available, low-wage workers may not be able to afford the premiums, copayments, or deductibles (Sherman and Addy 2018; Claxton, Rae, and Panchai 2015; Straw 2019). In 2018, workers with incomes below the federal poverty level had an overall coverage rate of only 15%; this contrasts with a coverage rate of 81% among those with incomes at or greater than 400% of the federal poverty level (Kaiser Family Foundation 2020b). The insurance coverage disparity also is seen along racial/ethnic lines, with 66% of White workers having employer-sponsored coverage, followed by Asian/Native Hawaiian and Pacific Islander (64%), Black (46%), Hispanic (41%), and Native American (36%) workers in 2018 (Kaiser Family Foundation 2020c). Workers in companies with at least 35% of workers earning $26,000 a year or less, moreover, are less likely to be eligible for health benefits than workers in firms with a relatively smaller share of lower-wage workers (Kaiser Family Foundation 2020a).

Low-income workers are more likely to suffer from chronic illness (Harris et al. 2011) and therefore have higher overall health care utilization rates (Pizzi et al. 2005; Sherman et al. 2017). Chronic conditions, especially without treatment, may interfere with low-wage workers' work productivity and chances of receiving a promotion.

Workplace-Based Health Promotion Programs

Workplace-based wellness and health promotion programs are employer initiatives directed at improving the health and well-being of workers and, in some cases, their dependents (Malik, Blake, and Suggs 2014; L. Wilson et al. 2016). Although most workplace-based wellness programs focus primarily on providing traditional health promotion (e.g., tobacco cessation programs, physical activities, and healthy eating programs), health screening, and disease management programs on-site, some model programs integrate on-site elements with health resources outside of the workplace and incorporate these benefits into health insurance plans. Larger worksites offer more health promotion programs, services, and screening programs and policies, but only 17.1% of employers in 2017 offered a comprehensive worksite health promotion program that incorporated five key elements defined in Healthy People 2010: health education, links to related employee services, supportive physical and social environments for health improvement, integration of health promotion into the organization's culture, and employee screenings with adequate treatment and follow-up. This was, however, an increase from 6.9% in 2004 (Linnan et al. 2019).

Paid Sick Leave

Overall, in the United States, approximately 78% of all civilian workers have paid sick leave. This varies markedly by occupation: 92% of workers in management, professional, and related occupations have paid sick leave compared to 62% of workers in service occupations (U.S. Bureau of Labor Statistics 2020b).

At the federal level, the Family Medical Leave Act (FMLA) enacted in 1993 provides eligible employees with at least 12 workweeks of unpaid, job-protected leave for circumstances such as childbirth; a serious personal medical condition; or care of a child, parent, or spouse with a serious medical condition. However, to be covered by FMLA, a worksite must be of a firm that has at least 50 employees. Most worksites are not covered by the FMLA, even those with more than half their employees being eligible (Klerman, Daley, and Pozniak 2012). Only approximately 17% of worksites are covered. Most employees receive some pay while on leave, but nearly half report not being able to afford financially to take more time off (Klerman, Daley, and Pozniak 2012).

Access to paid sick days can help workers recover from illnesses and provide care for sick family members, potentially preventing more severe illness and use of expensive hospital care. Although the Centers for Disease Control and Prevention (2020) recommends that workers who are ill stay home from work to prevent spread of disease in the workplace, following this advice may be difficult or impossible when sick days are unpaid. Lack of paid sick leave is likely to be a significant risk factor for coronavirus transmission (Pichler, Wen, and Ziebarth 2020).

Child Care Resources

Providing child and elder care assistance as a work benefit can be important for the health of workers and their dependents. In addition to the benefits of high-quality child care for children (see Chapter 6), reliable and stable child care can help parents secure and maintain steady employment and reduce workplace absenteeism (Montes and Halterman 2011). Parents of children with chronic health conditions are more likely to have child care-related employment issues (Montes and Halterman 2011; Harper et al. 2013). Finding and paying for high-quality child care can often be difficult for working parents, however, especially low-income parents, and can be a major source of lost productivity in the workplace and chronic stress with its accompanying health risks (Bigras, Lemay, and Brunson 2012).

Elder Care Resources

Providing or finding elder care can become an additional financial and emotional burden for a worker, especially one who also must work outside the home. Six in 10 people in the United States are employed while providing care; one in six employees have reported spending on average more than 20 hours per week providing assistance to a friend or relative (AARP Public Policy Institute 2015; AARP Family Caregiving 2020). These burdens can be greatest on workers in low-wage jobs, who are more likely to work for employers who do not provide paid family leave (Chen 2014). They are also more likely to have particularly limited access both to child and elder care resource and referral services and to employer-provided financial assistance for purchasing care (Lahaie, Earle, and Heymann 2013; Heymann et al. 2002). Stress from struggling to meet work and elderly caregiving responsibilities has been associated with numerous physical, mental, and emotional health problems, including fatigue, depression, and pain symptoms (Colin Reid, Stajduhar, and Chappell 2010; Honda et al. 2014; Kim and Gordon 2014).

Recognizing the implications for productivity, some employers have focused increasing attention on elder care, providing paid leave benefits or paid or unpaid time off for caregiving (AARP Family Caregiving 2020).

Retirement Benefits

Retirement benefits—including Social Security and employment-sponsored retirement plans such as the 401(k)—are a crucial source of steady income support for seniors. In 2020, Social Security was a major source of income for approximately 90% of American adults aged 65 years or older; its benefits represent approximately 33% of the income of the elderly (Social Security Administration 2020). This program has had positive health impacts by reducing poverty and increasing income among older Americans (Schoeni, Freedman, and Martin 2008). However, more recent findings from age-period-cohort models have demonstrated a reverse trend in health outcomes among younger U.S. cohorts who are not currently entering older adulthood (Seeman et al. 2010; Lin et al. 2012). In the United States, low-wage workers in general, and particularly low-wage Black and Latino workers, are less likely than others to be covered by employment-sponsored defined benefit or contribution plans (Rhee 2013); as a result, many low-wage workers enter retirement with very little savings, which can have serious adverse health consequences in the absence of adequate safety nets.

9.7. MAKING WORK HEALTHIER: EXAMPLES OF POLICIES AND PROGRAMS

Efforts to protect and promote workers' health and safety in the United States have historically focused on legislation and regulations intended to prevent work-related accidents and injuries by reducing physical hazards in the workplace. Although such measures remain important, dramatic changes in the nature of work during recent years—a shift from manufacturing to services and knowledge work—call for new strategies that will not only protect workers from major physical hazards but also promote healthier work.

Conclusive knowledge of the most effective and efficient interventions to make work healthier is limited; our current understanding of the health effects of both physical and psychosocial aspects of work and workplaces needs to be broadened and deepened. The existing knowledge base is, however, adequate to point to promising policies and programs that deserve to be carefully implemented and evaluated, using the strongest study designs that are appropriate and feasible, which will not always be randomized controlled trials.

Listed below are selected examples of strategies reflecting a range of approaches to making work healthier; many other examples also would be illustrative. Some, but not all, of the strategies have been evaluated with respect to health outcomes, with varying degrees of scientific rigor. These initiatives may be grouped roughly—with some overlap—into efforts to prevent workplace injury and work-related illness through improvements in worksites and conditions; efforts to prevent stress by changing the way work is organized; actions to promote healthy behaviors through workplace-based interventions;

and initiatives to expand workers' economic opportunities and resources. A final section acknowledges the role of labor unions in improving workers' health in various ways.

The examples below involve efforts by businesses and/or government agencies. Note that some voluntary initiatives by particularly socially responsible employers would be unnecessary if there were a stronger safety net of basic services—for example, free/affordable health care and child care, education benefits, or assurances of healthy conditions in workplaces—covering everyone in the population as a right.

Preventing Work-Related Illness and Injury

- As of August 15, 2020, 36 states, along with the District of Columbia, American Samoa, Guam, the Northern Mariana Islands, Puerto Rico, and the U.S. Virgin Islands, had 100% smoke-free workplace laws in place (American Nonsmokers' Rights Foundation 2020). Implementation of smoke-free workplace policies (prohibiting smoking in all enclosed areas within worksites) has been associated with reduced smoking rates, reduced number of cigarettes smoked by smokers (Titus et al. 2019), reduced exposure to environmental tobacco smoke among non-smokers (Su et al. 2019), and small but significant improvement in measures of cardiovascular health over time among the general population (Gao et al. 2019; Mayne et al. 2018).

- The National Institute for Occupational Safety and Health (NIOSH) is a federal agency created in 1970 to conduct research and make recommendations for the health and safety of workers. It conducts research, education, and training programs, making resources available to workers, employers, and the public. NIOSH also has some regulatory power; however, exercise of this power can be influenced by political conditions (NIOSH 2020a).

- The Ohio Bureau of Workers' Compensation's (2020) safety grant program provides financial and informational assistance to Ohio public and private employers to incorporate evidence-based best practices for ergonomic design in the workplace, such as redesigning video display terminal workstations and modifying methods of providing patient care in health care settings. Findings from data collected by companies before and after interventions indicate reductions in incidence of and days lost to cumulative trauma disorders (Schneider and Hamrick 2004; Hamrick 2001; Fujishiro et al. 2005; Lowe et al. 2019; Wurzelbacher et al. 2014).

Reducing Work-Related Stress

- A social intervention called STAR (Support. Transform. Achieve. Results.) trained supervisors to be more supportive of worker's work–family balance and developed new approaches to "increase employees' control over work time and focus on key results, rather than face-time." Reducing stress due to work–family conflict was a major goal. Researchers concluded that the intervention succeeded in reducing work–family conflict among those most vulnerable and did not adversely impact productivity (Kelly et al. 2014; Moen et al. 2016).

- The Results Only Work Environment (ROWE) strategy focuses on productivity and results of employees' work rather than hours or location worked (CultureRx 2020). Reducing work-related stress, including work–family conflict, without reducing productivity is a major goal. Workers rather than supervisors set work hours, schedules, and location (home versus office). ROWE has had mixed results, working very well in some places and not well in settings in which workers need ongoing supervision and support to be productive (Moen et al. 2011; Peek 2020).

Promoting Healthier Behaviors Through Improved Workplace Environments and Services

- Food Choice at Work (Food Choice 2020): Evidence from a 2016 study of this program indicates its potential for healthier eating and weight loss among participants (Geaney et al. 2016).
- Twenty-one states, Washington, DC, and Puerto Rico have laws related to breastfeeding in the workplace. In Colorado, for example, a law implemented in August 2008 protects an employee's right to breastfeed in a private room (other than a toilet stall) during break time for up to 2 years after giving birth; the law also requires the Department of Labor and Employment to provide information to employers on accommodating employees who breastfeed. At the federal level, Section 4207 of the ACA amends Section 7 of the Fair Labor Standards Act, with some limitations, to require employers to provide employees reasonable break time and a location other than a bathroom to express breast milk for 1 year after a child's birth (Hawkins, Dow-Fleisner, and Noble 2015).
- Goetzel et al. (2014) have reviewed the literature on multiple corporate- and university-sponsored workplace health promotion programs. These programs span a wide range of characteristics.
- Workplace-based interventions (i.e., workshops or trainings) to make work environments healthier also have included efforts to address racism, largely by increasing awareness of the history of racism and awareness of implicit bias among staff of all levels and professions. This approach is discussed in Chapter 5 (Abramovitz and Blitz 2015; Fix 2020).

Expanding Work-Related Economic Opportunities and Resources

Although the following are not generally thought of as initiatives to make work and workplaces healthier, if successful they would likely improve the health of many workers who have limited socioeconomic resources; the health improvement would occur through pathways involved in the health effects of socioeconomic factors.

- The *Job Corps*, created in 1964, is the nation's largest federally funded free job training and education program for disadvantaged youth ages 16–24 years. Under the Department of Labor, it provides career training, job placement, counseling services, and the opportunity to earn a high school diploma or GED (Job Corps 2020). Rigorous evaluations have documented positive impacts for Job

Corps participants, including higher paying jobs and increased levels of educational attainment and literacy (Schochet, Burghardt, and McConnell 2006; Flores et al. 2012).

- As of 2020, 28 states, the District of Columbia, New York City (Internal Revenue Service 2020), and San Francisco (City and County of San Francisco Human Services Agency 2020) offered programs that supplement the federal Earned Income Tax Credit (EITC). For example, the San Francisco Working Families Credit—San Francisco's city/county supplement to the federal EITC, created in 2004 through the efforts of a broad-based coalition of organizations from the public, private, and nonprofit sectors—administers tax credits for low-income workers with children, and it boosts participation of eligible recipients in the federal EITC. The federal EITC has been linked to a range of positive social and health-related outcomes, particularly among families with children (Hamad and Rehkopf 2016; Simon, McInerney, and Goodell 2018; Hoynes, Miller, and Simon 2015), although questions have been raised about its effectiveness in expanding employment (Meyer 2010).
- As of 2020, the following states had mandatory paid sick leave laws: Arizona, California, Colorado, Connecticut, Maine (implementation in 2021), Maryland, Massachusetts, Michigan, Nevada, New Jersey, Oregon, Rhode Island, Vermont, and Washington (National Conference of State Legislatures 2020). Several cities also have paid sick leave policies (National Partnership for Women & Families 2020).

Labor Unions and Workers' Health

Historically, unions have played a major role in protecting workers' health in ways that cut across all of the categories noted above. Labor unions led successful efforts resulting in the 8-hour workday (The Library of Congress 2020), the 5-day workweek, and a range of protections from highly hazardous conditions at work (Malinowski, Minkler, and Stock 2015). Unions have successfully advocated for legislation and enforced standards. They have informed members about their rights with respect to working conditions and about resources for addressing occupational illness/injury. They have helped members receive Workers' Compensation benefits for on-the-job injuries and aided them in disputes over workplace safety (Hagedorn et al. 2016). They have been instrumental in achieving better wages and benefits, including health insurance coverage, for a substantial proportion of the U.S. workforce (Malinowski et al. 2015).

Beginning in the 1970s, however, union membership began to decline, accompanied by declines in resources and bargaining power; in 2015, the union membership rate was approximately half the 1983 rate (Dunn and Walker 2016). Union membership and power have declined as many jobs have been moved outside the United States, where workers' pay and protections are far below U.S. standards. Employers' demands for concessions have correspondingly increased. Unions have become less likely to employ tactics (e.g., protest rallies and marches, strikes, and lawsuits) that historically have been powerful tools used to protect workers' health (Price and Burgard 2008; Malinowski et al. 2015).

9.8. KEY POINTS

- Psychosocial as well as physical aspects of work influence health. Work-related stress plays an important role.
- Organizational justice, the extent to which processes and outcomes in the workplace are perceived to be fair and just, is among the psychosocial influences associated with workers' health. Workplace discrimination based on race/ethnicity, gender, disability, sexual orientation or gender identity is an aspect of organizational injustice.
- Other psychosocial influences thought to influence workers' health include the balance between the demands made on a worker and the worker's degree of control over how the work is performed, and the balance between the level of effort a worker must put into work and the rewards (e.g., pay and recognition) received.
- In addition to earnings, work-related resources such as health care insurance, paid sick leave, and paid parenting/caregiver leave can influence health.

9.9. QUESTIONS FOR DISCUSSION

1. How plausible is the job demand–control model as an influence on health? How could it affect health? How could it affect health disparities by income or by race/ethnic group?
2. How could organizational justice affect workers' health?
3. How could racism in the workplace (a form of organizational injustice) affect health? Discuss at least one other form of discrimination in the workplace (e.g., gender-, disability-, or LGBTQ-related discrimination) and how it could affect health.
4. What are at least three examples of work-related resources (in addition to health insurance) and how could they plausibly affect health?

ACKNOWLEDGMENTS

This chapter builds on "Work Matters for Health," an issue brief supported by the Robert Wood Johnson Foundation, May 2011, by Jane An, Paula Braveman, Mercedes Dekker, Susan Egerter, and Rebecca Grossman-Kahn. Tram Nguyen and Nicole Holm also made contributions to the research for this chapter.

REFERENCES

AARP Family Caregiving. 2020. "2020 report: Caregiving in the U.S." AARP Family Caregiving and the National Alliance for Caregiving. https://www.aarp.org/content/dam/aarp/ppi/2020/05/full-report-caregiving-in-the-united-states.doi.10.26419-2Fppi.00103.001.pdf.

AARP Public Policy Institute. 2015. "2015 report: Caregiving in the U.S." AARP Public Policy Institute and National Alliance for Caregiving. https://www.aarp.org/content/dam/aarp/ppi/2015/caregiving-in-the-united-states-2015-report-revised.pdf.

Abramovitz, M., and L. V. Blitz. 2015. "Moving toward racial equity: The undoing Racism Workshop and organizational change." *Race Soc Problems* 7(2): 97–110. doi:10.1007/s12552-015-9147-4.

Adjei, N. K., and T. Brand. 2018. "Investigating the associations between productive house-work activities, sleep hours and self-reported health among elderly men and women in Western industrialised countries." *BMC Public Health* 18(1): 110. doi:10.1186/s12889-017-4979-z.

Alarcon, W. A. 2016. "Elevated blood lead levels among employed adults—United States, 1994–2013." *MMWR Morb Mortal Wkly Rep* 63(55): 59–65. doi:10.15585/mmwr.mm6355a5.

Aldana, S. G., D. R. Anderson, T. B. Adams, R. W. Whitmer, R. M. Merrill, V. George, and J. Noyce. 2012. "A review of the knowledge base on healthy worksite culture." *J Occup Environ Med* 54(4): 414–419. doi:10.1097/JOM.0b013e31824be25f.

Alves, M. G., Y. H. Hökerberg, and E. Faerstein. 2013. "Trends and diversity in the empirical use of Karasek's demand-control model (job strain): A systematic review." *Rev Bras Epidemiol* 16(1): 125–136. doi:10.1590/s1415-790x2013000100012.

American Nonsmokers' Rights Foundation. 2020. "Overview List—Number of smokefree and other tobacco-related laws." https://no-smoke.org/wp-content/uploads/pdf/mediaordlist.pdf.

Andersen, L. L., N. Fallentin, S. V. Thorsen, and A. Holtermann. 2016. "Physical workload and risk of long-term sickness absence in the general working population and among blue-collar workers: Prospective cohort study with register follow-up." *Occup Environ Med* 73(4): 246–253. doi:10.1136/oemed-2015-103314.

Araujo, M. Y. C., M. C. C. S. Norberto, A. M. Mantovani, B. C. Turi-Lynch, L. L. D. Santos, S. J. Ricardo, L. C. Morais, and J. S. Codogno. 2020. "Obesity increases costs with productivity loss due to disability retirements, independent of physical activity: A cohort study." *J Occup Environ Med* 62(5): 325–330. doi:10.1097/jom.0000000000001808.

Arlinghaus, A., P. Bohle, I. Iskra-Golec, N. Jansen, S. Jay, and L. Rotenberg. 2019. "Working Time Society consensus statements: Evidence-based effects of shift work and non-standard working hours on workers, family and community." *Ind Health* 57(2): 184–200. doi:10.2486/indhealth.SW-4.

Asay, G. R., K. Roy, J. E. Lang, R. L. Payne, and D. H. Howard. 2016. "Absenteeism and employer costs associated with chronic diseases and health risk factors in the US workforce." *Prev Chronic Dis* 13: E141. doi:10.5888/pcd13.150503.

Assari, S., and M. Moghani Lankarani. 2018. "Workplace racial composition explains high perceived discrimination of high socioeconomic status African American men." *Brain Sci* 8(8): 139. doi:10.3390/brainsci8080139.

Attell, B. K., K. Kummerow Brown, and L. A. Treiber. 2017. "Workplace bullying, perceived job stressors, and psychological distress: Gender and race differences in the stress process." *Soc Sci Res* 65: 210–221. https://doi.org/10.1016/j.ssresearch.2017.02.001.

Augustine, J. M. 2014. "Mothers' employment, education, and parenting." *Work Occupations* 41(2): 237–270. doi:10.1177/0730888413501342.

Autor, D. H. 2015. "Why are there still so many jobs? The history and future of workplace automation." *J Econ Perspect* 29(3): 3–30.

Bajwa, U., D. Gastaldo, E. Di Ruggiero, and L. Knorr. 2018. "The health of workers in the global gig economy." *Global Health* 14(1): 124. doi:10.1186/s12992-018-0444-8.

Bakker, A. B., and E. Demerouti. 2014. "Job demands–resources theory." In *Wellbeing: A Complete Reference Guide*, edited by Peter Y. Chen, Cary Cooper, 37–64. Malden, MA: Wiley.

Bannai, A., and A. Tamakoshi. 2014. "The association between long working hours and health: A systematic review of epidemiological evidence." *Scand J Work Environ Health* 40(1): 5–18. doi:10.5271/sjweh.3388.

Bartley, M., J. Ferrie, and S. M. Montgomery. 2006. "Health and labor market disadvantage: Unemployment, non-employment, and job insecurity." In *Social Determinants of Health*, edited by M. Marmot and R. G.

Wilkinson, 2nd ed., 78–95. Oxford: Oxford University Press.

Beckers, D. G. J., D. van der Linden, P. G. W. Smulders, M. A. J. Kompier, T. W. Taris, and S. A. E. Geurts. 2008. "Voluntary or involuntary? Control over overtime and rewards for overtime in relation to fatigue and work satisfaction." *Work Stress* 22(1): 33–50. doi:10.1080/02678370801984927.

Bell, C., D. Johnston, J. Allan, B. Pollard, and M. Johnston. 2017. "What do demand–control and effort–reward work stress questionnaires really measure? A discriminant content validity study of relevance and representativeness of measures." *Br J Health Psychol* 22(2): 295–329. doi:10.1111/bjhp.12232.

Bigras, N., L. Lemay, and L. Brunson. 2012. "Parental stress and daycare attendance: Does daycare quality and parental satisfaction with daycare moderate the relation between family income and stress level among parents of four years old children?" *Procedia* 55: 894–901. https://doi.org/10.1016/j.sbspro.2012.09.578.

Bisht, K., K. Sharma, and M.-È. Tremblay. 2018. "Chronic stress as a risk factor for Alzheimer's disease: Roles of microglia-mediated synaptic remodeling, inflammation, and oxidative stress." *Neurobiol Stress* 9: 9–21. https://doi.org/10.1016/j.ynstr.2018.05.003.

Boucher, P., M. Gilbert-Ouimet, X. Trudel, C. S. Duchaine, A. Milot, and C. Brisson. 2017. "Masked hypertension and effort–reward imbalance at work among 2369 white-collar workers." *J Hum Hypertens* 31(10): 620–626. doi:10.1038/jhh.2017.42.

Brauner, C., A. M. Wöhrmann, K. Frank, and A. Michel. 2019. "Health and work–life balance across types of work schedules: A latent class analysis." *Appl Ergon* 81: 102906. doi:10.1016/j.apergo.2019.102906.

Brewster, Z. W., and M. Lynn. 2014. "Black–White earnings gap among restaurant servers: A replication, extension, and exploration of consumer racial discrimination in tipping." *Sociol Inq* 84(4):545–569. https://doi.org/10.1111/soin.12056.

Bruns, A., and N. Pilkauskas. 2019. "Multiple job holding and mental health among low-income mothers." *Women's Health Issues* 29(3): 205–212. https://doi.org/10.1016/j.whi.2019.01.006.

Buehler, C., M. O'Brien, K. M. Swartout, and N. Zhou. 2014. "Maternal employment and parenting through middle childhood: Contextualizing factors." *J Marriage Fam* 76(5): 1025–1046. doi:10.1111/jomf.12130.

Burgard, S. A., and K. Y. Lin. 2013. "Bad jobs, bad health? How work and working conditions contribute to health disparities." *Am Behav Scientist* 57(8). doi:10.1177/0002764213487347.

Burns, R. A., P. Butterworth, and K. J. Anstey. 2016. "An examination of the long-term impact of job strain on mental health and wellbeing over a 12-year period." *Soc Psychiatry Psychiatr Epidemiol* 51(5): 725–733. doi:10.1007/s00127-016-1192-9.

Cantley, L. F., B. Tessier-Sherman, M. D. Slade, D. Galusha, and M. R. Cullen. 2016. "Expert ratings of job demand and job control as predictors of injury and musculoskeletal disorder risk in a manufacturing cohort." *Occup Environ Med* 73(4): 229–236. doi:10.1136/oemed-2015-102831.

Caruso, C. C. 2014. "Negative impacts of shiftwork and long work hours." *Rehabil Nursing* 39(1): 16–25. doi:10.1002/rnj.107.

Casetta, B., A. J. Videla, A. Bardach, P. Morello, N. Soto, K. Lee, P. A. Camacho, R. V. Hermoza Moquillaza, and A. Ciapponi. 2017. "Association between cigarette smoking prevalence and income level: A systematic review and meta-analysis." *Nicotine Tob Res* 19(12): 1401–1407. doi:10.1093/ntr/ntw266.

Celik, S., K. Celik, E. Dirimese, N. Taşdemir, T. Arik, and İ Büyükkara. 2018. "Determination of pain in musculoskeletal system reported by office workers and the pain risk factors." *Int J Occup Med Environ Health* 31(1): 91–111. doi:10.13075/ijomeh.1896.00901.

Centers for Disease Control and Prevention. 2020. "What to do if you are sick." Last modified September 11, 2020; accessed October 21, 2020. https://www.cdc.gov/coronavirus/2019-ncov/if-you-are-sick/steps-when-sick.html#:~:text=Take%20over%2Dthe%2Dcounter%20medicines,think%20it%20is%20an%20emergency.

Centers for Disease Control and Prevention, National Center for Chronic Disease Prevention and Health Promotion. 2017. *Workplace Health in America 2017*. Atlanta, GA: Centers for Disease Control and Prevention.

Champion, S. L., A. R. Rumbold, E. J. Steele, L. C. Giles, M. J. Davies, and V. M. Moore. 2012. "Parental work schedules and child overweight and obesity." *Int J Obes* 36(4): 573–580. doi:10.1038/ijo.2011.252.

Chavez, L. J., I. J. Ornelas, C. R. Lyles, and E. C. Williams. 2015. "Racial/ethnic workplace discrimination: Association with tobacco and alcohol use." *Am J Prev Med* 48(1): 42–49. doi:10.1016/j.amepre.2014.08.013.

Chen, M.-L. 2014. "The growing costs and burden of family caregiving of older adults: A review of paid sick leave and family leave policies." *The Gerontologist* 56(3): 391–396. doi:10.1093/geront/gnu093.

Chetty, R., M. Stepner, S. Abraham, S. Lin, B. Scuderi, N. Turner, A. Bergeron, and D. Cutler. 2016. "The association between income and life expectancy in the United States, 2001–2014." *JAMA* 315(16): 1750–1766. doi:10.1001/jama.2016.4226.

Cho, Y. 2018. "The effects of nonstandard work schedules on workers' health: A mediating role of work-to-family conflict." *Int J Soc Welfare* 27(1): 74–87. doi:10.1111/ijsw.12269.

Choi, B., P. L. Schnall, H. Yang, M. Dobson, P. Landsbergis, L. Israel, R. Karasek, and D. Baker. 2010. "Sedentary work, low physical job demand, and obesity in US workers." *Am J Ind Med* 53(11): 1088–1101. doi:10.1002/ajim.20886.

Choi, S. D., and K. Brings. 2015. "Work-related musculoskeletal risks associated with nurses and nursing assistants handling overweight and obese patients: A literature review." *Work* 53(2): 439–448. doi:10.3233/wor-152222.

Christie, N., and H. Ward. 2019. "The health and safety risks for people who drive for work in the gig economy." *J Transport Health* 13: 115–127. https://doi.org/10.1016/j.jth.2019.02.007.

City and County of San Francisco Human Services Agency. 2020. "Working families credit (WFC)." Accessed October 20, 2020. https://www.sfhsa.org/services/jobs-money/free-tax-help/how-get-working-families-credit-wfc#.

Claxton, G., M. Rae, and N. Panchai. 2015. "Consumer assets and patient cost sharing." Kaiser Family Foundation. Accessed October 21, 2020. https://www.kff.org/health-costs/issue-brief/consumer-assets-and-patient-cost-sharing.

Cohen-Charash, Y., and P. E. Spector. 2001. "The role of justice in organizations: A meta-analysis." *Organ Behav Hum Decis Process* 86(2): 278–321. doi:10.1006/obhd.2001.2958.

Colin Reid, R., K. I. Stajduhar, and N. L. Chappell. 2010. "The impact of work interferences on family caregiver outcomes." *J Appl Gerontol* 29(3): 267–289. doi:10.1177/0733464809339591.

Collins, C., L. C. Landivar, L. Ruppanner, and W. J. Scarborough. 2021. "COVID-19 and the gender gap in work hours." *Gend Work Organ* 28(S1): 101–112. doi:10.1111/gwao.12506.

Colquitt, J. A. 2001. "On the dimensionality of organizational justice: A construct validation of a measure." *J Appl Psychol* 86(3): 386–400. doi:10.1037/0021-9010.86.3.386.

Colquitt, J. A., D. E. Conlon, M. J. Wesson, C. O. L. H. Porter, and K. Y. Ng. 2001. "Justice at the millennium: A meta-analytic review of 25 years of organizational justice research." *J Appl Psychol* 86(3): 425–445. doi:10.1037/0021-9010.86.3.425.

Colquitt, J. A., J. Greenberg, and C. P. Zapata-Phelan. 2005. "What is organizational justice? A historical overview." In *Handbook of Organizational Justice*, edited by J. Greenberg and J. A. Colquitt, 3–56. Mahwah, NJ: Erlbaum.

Combs, G. M., and I. Milosevic. 2016. "Workplace discrimination and the wellbeing of minority women: Overview, prospects, and implications." In *Handbook on Well-Being of Working Women*, edited by M. L. Connerley and J. Wu, 17–31. Dordrecht, the Netherlands: Springer.

Cox, T. H., Jr. 1993. *Cultural Diversity in Organizations: Theory, Research & Practice*. Oakland, CA: Berrett-Koehler.

Craig, L., and A. Powell. 2011. "Non-standard work schedules, work–family balance and the gendered division of childcare."

Work Employment Society 25(2): 274–291. doi:10.1177/0950017011398894.

Crizzle, A. M., P. Bigelow, D. Adams, S. Gooderham, A. M. Myers, and P. Thiffault. 2017. "Health and wellness of long-haul truck and bus drivers: A systematic literature review and directions for future research." *J Transport Health* 7: 90–109. https://doi.org/10.1016/j.jth.2017.05.359.

CultureRx. 2020. "Results-Only Work Environment (ROWE)." Accessed October 20, 2020. https://www.gorowe.com.

da Costa, B. R., and E. R. Vieira. 2010. "Risk factors for work-related musculoskeletal disorders: A systematic review of recent longitudinal studies." *Am J Ind Med* 53(3): 285–323. doi:10.1002/ajim.20750.

Daly, M. C., G. J. Duncan, P. McDonough, and D. R. Williams. 2002. "Optimal indicators of socioeconomic status for health research." *Am J Public Health* 92(7): 1151–1157. doi:10.2105/ajph.92.7.1151.

Davis, M. E., and E. Hoyt. 2020. "A longitudinal study of piece rate and health: Evidence and implications for workers in the US gig economy." *Public Health* 180: 1–9. https://doi.org/10.1016/j.puhe.2019.10.021.

de Araújo, T. M., J. Siegrist, A. B. Moreno, M. de Jesus Mendes da Fonseca, S. M. Barreto, D. Chor, and R. H. Griep. 2019. "Effort–reward imbalance, over-commitment and depressive episodes at work: Evidence from the ELSA-Brasil Cohort Study." *Int J Environ Res Public Health* 16(17): 3025. doi:10.3390/ijerph16173025.

de Jonge, J., M. F. Dollard, C. Dormann, P. M. Le Blanc, and I. L. D. Houtman. 2000. "The demand–control model: Specific demands, specific control, and well-defined groups." *Int J Stress Manag* 7(4): 269–287. doi:10.1023/A:1009541929536.

de Lange, A. H., T. W. Taris, M. A. Kompier, I. L. Houtman, and P. M. Bongers. 2003. "'The very best of the millennium': Longitudinal research and the demand–control–(support) model." *J Occup Health Psychol* 8(4): 282–305. doi:10.1037/1076-8998.8.4.282.

de Lange, A. H., T. W. Taris, M. A. J. Kompier, I. L. D. Houtman, and P. M. Bongers. 2005. "Different mechanisms to explain the reversed effects of mental health on work

characteristics." *Scand J Work Environ Health* 31(1): 3–14.

Del-Pino-Casado, R., M. Rodríguez Cardosa, C. López-Martínez, and V. Orgeta. 2019. "The association between subjective caregiver burden and depressive symptoms in carers of older relatives: A systematic review and meta-analysis." *PLoS One* 14(5): e0217648. doi:10.1371/journal.pone.0217648.

Dettmers, J. 2017. "How extended work availability affects well-being: The mediating roles of psychological detachment and work–family conflict." *Work Stress* 31(1): 24–41. doi:10.1080/02678373.2017.1298164.

de Wolff, A. 2008. *Employment Insecurity and Health*. Antigonish, Nova Scotia: National Collaborating Centre for Determinants of Health.

Dickey, H., V. Watson, and A. Zangelidis. 2011. "Is it all about money? An examination of the motives behind moonlighting." *Appl Econ* 43(26): 3767–3774. doi:10.1080/00036841003724403.

Dragano, N., J. Siegrist, S. T. Nyberg, T. Lunau, E. I. Fransson, L. Alfredsson, J. B. Bjorner, et al. 2017. "Effort–reward imbalance at work and incident coronary heart disease: A multicohort study of 90,164 individuals." *Epidemiology* 28(4): 619–626. doi:10.1097/ede.0000000000000666.

Duni, A., V. Liakopoulos, S. Roumeliotis, D. Peschos, and E. Dounousi. 2019. "Oxidative stress in the pathogenesis and evolution of chronic kidney disease: Untangling Ariadne's thread." *Int J Mol Sci* 20(15): 3711. doi:10.3390/ijms20153711.

Dunn, M., and J. Walker. 2016. "Union membership in the United States." U.S. Bureau of Labor Statistics. Accessed October 20, 2020. https://www.bls.gov/spotlight/2016/union-membership-in-the-united-states/home.htm.

Dziak, E., B. L. Janzen, and N. Muhajarine. 2010. "Inequalities in the psychological well-being of employed, single and partnered mothers: The role of psychosocial work quality and work-family conflict." *Int J Equity Health* 9: 6. doi:10.1186/1475-9276-9-6.

Eddy, P., E. H. Wertheim, M. W. Hale, and B. J. Wright. 2018. "A systematic review and meta-analysis of the effort–reward imbalance model of workplace stress and hypothalamic–pituitary–adrenal axis measures of stress." *Psychosom Med* 80(1): 103–113. doi:10.1097/psy.0000000000000505.

Eliason, M. J., S. L. Dibble, and P. A. Robertson. 2011. "Lesbian, gay, bisexual, and transgender (LGBT) physicians' experiences in the workplace." *J Homosexuality* 58(10): 1355–1371. doi:10.1080/00918369.2011.614902.

Eliason, M. J., C. Streed, and M. Henne. 2018. "Coping with stress as an LGBTQ+ health care professional." *J Homosexuality* 65(5): 561–578. doi:10.1080/00918369.2017.1328224.

Elovainio, M., T. Heponiemi, H. Kuusio, M. Jokela, A. M. Aalto, L. Pekkarinen, A. Noro, H. Finne-Soveri, M. Kivimäki, and T. Sinervo. 2015. "Job demands and job strain as risk factors for employee wellbeing in elderly care: An instrumental-variables analysis." *Eur J Public Health* 25(1): 103–108. doi:10.1093/eurpub/cku115.

Elovainio, M., A. Linna, M. Virtanen, T. Oksanen, M. Kivimäki, J. Pentti, and J. Vahtera. 2013. "Perceived organizational justice as a predictor of long-term sickness absence due to diagnosed mental disorders: Results from the prospective longitudinal Finnish Public Sector Study." *Soc Sci Med* 91: 39–47. https://doi.org/10.1016/j.socscimed.2013.05.008.

Eskenazi, B., J. Chevrier, S. A. Rauch, K. Kogut, K. G. Harley, C. Johnson, C. Trujillo, A. Sjödin, and A. Bradman. 2013. "In utero and childhood polybrominated diphenyl ether (PBDE) exposures and neurodevelopment in the CHAMACOS study." *Environ Health Perspect* 121(2): 257–262. doi:10.1289/ehp.1205597.

Estill, C. F., C. H. Rice, T. Morata, and A. Bhattacharya. 2017. "Noise and neurotoxic chemical exposure relationship to workplace traumatic injuries: A review." *J Safety Res* 60: 35–42. doi:10.1016/j.jsr.2016.11.005.

Fagundes, C. P., R. Glaser, and J. K. Kiecolt-Glaser. 2013. "Stressful early life experiences and immune dysregulation across the lifespan." *Brain Behav Immun* 27(1): 8–12. doi:10.1016/j.bbi.2012.06.014.

Fan, W., P. Moen, E. L. Kelly, L. B. Hammer, and L. F. Berkman. 2019. "Job strain, time strain, and well-being: A longitudinal, person-centered approach in two industries." *J Vocat Behav* 110(Pt A): 102–116. doi:10.1016/j.jvb.2018.10.017.

Fana, M., S. Torrejón Pérez, and E. Fernández-Macías. 2020. "Employment impact of COVID-19 crisis: From short term effects to long terms prospects." *J Ind Bus Econ* 47: 391–410. doi:10.1007/s40812-020-00168-5.

Fernandez, R. C., J. L. Marino, T. J. Varcoe, S. Davis, L. J. Moran, A. R. Rumbold, H. M. Brown, M. J. Whitrow, M. J. Davies, and V. M. Moore. 2016. "Fixed or rotating night shift work undertaken by women: Implications for fertility and miscarriage." *Semin Reprod Med* 34(2): 74–82. doi:10.1055/s-0036-1571354.

Fischer, F. M., A. Silva-Costa, R. H. Griep, M. H. Smolensky, P. Bohle, and L. Rotenberg. 2019. "Working Time Society consensus statements: Psychosocial stressors relevant to the health and wellbeing of night and shift workers." *Ind Health* 57(2): 175–183. doi:10.2486/indhealth.SW-3.

Fishwick, D. 2014. "Work aggravated asthma; A review of the recent evidence." *Br Med Bull* 110(1): 77–88. doi:10.1093/bmb/ldu004.

Fix, R. L. 2020. "Justice is not blind: A preliminary evaluation of an implicit bias training for justice professionals." *Race Social Problems* 12(4): 362–374. doi:10.1007/s12552-020-09297-x.

Fleischer, N. L., H. M. Tiesman, J. Sumitani, T. Mize, K. Kartik Amarnath, A. Rana Bayakly, and M. W. Murphy. 2013. "Public health impact of heat-related illness among migrant farmworkers." *Am J Prev Med* 44(3): 199–206. https://doi.org/10.1016/j.amepre.2012.10.020.

Flores, C. A., A. Flores-Lagunes, A. Gonzalez, and T. C. Neumann. 2012. "Estimating the effects of length of exposure to instruction in a training program: The case of Job Corps." *Rev Econ Stat* 94(1): 153–171. doi:10.1162/REST_a_00177.

Food Choice. 2020. "Food choice at work." Accessed October 20, 2020. https://www.foodchoiceatwork.com/about-us.

Fouad, A. M., A. Waheed, A. Gamal, S. A. Amer, R. F. Abdellah, and F. M. Shebl. 2017. "Effect of chronic diseases on work productivity: A propensity score analysis." *J Occup Environ Med* 59(5): 480–485. doi:10.1097/jom.0000000000000981.

Friedman, L. S., K. S. Almberg, and R. A. Cohen. 2019. "Injuries associated with long working hours among employees in the US mining industry: Risk factors and adverse outcomes." *Occup Environ Med* 76(6): 389–395. doi:10.1136/oemed-2018-105558.

Fujishiro, K., J. L. Weaver, C. A. Heaney, C. A. Hamrick, and W. S. Marras. 2005. "The effect of ergonomic interventions in healthcare facilities on musculoskeletal disorders." *Am J Ind Med* 48(5): 338–347. doi:10.1002/ajim.20225.

Galupo, M. P., and C. A. Resnick. 2016. "Experiences of LGBT microaggressions in the workplace: Implications for policy." In *Sexual Orientation and Transgender Issues in Organizations: Global Perspectives on LGBT Workforce Diversity*, edited by T. Köllen, 271–287. Cham, Switzerland: Springer.

Gany, F., P. Novo, R. Dobslaw, and J. Leng. 2014. "Urban occupational health in the Mexican and Latino/Latina immigrant population: A literature review." *J Immigr Minor Health* 16(5): 846–855. doi:10.1007/s10903-013-9806-8.

Gao, M., Y. Li, F. Wang, S. Zhang, Z. Qu, X. Wan, X. Wang, J. Yang, D. Tian, and W. Zhang. 2019. "The effect of smoke-free legislation on the mortality rate of acute myocardial infarction: a meta-analysis." *BMC Public Health* 19(1): 1269. doi:10.1186/s12889-019-7408-7.

Geaney, F., C. Kelly, J. Scotto Di Marrazzo, J. M. Harrington, A. P. Fitzgerald, B. A. Greiner, and I. J. Perry. 2016. "The effect of complex workplace dietary interventions on employees' dietary intakes, nutrition knowledge and health status: A cluster controlled trial." *Prev Med* 89: 76–83. https://doi.org/10.1016/j.ypmed.2016.05.005.

Gilbert-Ouimet, M., X. Trudel, C. Brisson, A. Milot, and M. Vézina. 2014. "Adverse effects of psychosocial work factors on blood pressure: Systematic review of studies on demand–control–support and effort–reward imbalance models." *Scand J Work Environ Health* 40(2): 109–132. doi:10.5271/sjweh.3390.

Goetzel, R. Z., R. M. Henke, M. Tabrizi, K. R. Pelletier, R. Loeppke, D. W. Ballard, J. Grossmeier, et al. 2014. "Do workplace health promotion (wellness) programs work?" *J Occup Environ Med* 56(9): 927–934. doi:10.1097/jom.0000000000000276.

Greenberg, J. 1987. "A taxonomy of organizational justice theories." *Acad Manag Rev* 12(1): 9–22. doi:10.5465/amr.1987.4306437.

Greenhaus, J. H., and N. J. Beutell. 1985. "Sources of conflict between work and family roles." *Acad Manag Rev* 10(1): 76–88. doi:10.5465/amr.1985.4277352.

Grineski, S. E., T. W. Collins, and D. X. Morales. 2017. "Asian Americans and disproportionate exposure to carcinogenic hazardous air pollutants: A national study." *Soc Sci Med* 185: 71–80. https://doi.org/10.1016/j.socscimed.2017.05.042.

Haar, J. M., M. Russo, A. Suñe, and A. Ollier-Malaterre. 2014. "Outcomes of work–life balance on job satisfaction, life satisfaction and mental health: A study across seven cultures." *J Vocat Behav* 85(3): 361–373. https://doi.org/10.1016/j.jvb.2014.08.010.

Hagedorn, J., C. A. Paras, H. Greenwich, and A. Hagopian. 2016. "The role of labor unions in creating working conditions that promote public health." *Am J Public Health* 106(6):989–995. doi:10.2105/ajph.2016.303138.

Hall, J. V., and A. B. Krueger. 2018. "An analysis of the labor market for Uber's driver-partners in the United States." *ILR Rev* 71(3): 705–732. doi:10.1177/0019793917717222.

Halonen, J. I., A. Pulakka, J. Vahtera, J. Pentti, H. Laström, S. Stenholm, and L. Magnusson Hanson. 2020. "Commuting time to work and behaviour-related health: A fixed-effect analysis." *Occup Environ Med* 77(2): 77–83. doi:10.1136/oemed-2019-106173.

Hamad, R., and D. H. Rehkopf. 2016. "Poverty and child development: A longitudinal study of the impact of the Earned Income Tax Credit." *Am J Epidemiol* 183(9): 775–784. doi:10.1093/aje/kwv317.

Hammond, W. P., M. Gillen, and I. H. Yen. 2010. "Workplace discrimination and depressive symptoms: A study of multi-ethnic hospital employees." *Race Soc Probl* 2(1): 19–30. doi:10.1007/s12552-010-9024-0.

Hamrick, C. A. 2001. "Proof that ergonomics works: Combined results of over 100 independent ergonomic intervention studies." *Proc Hum Factors Ergonom Soc Annu Meeting* 45(14): 987–991. doi:10.1177/154193120104501442.

Harley, K. G., R. Aguilar Schall, J. Chevrier, K. Tyler, H. Aguirre, A. Bradman, N. T. Holland, R. H. Lustig, A. M. Calafat, and B. Eskenazi. 2013. "Prenatal and postnatal bisphenol A exposure and body mass index in childhood in the CHAMACOS cohort." *Environ Health Perspect* 121(4): 514–520. doi:10.1289/ehp.1205548.

Harnois, C. E., and J. L. Bastos. 2018. "Discrimination, harassment, and gendered health inequalities: Do perceptions of workplace mistreatment contribute to the gender gap in self-reported health?" *J Health Soc Behav* 59(2): 283–299. doi:10.1177/0022146518767407.

Harper, A., T. Taylor Dyches, J. Harper, S. Olsen Roper, and M. South. 2013. "Respite care, marital quality, and stress in parents of children with autism spectrum disorders." *J Autism Dev Disord* 43(11): 2604–2616. doi:10.1007/s10803-013-1812-0.

Harris, J. R., Y. Huang, P. A. Hannon, and B. Williams. 2011. "Low-socioeconomic status workers: Their health risks and how to reach them." *J Occup Environ Med* 53(2): 132–138. doi:10.1097/JOM.0b013e3182045f2c.

Häusser, J. A., A. Mojzisch, M. Niesel, and S. Schulz-Hardt. 2010. "Ten years on: A review of recent research on the job demand–control (–support) model and psychological well-being." *Work Stress* 24(1): 1–35. doi:10.1080/02678371003683747.

Hawkins, S. S., S. Dow-Fleisner, and A. Noble. 2015. "Breastfeeding and the Affordable Care Act." *Pediatr Clin North Am* 62(5): 1071–1091. doi:10.1016/j.pcl.2015.05.002.

Heikkilä, K., E. I. Fransson, S. T. Nyberg, M. Zins, H. Westerlund, P. Westerholm, M. Virtanen, et al.; PD-Work Consortium. 2013. "Job strain and health-related lifestyle: Findings from an individual-participant meta-analysis of 118,000 working adults." *Am J Public Health* 103(11): 2090–2097. doi:10.2105/AJPH.2012.301090.

Henneberger, P. K., M. C. Mirabelli, M. Kogevinas, J. M. Antó, E. Plana, A. Dahlman-Höglund, D. L. Jarvis, et al. 2010. "The occupational contribution to severe exacerbation of asthma." *Eur Respir J* 36(4): 743–750. doi:10.1183/09031936.00135109.

Herber, G.-C., A. Ruijsbroek, M. Koopmanschap, K. Proper, F. van der Lucht, H. Boshuizen, J. Polder, and E. Uiters. 2019. "Single transitions and persistence of unemployment are associated with poor health outcomes." *BMC Public Health* 19(1): 740. doi:10.1186/s12889-019-7059-8.

Herman, J. P., J. M. McKlveen, S. Ghosal, B. Kopp, A. Wulsin, R. Makinson, J. Scheimann, and B. Myers. 2016. "Regulation of the hypothalamic–pituitary–adrenocortical stress response." *Compr Physiol* 6(2): 603–621. doi:10.1002/cphy.c150015.

Herring, C., and L. Henderson. 2016. "Wealth inequality in black and white: Cultural and structural sources of the racial wealth gap." *Race Social Problems* 8(1): 4–17. doi:10.1007/s12552-016-9159-8.

Heymann, J., R. Boynton-Jarrett, P. Carter, J. T. Bond, and E. Galinsky. 2002. *Work–Family Issues and Low-Income Families*. New York, NY: Project on Work, Family, and Democracy at Harvard University.

Hoehner, C. M., C. E. Barlow, P. Allen, and M. Schootman. 2012. "Commuting distance, cardiorespiratory fitness, and metabolic risk." *Am J Prev Med* 42(6): 571–578. doi:10.1016/j.amepre.2012.02.020.

Honda, A., Y. Date, Y. Abe, K. Aoyagi, and S. Honda. 2014. "Work-related stress, caregiver role, and depressive symptoms among Japanese workers." *Saf Health Work* 5(1): 7–12. doi:10.1016/j.shaw.2013.11.002.

Hoynes, H., D. Miller, and D. Simon. 2015. "Income, the Earned Income Tax Credit, and infant health." *Am Econ J Econ Policy* 7(1): 172–211. doi:10.1257/pol.20120179.

Hsieh, N.-H., S.-H. Chung, S.-C. Chen, W.-Y. Chen, Y.-H. Cheng, Y.-J. Lin, S.-H. You, and C.-M. Liao. 2017. "Anemia risk in relation to lead exposure in lead-related manufacturing." *BMC Public Health* 17(1): 389. doi:10.1186/s12889-017-4315-7.

Hu, M., H. Lin, J. Wang, C. Xu, A. J. Tatem, B. Meng, X. Zhang, et al. 2021. "Risk of coronavirus disease 2019 transmission in train passengers: An epidemiological and modeling study." *Clin Infect Dis* 72(4): 604–610. doi:10.1093/cid/ciaa1057.

Internal Revenue Service. 2020. "States and local governments with Earned Income Tax Credit." Accessed October 20, 2020. https://www.irs.gov/credits-deductions/individuals/

earned-income-tax-credit/states-and-local-governments-with-earned-income-tax-credit.

International Labour Organization. 2018. *ILO Global Estimates on International Migrant Workers—Results and Methodology.* Geneva, Switzerland: International Labour Organization.

Jaakkola, M. S., T. K. Lajunen, and J. J. K. Jaakkola. 2020. "Indoor mold odor in the workplace increases the risk of asthma–COPD overlap syndrome: A population-based incident case–control study." *Clin Transl Allergy* 10: 3. doi:10.1186/s13601-019-0307-2.

Jacobsen, H. B., S. E. Reme, G. Sembajwe, K. Hopcia, A. M. Stoddard, C. Kenwood, T. C. Stiles, G. Sorensen, and O. M. Buxton. 2014. "Work–family conflict, psychological distress, and sleep deficiency among patient care workers." *Workplace Health Saf* 62(7): 282–291. doi:10.1177/216507991406200703.

James-Todd, T. M., Y.-H. Chiu, and A. R. Zota. 2016. "Racial/ethnic disparities in environmental endocrine disrupting chemicals and women's reproductive health outcomes: Epidemiological examples across the life course." *Curr Epidemiol Rep* 3(2): 161–180. doi:10.1007/s40471-016-0073-9.

Janlert, U., A. H. Winefield, and A. Hammarström. 2015. "Length of unemployment and health-related outcomes: A life-course analysis." *Eur J Public Health* 25(4): 662–667. doi:10.1093/eurpub/cku186.

Job Corps. 2020. "Job Corps." Accessed October 20, 2020. https://www.jobcorps.gov.

Jolly, S., K. A. Griffith, R. DeCastro, A. Stewart, P. Ubel, and R. Jagsi. 2014. "Gender differences in time spent on parenting and domestic responsibilities by high-achieving young physician-researchers." *Ann Intern Med* 160(5): 344–353. doi:10.7326/M13-0974.

Jost, T. 2012, December 29. "Implementing health reform: The employer mandate." Health Affairs. https://www.healthaffairs.org/do/10.1377/hblog20121229.026707/full.

Jung, A.-K., and K. M. O'Brien. 2019. "The profound influence of unpaid work on women's lives: An overview and future directions." *J Career Dev* 46(2): 184–200. doi:10.1177/0894845317734648.

Kaiser Family Foundation. 2019. "Employer responsibility under the Affordable Care Act."

Accessed October 21, 2020. https://www.kff.org/infographic/employer-responsibility-under-the-affordable-care-act.

Kaiser Family Foundation. 2020a. "2020 Employer Health Benefits Survey." https://www.kff.org/health-costs/report/2020-employer-health-benefits-survey.

Kaiser Family Foundation. 2020b. "Employer-sponsored coverage rates for the nonelderly by Federal Poverty Level (FPL)." Accessed October 21, 2020. https://www.kff.org/other/state-indicator/rate-by-fpl-2.

Kaiser Family Foundation. 2020c. "Employer-sponsored coverage rates for the nonelderly by race/ethnicity." Accessed October 21, 2020. https://www.kff.org/other/state-indicator/rate-by-raceethnicity-2.

Karasek, R., D. Baker, F. Marxer, A. Ahlbom, and T. Theorell. 1981. "Job decision latitude, job demands, and cardiovascular disease: A prospective study of Swedish men." *Am J Public Health* 71(7): 694–705. doi:10.2105/ajph.71.7.694.

Karasek, R. A. 1979. "Job demands, job decision latitude, and mental strain: Implications for job redesign." *Admin Sci Q* 24(2): 285–308. doi:10.2307/2392498.

Karatsoreos, I. N., and B. S. McEwen. 2013. "Resilience and vulnerability: A neurobiological perspective." *F1000prime Rep* 5: 13–13. doi:10.12703/P5-13.

Kelly, E. L., P. Moen, J. M. Oakes, W. Fan, C. Okechukwu, K. D. Davis, L. B. Hammer, et al. 2014. "Changing work and work–family conflict: Evidence from the Work, Family, and Health Network." *Am Sociol Rev* 79(3): 485–516. doi:10.1177/0003122414531435.

Kervezee, L., A. Shechter, and D. B. Boivin. 2018. "Impact of shift work on the circadian timing system and health in women." *Sleep Med Clin* 13(3): 295–306. https://doi.org/10.1016/j.jsmc.2018.04.003.

Khubchandani, J., and J. H. Price. 2017. "Association of job insecurity with health risk factors and poorer health in American workers." *J Community Health* 42(2): 242–251. doi:10.1007/s10900-016-0249-8.

Kim, N., and J. R. Gordon. 2014. "Addressing the stress of work and elder caregiving of the graying workforce: The moderating effects of financial strain on the relationship between work–caregiving conflict and psychological well-being." *Hum Resour Manag* 53(5): 723–747. doi:10.1002/hrm.21582.

King, D. M., and S. H. Jacobson. 2017. "What is driving obesity? A review on the connections between obesity and motorized transportation." *Curr Obes Rep* 6(1): 3–9. doi:10.1007/s13679-017-0238-y.

Kivimäki, M., S. T. Nyberg, G. D. Batty, E. I. Fransson, K. Heikkilä, L. Alfredsson, J. B. Bjorner, et al. 2012. "Job strain as a risk factor for coronary heart disease: A collaborative meta-analysis of individual participant data." *Lancet* 380(9852): 1491–1497. https://doi.org/10.1016/S0140-6736(12)60994-5.

Kivimäki, M., and A. Steptoe. 2018. "Effects of stress on the development and progression of cardiovascular disease." *Nat Rev Cardiol* 15(4): 215–229. doi:10.1038/nrcardio.2017.189.

Klerman, J., K. Daley, and A. Pozniak. 2012. *Family and Medical Leave in 2012: Technical Report*. Atlanta, GA: Abt Associates.

Kobayashi, Y., and N. Kondo. 2019. "Organizational justice, psychological distress, and stress-related behaviors by occupational class in female Japanese employees." *PLoS One* 14(4): e0214393. doi:10.1371/journal.pone.0214393.

Krieger, N. 2014. "Discrimination and health inequities." *Int J Health Services* 44(4): 643–710. doi:10.2190/HS.44.4.b.

Kristenson, M., H. R. Eriksen, J. K. Sluiter, D. Starke, and H. Ursin. 2004. "Psychobiological mechanisms of socioeconomic differences in health." *Soc Sci Med* 58(8): 1511–1522. https://doi.org/10.1016/S0277-9536(03)00353-8.

Lachapelle, U., L. Frank, B. E. Saelens, J. F. Sallis, and T. L. Conway. 2011. "Commuting by public transit and physical activity: Where you live, where you work, and how you get there." *J Phys Act Health* 8(Suppl 1): S72–S82. doi:10.1123/jpah.8.s1.s72.

Lahaie, C., A. Earle, and J. Heymann. 2013. "An uneven burden: Social disparities in adult caregiving responsibilities, working conditions, and caregiver outcomes." *Res Aging* 35(3): 243–274. doi:10.1177/0164027512446028.

Lallukka, T., L. Kaila-Kangas, M. Mänty, S. Koskinen, E. Haukka, J. Kausto, P. Leino-Arjas, R. Kaikkonen, J. I. Halonen, and R. Shiri. 2019. "Work-related exposures and sickness absence trajectories: A nationally representative follow-up study among Finnish working-aged people." *Int J Environ Res Public Health* 16(12): 2099. doi:10.3390/ijerph16122099.

Landsbergis, P. A., A. V. Diez-Roux, K. Fujishiro, S. Baron, J. D. Kaufman, J. D. Meyer, G. Koutsouras, et al. 2015. "Job strain, occupational category, systolic blood pressure, and hypertension prevalence: The Multi-Ethnic Study of Atherosclerosis." *J Occup Environ Med* 57(11): 1178–1184. doi:10.1097/jom.0000000000000533.

Landsbergis, P. A., J. G. Grzywacz, and A. D. LaMontagne. 2014. "Work organization, job insecurity, and occupational health disparities." *Am J Ind Med* 57(5): 495–515. doi:10.1002/ajim.22126.

Lee, Y., and F. Tang. 2015. "More caregiving, less working: Caregiving roles and gender difference." *J Appl Gerontol* 34(4): 465–483. doi:10.1177/0733464813508649.

Legrain, A., N. Eluru, and A. M. El-Geneidy. 2015. "Am stressed, must travel: The relationship between mode choice and commuting stress." *Transport Res F Traffic Psychol Behav* 34: 141–151. https://doi.org/10.1016/j.trf.2015.08.001.

Leigh, J. P. 2011. "Economic burden of occupational injury and illness in the United States." *Milbank Q* 89(4): 728–772. doi:10.1111/j.1468-0009.2011.00648.x.

Leineweber, C., M. Baltzer, L. L. Magnusson Hanson, and H. Westerlund. 2012. "Work–family conflict and health in Swedish working women and men: A 2-year prospective analysis (the SLOSH study)." *Eur J Public Health* 23(4): 710–716. doi:10.1093/eurpub/cks064.

Lewis, T. T., C. D. Cogburn, and D. R. Williams. 2015. "Self-reported experiences of discrimination and health: Scientific advances, ongoing controversies, and emerging issues." *Annu Rev Clin Psychol* 11(1): 407–440. doi:10.1146/annurev-clinpsy-032814-112728.

Li, J., S. E. Johnson, W.-J. Han, S. Andrews, G. Kendall, L. Strazdins, and A. Dockery. 2014. "Parents' nonstandard work schedules and child well-being: A critical review of the literature." *J Primary Prev* 35(1): 53–73. doi:10.1007/s10935-013-0318-z.

Liguori, I., G. Russo, F. Curcio, G. Bulli, L. Aran, D. Della-Morte, G. Gargiulo, G. Testa, F. Cacciatore, D. Bonaduce, and P. Abete. 2018. "Oxidative stress, aging, and diseases." *Clin Interv Aging* 13: 757–772. doi:10.2147/cia.S158513.

Lin, S.-F., A. N. Beck, B. K. Finch, R. A. Hummer, and R. K. Master. 2012. "Trends in US older adult disability: Exploring age, period, and cohort effects." *Am J Public Health* 102(11): 2157–2163. doi:10.2105/ajph.2011.300602.

Linnan, L. A., L. Cluff, J. E. Lang, M. Penne, and M. S. Leff. 2019. "Results of the Workplace Health in America Survey." *Am J Health Promot* 33(5): 652–665. doi:10.1177/0890117119842047.

Litchfield, P., C. Cooper, C. Hancock, and P. Watt. 2016. "Work and wellbeing in the 21st century." *Int J Environ Res Public Health* 13(11): 1065. doi:10.3390/ijerph13111065.

Lloren, A., and L. Parini. 2017. "How LGBT-supportive workplace policies shape the experience of lesbian, gay men, and bisexual employees." *Sex Res Soc Policy* 14(3): 289–299. doi:10.1007/s13178-016-0253-x.

Lo, J. C., J. A. Groeger, G. H. Cheng, D. J. Dijk, and M. W. Chee. 2016. "Self-reported sleep duration and cognitive performance in older adults: A systematic review and meta-analysis." *Sleep Med* 17: 87–98. doi:10.1016/j.sleep.2015.08.021.

Lowe, B., J. Albers, M. Hayden, M. Lampl, S. Naber, and S. Wurzelbacher. 2019. *Equipment Interventions to Improve Construction Industry Safety and Health: A Review of Case Studies.* Cham, Switzerland: Springer.

Malik, S. H., H. Blake, and L. S. Suggs. 2014. "A systematic review of workplace health promotion interventions for increasing physical activity." *Br J Health Psychol* 19(1): 149–180. doi:10.1111/bjhp.12052.

Malinowski, B., M. Minkler, and L. Stock. 2015. "Labor unions: A public health institution." *Am J Public Health* 105(2): 261–271. doi:10.2105/ajph.2014.302309.

Malos, S., G. V. Lester, and M. Virick. 2018. "Uber drivers and employment status in the gig economy: Should corporate social responsibility tip the scales?" *Employee Responsibilities Rights J* 30(4): 239–251. doi:10.1007/s10672-018-9325-9.

Mandel, H., and M. Semyonov. 2014. "Gender pay gap and employment sector: Sources of earnings disparities in the United States, 1970–2010." *Demography* 51(5): 1597–1618. doi:10.1007/s13524-014-0320-y.

Marmot, M. G., H. Bosma, H. Hemingway, E. Brunner, and S. Stansfeld. 1997. "Contribution of job control and other risk factors to social variations in coronary heart disease incidence." *Lancet* 350(9073): 235–239. doi:10.1016/s0140-6736(97)04244-x.

Marucci-Wellman, H. R., D. A. Lombardi, and J. L. Willetts. 2016. "Working multiple jobs over a day or a week: Short-term effects on sleep duration." *Chronobiol Int* 33(6): 630–649. doi:10.3109/07420528.2016.1167717.

Marucci-Wellman, H. R., J. L. Willetts, T.-C. Lin, M. J. Brennan, and S. K. Verma. 2014. "Work in multiple jobs and the risk of injury in the US working population." *Am J Public Health* 104(1): 134–142. doi:10.2105/AJPH.2013.301431.

Matilla-Santander, N., J. C. Martín-Sánchez, A. González-Marrón, À. Cartanyà-Hueso, C. Lidón-Moyano, and J. M. Martínez-Sánchez. 2021. "Precarious employment, unemployment and their association with health-related outcomes in 35 European countries: A cross-sectional study." *Crit Public Health* 31(4): 404–415. doi:10.1080/09581596.2019.1701183.

Mausner-Dorsch, H., and W. W. Eaton. 2000. "Psychosocial work environment and depression: Epidemiologic assessment of the demand–control model." *Am J Public Health* 90(11): 1765–1770. doi:10.2105/ajph.90.11.1765.

Mayne, S. L., D. R. Jacobs, P. J. Schreiner, R. Widome, P. Gordon-Larsen, and K. N. Kershaw. 2018. "Associations of smoke-free policies in restaurants, bars, and workplaces with blood pressure changes in the CARDIA study." *J Am Heart Assoc* 7(23): e009829. doi:10.1161/JAHA.118.009829.

McCauley, L. A., W. K. Anger, M. Keifer, R. Langley, M. G. Robson, and D. Rohlman. 2006. "Studying health outcomes in farmworker populations exposed to pesticides." *Environ Health Perspect* 114(6): 953–960. doi:10.1289/ehp.8526.

McCord, M. A., D. L. Joseph, L. Y. Dhanani, and J. M. Beus. 2018. "A meta-analysis of sex and race differences in perceived workplace mistreatment." *J Appl Psychol* 103(2): 137–163. doi:10.1037/apl0000250.

McEwen, B. S. 2013. "The brain on stress: Toward an integrative approach to brain, body, and behavior." *Perspect Psychol Sci* 8(6): 673–675. doi:10.1177/1745691613506907.

McEwen, B. S. 2017. "Neurobiological and systemic effects of chronic stress." *Chronic Stress* 1: 2470547017692328. doi:10.1177/2470547017692328.

Mellor, S., and R. E Decker. 2020. "Multiple jobholders with families: A path from jobs held to psychological stress through work–family conflict and performance quality." *Employee Responsibilities Rights J* 32: 1–21.

Ménard, C., M. L. Pfau, G. E. Hodes, and S. J. Russo. 2017. "Immune and neuroendocrine mechanisms of stress vulnerability and resilience." *Neuropsychopharmacology* 42(1): 62–80. doi:10.1038/npp.2016.90.

Mensah, A., and N. K. Adjei. 2020. "Work–life balance and self-reported health among working adults in Europe: A gender and welfare state regime comparative analysis." *BMC Public Health* 20(1): 1052. doi:10.1186/s12889-020-09139-w.

Meyer, B. D. 2010. "The effects of the Earned Income Tax Credit and recent reforms." *Tax Policy Econ* 24(1):153–180. doi:10.1086/649831.

Miller, S. 2020. "Black workers still earn less than their White counterparts." https://www.shrm.org/resourcesandtools/hr-topics/compensation/pages/racial-wage-gaps-persistence-poses-challenge.aspx

Moen, P., E. L. Kelly, W. Fan, S.-R. Lee, D. Almeida, E. E. Kossek, and O. M. Buxton. 2016. "Does a flexibility/support organizational initiative improve high-tech employees' well-being? Evidence from the Work, Family, and Health Network." *Am Sociol Rev* 81(1): 134–164. doi:10.1177/0003122415622391.

Moen, P., E. L. Kelly, E. Tranby, and Q. Huang. 2011. "Changing work, changing health: Can real work-time flexibility promote health behaviors and well-being?" *J Health Soc Behav* 52(4): 404–429. doi:10.1177/0022146511418979.

Montes, G., and J. S. Halterman. 2011. "The impact of child care problems on employment: Findings from a national survey of US parents." *Acad Pediatr* 11(1): 80–87. doi:10.1016/j.acap.2010.11.005.

Moyce, S. C., and M. Schenker. 2018. "Migrant workers and their occupational health and safety." *Annu Rev Public Health* 39(1): 351–365. doi:10.1146/annurev-publhealth-040617-013714.

Mravec, B., L. Horvathova, and A. Padova. 2018. "Brain under stress and Alzheimer's disease." *Cell Mol Neurobiol* 38(1): 73–84. doi:10.1007/s10571-017-0521-1.

Muntaner, C. 2018. "Digital platforms, gig economy, precarious employment, and the invisible hand of social class." *Int J Health Serv* 48(4): 597–600. doi:10.1177/0020731418801413.

National Conference of State Legislatures. 2020. "Paid sick leave." Accessed October 20, 2020. https://www.ncsl.org/research/labor-and-employment/paid-sick-leave.aspx.

National Partnership for Women & Families. 2020. "Current sick days laws." Accessed October 20, 2020. http://paidsickdays.org/research-resources/current-sick-days-laws.html.

National Research Council. 2011. *Assessing 21st Century Skills: Summary of a Workshop*, edited by J. Anderson Koenig. Washington, DC: National Academies Press.

National Research Council. 2012. *Education for Life and Work: Developing Transferable Knowledge and Skills in the 21st Century*, edited by J. W. Pellegrino and M. L. Hilton. Washington, DC: National Academies Press.

Ndjaboué, R., C. Brisson, and M. Vézina. 2012. "Organisational justice and mental health: A systematic review of prospective studies." *Occup Environ Med* 69(10): 694–700. doi:10.1136/oemed-2011-100595.

Nielsen, M. K., M. A. Neergaard, A. B. Jensen, F. Bro, and M.-B. Guldin. 2016. "Psychological distress, health, and socio-economic factors in caregivers of terminally ill patients: A nationwide population-based cohort study." *Support Care Cancer* 24 (7): 3057–3067. doi:10.1007/s00520-016-3120-7.

Norström, F., A.-K. Waenerlund, L. Lindholm, R. Nygren, K.-G. Sahlén, and A. Brydsten. 2019.

"Does unemployment contribute to poorer health-related quality of life among Swedish adults?" *BMC Public Health* 19(1): 457. doi:10.1186/s12889-019-6825-y.

Notelaers, G., M. Törnroos, and D. Salin. 2019. "Effort–reward imbalance: A risk factor for exposure to workplace bullying." *Front Psychol* 10: 386. doi:10.3389/fpsyg.2019.00386.

Nyberg, S. T., E. I. Fransson, K. Heikkilä, L. Alfredsson, A. Casini, E. Clays, D. De Bacquer, et al. 2013. "Job strain and cardiovascular disease risk factors: Meta-analysis of individual-participant data from 47,000 men and women." *PLoS One* 8(6): e67323. doi:10.1371/journal.pone.0067323.

Obeng-Gyasi, E. 2019. "Lead exposure and cardiovascular disease among young and middle-aged adults." *Med Sci* 7(11): 103. doi:10.3390/medsci7110103.

Ogden, C. L., T. H. Fakhouri, M. D. Carroll, C. M. Hales, C. D. Fryar, X. Li, and D. S. Freedman. 2017. "Prevalence of obesity among adults, by household income and education—United States, 2011–2014." *MMWR Morb Mortal Wkly Rep* 66(50): 1369–1373. doi:10.15585/mmwr.mm6650a1.

Ohio Bureau of Workers' Compensation. 2020. Accessed October 20, 2020. https://info.bwc.ohio.gov/wps/portal/gov/bwc/home.

Okechukwu, C. A., K. Souza, K. D. Davis, and A. B. de Castro. 2014. "Discrimination, harassment, abuse, and bullying in the workplace: Contribution of workplace injustice to occupational health disparities." *Am J Ind Med* 57(5): 573–586. doi:10.1002/ajim.22221.

Oliveira, B. S., M. V. Zunzunegui, J. Quinlan, H. Fahmi, M. T. Tu, and R. O. Guerra. 2016. "Systematic review of the association between chronic social stress and telomere length: A life course perspective." *Ageing Res Rev* 26: 37–52. doi:10.1016/j.arr.2015.12.006.

Ostry, A. S., S. Kelly, P. A. Demers, C. Mustard, and C. Hertzman. 2003. "A comparison between the effort–reward imbalance and demand control models." *BMC Public Health* 3(1): 10. doi:10.1186/1471-2458-3-10.

Payne, J., L. Cluff, J. Lang, D. Matson-Koffman, and A. Morgan-Lopez. 2018. "Elements of a workplace culture of health, perceived organizational support for health, and lifestyle risk." *Am J Health Promot* 32(7): 1555–1567. doi:10.1177/0890117118758235.

Peek, S. 2020. "Do results-only workplaces really work?" business.com. Last modified April 6, 2020. Accessed October 20, 2020. https://www.business.com/articles/do-results-only-workplaces-really-work.

Perreault, M., E. H. Touré, N. Perreault, and J. Caron. 2017. "Employment status and mental health: Mediating roles of social support and coping strategies." *Psychiatr Q* 88(3): 501–514. doi:10.1007/s11126-016-9460-0.

Pew Research Center. 2013. "On pay gap, millennial women near parity—for now: Despite gains, many see roadblocks ahead. https://www.pewresearch.org/social-trends/2013/12/11/on-pay-gap-millennial-women-near-parity-for-now.

Pew Research Center. 2015a. "Parenting in America: Outlook, worries, aspirations are strongly linked to financial situation." https://www.pewresearch.org/social-trends/2015/12/17/parenting-in-america.

Pew Research Center. 2015b. "Raising kids and running a household: How working parents share the load." https://www.pewresearch.org/social-trends/2015/11/04/raising-kids-and-running-a-household-how-working-parents-share-the-load.

Pichler, S., K. Wen, and N. Ziebarth. 2020. "COVID-19 emergency sick leave has helped flatten the curve in the United States." *Health Affairs* 39 (12). doi:10.1377/hlthaff.2020.00863.

Pietiläinen, M., J. Nätti, and S. Ojala. 2020. "Perceived gender discrimination at work and subsequent long-term sickness absence among Finnish employed women." *Eur J Public Health* 30(2): 311–316. doi:10.1093/eurpub/ckz156.

Pizzi, L. T., C. T. Carter, J. B. Howell, S. M. Vallow, A. G. Crawford, and E. D. Frank. 2005. "Work loss, healthcare utilization, and costs among US employees with chronic pain." *Dis Manag Health Outcomes* 13(3): 201–208. doi:10.2165/00115677-200513030-00005.

Polachek, A. J., and J. E. Wallace. 2015. "Unfair to me or unfair to my spouse: Men's and women's perceptions of domestic equity and how they relate to mental and physical health." *Marriage Fam Rev* 51(3): 205–228. doi:10.1080/01494929.2015.1031420.

Powell, N. D., A. J. Tarr, and J. F. Sheridan. 2013. "Psychosocial stress and inflammation in cancer." *Brain Behav Immun* 30(Suppl): S41–S47. doi:10.1016/j.bbi.2012.06.015.

Power, K. 2020. "The COVID-19 pandemic has increased the care burden of women and families." *Sustainability* 16(1): 67–73. doi:10.1080/15487733.2020.1776561.

Prasad, K. N., M. Wu, and S. C. Bondy. 2017. "Telomere shortening during aging: Attenuation by antioxidants and anti-inflammatory agents." *Mech Ageing Dev* 164: 61–66. https://doi.org/10.1016/j.mad.2017.04.004.

Price, R., and S. Burgard. 2008. "The new employment contract and worker health in the United States." In *Making Americans Healthier: Social and Economic Policy as Health Policy*, edited by R. Schoeni, J. House, G. Kaplan, and H. Pollack, 173–199. New York, NY: Russell Sage Foundation.

Ranasinghe, P., Y. S. Perera, D. A. Lamabadusuriya, S. Kulatunga, N. Jayawardana, S. Rajapakse, and P. Katulanda. 2011. "Work related complaints of neck, shoulder and arm among computer office workers: A cross-sectional evaluation of prevalence and risk factors in a developing country." *Environ Health* 10: 70. doi:10.1186/1476-069X-10-70.

Revenson, T., K. Griva, A. Luszczynska, V. Morrison, E. Panagopoulou, N. Vilchinsky, and M. Hagedoorn. 2016. "Gender and caregiving: The costs of caregiving for women." In *Caregiving in the Illness Context*, 48–63. London, UK: Palgrave Pivot.

Rhee, N. 2013. "Race and retirement insecurity in the United States." National Institute on Retirement Security. https://www.nirsonline.org/reports/race-and-retirement-insecurity-in-the-united-states.

Rocco, P. T. P., I. M. Bensenor, R. H. Griep, A. B. Moreno, A. P. Alencar, P. A. Lotufo, and I. S. Santos. 2017. "Job strain and cardiovascular health score (from the Brazilian Longitudinal Study of Adult Health [ELSA-Brasil] Baseline)." *Am J Cardiol* 120(2): 207–212. doi:10.1016/j.amjcard.2017.04.008.

Rosenthal, L., A. Carroll-Scott, V. A. Earnshaw, A. Santilli, and J. R. Ickovics. 2012. "The importance of full-time work for urban adults' mental and physical health." *Soc Sci Med* 75(9): 1692–1696. https://doi.org/10.1016/j.socscimed.2012.07.003.

Rothstein, R. 2017. *The Color of Law: A Forgotten History of How Our Government Segregated America*. New York, NY: Liveright.

Rubin, R. 2016. "Despite potential health benefits of maternity leave, US lags behind other industrialized countries." *JAMA* 315(7): 643–645. doi:10.1001/jama.2015.18609.

Russell, G., and S. Lightman. 2019. "The human stress response." *Nat Rev Endocrinol* 15(9): 525–534. doi:10.1038/s41574-019-0228-0.

Sabbath, E. L., I. Mejía-Guevara, C. Noelke, and L. F. Berkman. 2015. "The long-term mortality impact of combined job strain and family circumstances: A life course analysis of working American mothers." *Soc Sci Med* 146: 111–119. doi:10.1016/j.socscimed.2015.10.024.

Sareen, J., T. O. Afifi, K. A. McMillan, and G. J. G. Asmundson. 2011. "Relationship between household income and mental disorders: Findings from a population-based longitudinal study." *Arch Gen Psychiatry* 68(4): 419–427. doi:10.1001/archgenpsychiatry.2011.15.

Schaufeli, W. B., and T. W. Taris. 2014. "A critical review of the job demands–resources model: Implications for improving work and health." In *Bridging Occupational, Organizational and Public Health: A Transdisciplinary Approach*, 43–68. Dordrecht, the Netherlands: Springer.

Schneider, S., and C. A. Hamrick. 2004. "Ergonomics." *J Occup Environ Hygiene* 1(4): D42–D46. doi:10.1080/15459620490432051.

Schnettler, B., E. Miranda-Zapata, G. Lobos, M. Saracostti, M. Denegri, M. Lapo, and C. Hueche. 2018. "The mediating role of family and food-related life satisfaction in the relationships between family support, parent work–life balance and adolescent life satisfaction in dual-earner families." *Int J Environ Res Public Health* 15(11): 2549. doi:10.3390/ijerph15112549.

Schochet, P. Z., J. Burghardt, and S. McConnell. 2006. "National Job Corps Study and longer-term follow-up study: Impact and benefit–cost findings using survey and summary earnings records data—Final report." Princeton, NJ: Mathematica Policy Research.

Schoeni, R. F., V. A. Freedman, and L. G. Martin. 2008. "Why is late-life disability declining?" *Milbank Q* 86(1): 47–89. doi:10.1111/j.1468-0009.2007.00513.x.

Sears, J. M., A. T. Edmonds, and N. B. Coe. 2020. "Coverage gaps and cost-shifting for work-related injury and illness: Who bears the financial burden?" *Med Care Res Rev* 77(3): 223–235. doi:10.1177/1077558719845726.

Seeman, T. E., S. S. Merkin, E. M. Crimmins, and A. S. Karlamangla. 2010. "Disability trends among older Americans: National Health and Nutrition Examination Surveys, 1988–1994 and 1999–2004." *Am J Public Health* 100(1): 100–107. doi:10.2105/ajph.2008.157388.

Seeman, T. E., D. Thomas, S. Stein Merkin, K. Moore, K. Watson, and A. Karlamangla. 2018. "The Great Recession worsened blood pressure and blood glucose levels in American adults." *Proc Natl Acad Sci USA* 115(13): 3296. doi:10.1073/pnas.1710502115.

Semega, J., M. Kollar, J. Creamer, and A. Mohanty. 2019. "Income and Poverty in the United States: 2018." U.S. Census Bureau. https://www.census.gov/library/publications/2019/demo/p60-266.html.

Shammas, M. A. 2011. "Telomeres, lifestyle, cancer, and aging." *Curr Opin Clin Nutr Metab Care* 14(1): 28–34. doi:10.1097/MCO.0b013e32834121b1.

Shan, Z., Y. Li, G. Zong, Y. Guo, J. Li, J. E. Manson, F. B. Hu, W. C. Willett, E. S. Schernhammer, and S. N. Bhupathiraju. 2018. "Rotating night shift work and adherence to unhealthy lifestyle in predicting risk of type 2 diabetes: Results from two large US cohorts of female nurses." *BMJ* 363: k4641. doi:10.1136/bmj.k4641.

Sherman, B. W., and C. Addy. 2018. "Low-wage workers and health benefits use: Are we missing an opportunity?" *Popul Health Manag* 21(6): 435–437. doi:10.1089/pop.2017.0191.

Sherman, B. W., T. B. Gibson, W. D. Lynch, and C. Addy. 2017. "Health care use and spending patterns vary by wage level

in employer-sponsored plans." *Health Affairs* 36(2): 250–257. doi:10.1377/hlthaff.2016.1147.

Siegrist, J. 1996. "Adverse health effects of high-effort/low-reward conditions." *J Occup Health Psychol* 1(1): 27–41. doi:10.1037/1076-8998.1.1.27.

Siegrist, J., and J. Li. 2016. "Associations of extrinsic and intrinsic components of work stress with health: A systematic review of evidence on the effort–reward imbalance model." *Int J Environ Res Public Health* 13(4): 432. doi:10.3390/ijerph13040432.

Siegrist, J., K. Siegrist, and I. Weber. 1986. "Sociological concepts in the etiology of chronic disease: The case of ischemic heart disease." *Soc Sci Med* 22(2): 247–253. https://doi.org/10.1016/0277-9536(86)90073-0.

Simon, D., M. McInerney, and S. Goodell. 2018. *The Earned Income Tax Credit, Poverty, and Health*. Bethesda, MD: Health Affairs.

Slopen, N., R. J. Glynn, J. E. Buring, T. T. Lewis, D. R. Williams, and M. A. Albert. 2012. "Job strain, job insecurity, and incident cardiovascular disease in the Women's Health Study: Results from a 10-year prospective study." *PLoS One* 7(7): e40512. doi:10.1371/journal.pone.0040512.

Social Security Administration. 2020. "Fact sheet: Social Security." Accessed October 22, 2020. https://www.ssa.gov/news/press/factsheets/basicfact-alt.pdf.

Sojo, V. E., R. E. Wood, and A. E. Genat. 2016. "Harmful workplace experiences and women's occupational well-being: A meta-analysis." *Psychol Women Q* 40(1): 10–40. doi:10.1177/0361684315599346.

Stanbury, M., and K. D. Rosenman. 2014. "Occupational health disparities: A state public health-based approach." *Am J Ind Med* 57(5): 596–604. doi:10.1002/ajim.22292.

Straw, T. 2019, December 3. "Beyond the firewall: Pathways to affordable health coverage for low-income workers." Health Affairs. https://www.healthaffairs.org/do/10.1377/hblog20191127.362854/full.

Su, C. P., G. Syamlal, S. Tamers, J. Li, and S. E. Luckhaupt. 2019. "Workplace secondhand tobacco smoke exposure among U.S. non-smoking workers, 2015." *MMWR Morb Mortal*

Wkly Rep 68(27): 604–607. doi:10.15585/mmwr.mm6827a2.

Sundell, J., H. Levin, W. W. Nazaroff, W. S. Cain, W. J. Fisk, D. T. Grimsrud, F. Gyntelberg, et al. 2011. "Ventilation rates and health: Multidisciplinary review of the scientific literature." *Indoor Air* 21(3): 191–204. doi:10.1111/j.1600-0668.2010.00703.x.

Supreme Court of the United States. 2020. "Bostock v. Clayton County, Georgia: Certiorari to the United States Court of Appeals for the Eleventh Circuit." Washington, DC: Supreme Court of the United States.

Tamborini, C. R., C. H. Kim, and A. Sakamoto. 2015. "Education and lifetime earnings in the United States." *Demography* 52(4): 1383–1407. doi:10.1007/s13524-015-0407-0.

Tang, K. 2014. "A reciprocal interplay between psychosocial job stressors and worker well-being? A systematic review of the 'reversed' effect." *Scand J Work Environ Health* 40(5): 441–456. doi:10.5271/sjweh.3431.

Tao, W., B. L. Janzen, and S. Abonyi. 2010. "Gender, division of unpaid family work and psychological distress in dual-earner families." *Clin Pract Epidemiol Ment Health* 6: 36–46. doi:10.2174/1745017901006010036.

The Commonwealth Fund. 2019. "Underinsured rate rose from 2014–2018, with greatest growth among people in employer health plans." Accessed October 21, 2020. https://www.commonwealthfund.org/press-release/2019/underinsured-rate-rose-2014-2018-greatest-growth-among-people-employer-health.

The Library of Congress. 2020. "8-Hour work day." Accessed October 20, 2020. https://www.loc.gov/item/today-in-history/august-20.

The National Institute for Occupational Safety and Health. 2020a. Accessed October 19, 2020. https://www.cdc.gov/niosh/index.htm.

The National Institute for Occupational Safety and Health. 2020b. "Severe nonfatal injuries and illnesses charts." Centers for Disease Control and Prevention. Accessed October 13, 2020. https://wwwn.cdc.gov/NIOSH-WHC/chart/bls-ch/illness?T=ZS&V=C&D=RANGE&Y1=2018&Y2=2018.

Theorell, T., A. Hammarström, G. Aronsson, L. Träskman Bendz, T. Grape, C. Hogstedt, I. Marteinsdottir, I. Skoog, and C. Hall. 2015. "A systematic review including meta-analysis of work environment and depressive symptoms." *BMC Public Health* 15: 738. doi:10.1186/s12889-015-1954-4.

Thomas, C. L., E. Laguda, F. Olufemi-Ayoola, S. Netzley, J. Yu, and C. Spitzmueller. 2018. "Linking job work hours to women's physical health: The role of perceived unfairness and household work hours." *Sex Roles* 79(7): 476–488. doi:10.1007/s11199-017-0888-y.

Titus, A. R., L. Kalousova, R. Meza, D. T. Levy, J. F. Thrasher, M. R. Elliott, P. M. Lantz, and N. L. Fleischer. 2019. "Smoke-free policies and smoking cessation in the United States, 2003–2015." *Int J Environ Res Public Health* 16(17): 3200. doi:10.3390/ijerph16173200.

Toossi, M., and T. Morisi. 2017. "Women in the workforce before, during, and after the Great Recession." U.S. Bureau of Labor Statistics. Accessed October 13, 2020. https://www.bls.gov/spotlight/2017/women-in-the-workforce-before-during-and-after-the-great-recession/home.htm.

Toossi, M., and E. Torpey. 2017. "Older workers: Labor force trends and career options." U.S. Bureau of Labor Statistics. Accessed October 13, 2020. https://www.bls.gov/careeroutlook/2017/article/older-workers.htm.

Tran, M., and R. K. Sokas. 2017. "The gig economy and contingent work: An occupational health assessment." *J Occup Environ Med* 59(4): e63–e66. doi:10.1097/jom.0000000000000977.

Triana, M. C., M. Jayasinghe, and J. R. Pieper. 2015. "Perceived workplace racial discrimination and its correlates: A meta-analysis." *J Organ Behav* 36(4):491–513. doi:10.1002/job.1988.

Trudel, X., A. Milot, M. Gilbert-Ouimet, C. Duchaine, L. Guénette, V. Dalens, and C. Brisson. 2017. "Effort–reward imbalance at work and the prevalence of unsuccessfully treated hypertension among white-collar workers." *Am J Epidemiol* 186(4): 456–462. doi:10.1093/aje/kwx116.

Tsutsumi, A., and N. Kawakami. 2004. "A review of empirical studies on the model of effort–reward imbalance at work: Reducing occupational stress by implementing a new theory."

Soc Sci Med 59(11): 2335–2359. https://doi.org/10.1016/j.socscimed.2004.03.030.

U.S. Bureau of Labor Statistics. 2017. "Women in the labor force: A databook." *BLS Reports*. https://www.bls.gov/opub/reports/womens-databook/2021/home.htm.

U.S. Bureau of Labor Statistics. 2018. "Contingent and alternative employment arrangements—May 2017.". https://www.bls.gov/news.release/pdf/conemp.pdf.

U.S. Bureau of Labor Statistics. 2019a. "Census of fatal occupational injuries: News release.". https://www.bls.gov/news.release/archives/cfoi_12162020.htm.

U.S. Bureau of Labor Statistics. 2019b. "Employer-reported workplace injuries and illnesses (annual): News release." https://www.bls.gov/news.release/archives/osh_11032021.htm.

U.S. Bureau of Labor Statistics. 2019c. "Injuries, illnesses, and fatalities." Accessed October 13, 2020. https://www.bls.gov/iif/soii-chart-data-2018.htm.

U.S. Bureau of Labor Statistics. 2019d. "Labor force characteristics by race and ethnicity, 2018." *BLS Reports*. https://www.bls.gov/opub/reports/race-and-ethnicity/2018/home.htm.

U.S. Bureau of Labor Statistics. 2019e. "A profile of the working poor, 2017." BLS Reports. https://www.bls.gov/opub/reports/working-poor/2017/home.htm.

U.S. Bureau of Labor Statistics. 2020a. "American time use survey news release." https://www.bls.gov/news.release/archives/atus_06232022.htm.

U.S. Bureau of Labor Statistics. 2020b. "Employee benefits in the United States—March 2020." https://www.bls.gov/ncs/ebs/benefits/2020/employee-benefits-in-the-united-states-march-2020.pdf.

U.S. Bureau of Labor Statistics. 2020c. "Employee benefits in the United States news release." https://www.bls.gov/news.release/ebs2.htm.

U.S. Bureau of Labor Statistics. 2020d. "Projections overview and highlights: 2019–29." https://www.bls.gov/mlr/2020/article/projections-overview-and-highlights-2019-29.htm.

U.S. Bureau of Labor Statistics. 2020e. "Frequently asked questions about data on contingent and alternative employment arrangements." Accessed October 19, 2020. https://www.bls.gov/cps/contingent-and-alternative-arrangements-faqs.htm#contingent.

U.S. Bureau of Labor Statistics. 2020f. "Labor force characteristics of foreign-born workers news release." https://www.bls.gov/news.release/forbrn.htm.

U.S. Bureau of Labor Statistics. 2020g. "Labor force statistics from the current population survey." Last modified January 22, 2020. Accessed October 13, 2020. https://www.bls.gov/cps/cpsaat03.htm.

U.S. Bureau of Labor Statistics. 2021. "Unemployment rises in 2020, as the country battles the COVID-19 pandemic." https://www.bls.gov/opub/mlr/2021/article/unemployment-rises-in-2020-as-the-country-battles-the-covid-19-pandemic.htm.

U.S. Census Bureau. 2018. "2014–2018 ACS 5-year data profile." Accessed October 13, 2020. https://data.census.gov/cedsci/table?d=ACS%205-Year%20Estimates%20Data%20Profiles&tid=ACSDP5Y2018.DP05.

U.S. Census Bureau. 2019. "American Community Survey: Selected economic characteristics." Accessed October 13, 2020. https://data.census.gov/cedsci/table?d=ACS%201-Year%20Estimates%20Data%20Profiles&tid=ACSDP1Y2019.DP03.

U.S. Census Bureau. 2022. "Stats for stories: Equal pay day: March 21, 2020.". https://www.census.gov/library/stories/2020/03/equal-pay-day-is-march-31-earliest-since-1996.html

U.S. Department of Health and Human Services. 2011. "The Surgeon General's call to action to support breastfeeding." https://www.cdc.gov/breastfeeding/resources/calltoaction.htm.

U.S. Equal Employment Opportunity Commission. 2020. "Charge statistics (charges filed with EEOC) FY 1997 through FY 2019." Accessed October 15, 2020. https://www.eeoc.gov/statistics/charge-statistics-charges-filed-eeoc-fy-1997-through-fy-2019.

Van der Doef, M., and S. Maes. 1999. "The job demand–control (–support) model and psychological well-being: A review of 20 years of empirical research." *Work Stress* 13(2): 87–114. doi:10.1080/026783799296084.

van Vegchel, N., J. de Jonge, H. Bosma, and W. Schaufeli. 2005. "Reviewing the effort–reward imbalance model: Drawing up the balance of 45 empirical studies." *Soc Sci Med* 60(5): 1117–1131. https://doi.org/10.1016/j.socscimed.2004.06.043.

Velez, B. L., R. Cox, C. J. Polihronakis, and B. Moradi. 2018. "Discrimination, work outcomes, and mental health among women of color: The protective role of womanist attitudes." *J Couns Psychol* 65(2): 178–193. doi:10.1037/cou0000274.

Vetter, C., E. E. Devore, L. R. Wegrzyn, J. Massa, F. E. Speizer, I. Kawachi, B. Rosner, M. J. Stampfer, and E. S. Schernhammer. 2016. "Association between rotating night shift work and risk of coronary heart disease among women." *JAMA* 315(16): 1726–1734. doi:10.1001/jama.2016.4454.

Wang, L. J., A. Tanious, C. Go, D. M. Coleman, S. K. McKinley, M. J. Eagleton, W. D. Clouse, and M. F. Conrad. 2020. "Gender-based discrimination is prevalent in the integrated vascular trainee experience and serves as a predictor of burnout." *J Vasc Surg* 71(1): 220–227. doi:10.1016/j.jvs.2019.02.064.

Wang, M.-J., A. Mykletun, E. I. Møyner, S. Øverland, M. Henderson, S. Stansfeld, M. Hotopf, and S. B. Harvey. 2014. "Job strain, health and sickness absence: Results from the Hordaland Health Study." *PLoS One* 9(4): e96025. doi:10.1371/journal.pone.0096025.

Weiss, E., G. Murphy, and L. Boden. 2019. Workers' compensation: Benefits, costs, and coverage—2017 data. In *Workers' Compensation Benefits, Costs, and Coverage*. Washington, DC: National Academy of Social Insurance. https://www.nasi.org/sites/default/files/nasi RptWkrsComp2017%20Final.pdf

Whitney, P., J. M. Hinson, B. C. Satterfield, D. A. Grant, K. A. Honn, and H. P. A. Van Dongen. 2017. "Sleep deprivation diminishes attentional control effectiveness and impairs flexible adaptation to changing conditions." *Sci Rep* 7(1): 16020. doi:10.1038/s41598-017-16165-z.

Wilson, L., D. Lero, A. Smofsky, D. Gross, and J. Haines. 2016. "Parents working together: Development and feasibility trial of a workplace-based program for parents that incorporates general parenting and health behaviour messages." *BMC Public Health* 16(1): 1154. doi:10.1186/s12889-016-3817-z.

Wilson, V., and W. M. Rodgers, III. 2016. "Black–White wage gaps expand with rising wage inequality." Economic Policy Institute. https://www.epi.org/publication/black-white-wage-gaps-expand-with-rising-wage-inequality.

Wirtz, P. H., and R. von Känel. 2017. "Psychological stress, inflammation, and coronary heart disease." *Curr Cardiol Rep* 19(11): 111. doi:10.1007/s11886-017-0919-x.

Wolff, J. M., K. M. Rospenda, J. A. Richman, L. Liu, and L. A. Milner. 2013. "Work–family conflict and alcohol use: Examination of a moderated mediation model." *J Addict Dis* 32(1): 85–98. doi:10.1080/10550887.2012.759856.

Wong, K., A. H. S. Chan, and S. C. Ngan. 2019. "The effect of long working hours and over-time on occupational health: A meta-analysis of evidence from 1998 to 2018." *Int J Environ Res Public Health* 16(12): 2102. doi:10.3390/ijerph16122102.

World Health Organization. 2019. "Commission on Social Determinants of Health, 2005–2008." Accessed August 14, 2019. https://www.who.int/teams/social-determinants-of-health/equity-and-health/commission-on-social-determinants-of-health.

Wurzelbacher, S. J., S. J. Bertke, M. P. Lampl, P. T. Bushnell, A. R. Meyers, D. C. Robins, and I. S. Al-Tarawneh. 2014. "The effectiveness of insurer-supported safety and health engineering controls in reducing workers' compensation claims and costs." *Am J Ind Med* 57(12): 1398–1412. doi:10.1002/ajim.22372.

Xiao, H., S. A. McCurdy, M. T. Stoecklin-Marois, C.-S. Li, and M. B. Schenker. 2013. "Agricultural work and chronic musculoskeletal pain among Latino farm workers: The MICASA study." *Am J Ind Med* 56(2): 216–225. https://doi.org/10.1002/ajim.22118.

Yanar, B., A. Kosny, and P. M. Smith. 2018. "Occupational health and safety vulnerability of recent immigrants and refugees." *Int J Environ Res Public Health* 15(9): 2004. doi:10.3390/ijerph15092004.

Ybema, J. F., and K. van den Bos. 2010. "Effects of organizational justice on depressive symptoms and sickness absence: A longitudinal perspective." *Soc Sci Med* 70(10): 1609–1617. doi:10.1016/j.socscimed.2010.01.027.

Yean, T. F., and A. A. Yusof. 2016. "Organizational justice: A conceptual discussion." *Procedia* 219: 798–803. https://doi.org/10.1016/j.sbs pro.2016.05.082.

Yearby, R. 2019. "The impact of structural racism in employment and wages on minority women's health." America Bar Association. Accessed February 15, 2021. https://www.americanbar.org/groups/crsj/publications/human_rights_magazine_h

ome/the-state-of-healthcare-in-the-united-states/minority-womens-health.

Zapf, D., C. Dormann, and M. Frese. 1996. "Longitudinal studies in organizational stress research: A review of the literature with reference to methodological issues." *J Occup Health Psychol* 1(2): 145–169. doi:10.1037//1076-8998.1.2.145.

Zheng, R., Y. Xu, W. Wang, G. Ning, and Y. Bi. 2020. "Spatial transmission of COVID-19 via public and private transportation in China." *Travel Med Infect Dis* 34: 101626. doi:10.1016/j.tmaid.2020.101626.

CHAPTER 10

Behaviors Influence Health

What Influences Behaviors?

10.1. INTRODUCTION

Since the latter half of the 20th century, scientists have documented how our behaviors can protect us from—or put us at risk for—ill health. There is wide consensus that behaviors contribute significantly to poor health and premature death (Ma et al. 2018; Young et al. 2016; Lortet-Tieulent et al. 2016, 2017). Most of us know what we should do to be healthier: exercise more, eat a more nutritious diet, and abstain from smoking, excessive alcohol, and other harmful substances. Despite increased awareness, however, many of us continue to practice unhealthy behaviors. In 2017, for example, 43% of U.S. adults did not meet federal guidelines for leisure-time physical activity, and one in seven was a current smoker (National Center for Health Statistics 2019).

Behaviors are well known to influence health in many ways. Physical activity, for example, reduces the risk of obesity (Hills, Andersen, and Byrne 2011; Hong et al. 2016), improves muscle strength (Chan et al. 2018), and has been linked with mental health benefits (Biddle 2016). A healthy diet is needed for optimal functioning of bodily systems and can influence susceptibility to infections through effects on immune system functioning; nutrition can alter the microbiota—the microscopic microorganisms that inhabit our bodies and have been shown to influence many health conditions (Singh et al. 2017). Inadequate sleep can adversely affect both mental and physical health (Fernandez-Mendoza and Vgontzas 2013). Prolonged excessive alcohol intake leads to liver disease that can be fatal (Osna, Donohue, and Kharbanda 2017). Smoking cigarettes causes lung cancer (Ozlü and Bülbül 2005; O'Keeffe et al. 2018) and chronic obstructive pulmonary disease (emphysema) (Laniado-Laborín 2009; Rycroft et al. 2012). Opioid use takes a large toll in death (Bech et al. 2019) and loss of productivity (Florence, Luo, and Rice 2021).

Until the early 2000s, most efforts to improve health-related behaviors focused on health education to inform people about the importance of making healthier decisions and urge them to adopt healthier behaviors. Over time, however, evidence has accumulated and awareness has increased of how health and health-related behaviors are powerfully shaped by the conditions in which we live, learn, work, and play—that is,

The Social Determinants of Health and Health Disparities. Paula Braveman, Oxford University Press. © Oxford University Press 2023. DOI: 10.1093/oso/9780190624118.003.0010

the social determinants of health (World Health Organization 2008; Woolf et al. 2011; Yen and Syme 1999; Lynch, Kaplan, and Salonen 1997; Frieden 2010; Nathan et al. 2018; Petrovic et al. 2018; Turecki and Meaney 2016). For example, many Americans cannot afford to purchase a nutritious diet; cannot afford to live in neighborhoods without heavy air pollution and with access to safe places to exercise; and experience nearly constant stress due to having inadequate resources to pay for child care, housing, and food for their families and transportation to and from work for themselves. Each of these situations represents a significant obstacle to making healthy choices for oneself and one's family. Indeed, in these circumstances, people cannot make healthy choices because healthy choices are not accessible to them.

Although most approaches to improving health-related behaviors have focused on individual responsibility, a large and growing body of knowledge indicates that people's living and working conditions—and key factors such as education, income, and racism that shape those conditions—play a fundamental role as obstacles to or facilitators of healthy behaviors. "Education," as used in this book and widely, refers to schooling or educational attainment, measured in years or more meaningfully in credentials or levels of completed schooling—for example, less than high school, high school, and college graduate. This chapter summarizes current knowledge about factors that shape health-related behaviors (often called "health behaviors") and suggests promising approaches based on that knowledge.

10.2. HEALTH-RELATED BEHAVIORS ARE STRONGLY SHAPED BY SOCIAL FACTORS

Presumably, we all want to be healthy. If that is true, why do some people practice healthy behaviors, while others—including many who have the relevant information—do not? A person's behaviors can be affected in part by their genetic makeup; for example, individuals who are genetically disposed to become symptomatically sick when they drink alcohol are unlikely to become alcoholics. Extensive evidence indicates, however, that generally, the social and physical environments in which people grow up, learn, and adopt and maintain behaviors are likely to play a more important role (Lynch et al. 1997; Woolf et al. 2011; Braveman and Egerter 2013; Glass and McAtee 2006; Nathan et al. 2018; Artiga and Hinton 2018). Epigenetic effects (gene–environment interactions), furthermore, can be affected by a person's exposures and experiences, which determine whether or not a specific gene is expressed or suppressed. This means that one's genetic makeup is not necessarily one's destiny.

Figure 10.1—a slightly modified version of the conceptual framework diagram presented in Chapter 1—highlights key influences on health-related behaviors as well as the relationship between health-related behaviors and health. As discussed in Chapter 1, using the metaphor of a stream flowing down from its source in the mountains, "upstream" denotes a causal/contributory factor that is at or near the origin or source of a causal chain. Upstream factors are distinguished from "downstream" factors, which have their effects near the end of a causal chain, close to the outcome. Figure 10.1 traces the determinants of health-related behaviors from their upstream sources in systems, laws, policies, and widely established practices and beliefs (depicted in the first column on

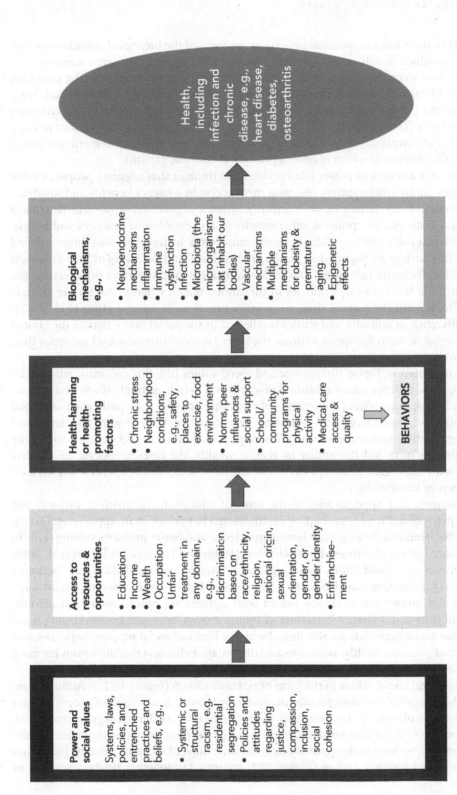

FIGURE 10.1 Behaviors influence health. What influences health-related behaviors (and disparities in health-related behaviors)?

the left) to their most downstream effects in the form of the biological mechanisms that directly produce health outcomes. This causal chain happens through a succession of intermediate steps that, in some cases, include health-related behaviors. The upstream sources of health-related behaviors (in the box to the far left in Figure 10.1) include laws, policies, and entrenched attitudes and beliefs regarding poverty, justice, social cohesion and solidarity (connectedness with, caring about, and willingness to help others in one's society), and compassion. They include systemic racism and enfranchisement (the power to vote, the absence of which is often a product of systemic racism).

Racism is a system of power relationships and thought that relegates people of color to inferior status and treatment, denying them access to society's benefits and justifying this with beliefs about their innate inferiority. *Systemic* or *structural racism* is racism that is built into systems, laws, policies, other structures, and established practices and beliefs. Attitudes toward poverty, solidarity, and compassion include whether impoverished people in a society are regarded as "down on their luck" and deserving of help or viewed as lazy, insufficiently motivated, and/or less intelligent, and therefore undeserving; the latter attitude has permeated policies in the United States, whereas the former attitude has, at least until the present time, been more prevalent in Europe (Toro et al. 2007). This difference in attitudes and values is reflected in the social safety nets of the United States versus western European nations, the latter far more extensive and generous than the former (Woolf and Aron 2013).

As indicated in Figure 10.1, power and social values (the first column), reflected by systems, laws, policies, and established practices and beliefs, strongly shape access to resources and opportunities (the second column) that are vital for health, such as a good education and, based largely on education, an occupation with good pay, benefits, and working conditions. For the vast majority of people, education and occupation heavily determine income and the ability to acquire wealth; the rare exceptions are the few people with substantial inherited wealth, whose income does not depend solely on their education or occupation.

Resources and opportunities in the form of education, occupation, income, and wealth play powerful roles in shaping health-related behaviors, in multiple ways. Having more education can mean greater health knowledge and better problem-solving skills to make more informed choices about behaviors (Hahn and Truman 2015; Friis et al. 2016; Zimmerman and Woolf 2014), including those related to seeking medical care (Berkman et al. 2011). Education can also shape health-related behaviors in other important ways. Educational attainment is closely linked with options for employment and income, which in turn can influence behaviors in multiple ways, as noted below. Having more education and a better job are also linked with the kinds of social support, networks, and norms that promote healthy behaviors and discourage behaviors that are health-harming (Hahn and Truman 2015; Umberson, Crosnoe, and Reczek 2010).

Power and social values in the form of systemic racism (Figure 10.1, column 1) constrain the education and therefore the occupations, income, and wealth of people of color (Figure 10.1, column 2); this occurs partly through racial residential segregation, which tracks people of color into residential areas with low economic opportunity due to inferior schools, few decent job opportunities, and little hope of escaping poverty. The beliefs that undergird systemic racism (Figure 10.1, column 1)—whether held consciously or unconsciously—have an insidious effect as they perpetuate myths about innate inferiority that produce and condone unfair treatment, including both interpersonal and internalized racism (Figure 10.1, column 2; see also Chapter 5).

> Racism and its product, race-based unfair treatment, constrain the access that people of color have to resources and opportunities that shape health-related behaviors and health itself.

Unfair treatment—for example, discrimination in housing, employment (hiring, pay, and promotions), education, policing, sentencing, and medical care—diminishes access to resources and opportunities. The mass incarceration of Black men has wreaked economic havoc not only on the men but also on their families and communities because the stigma of having been incarcerated is a daunting, often permanent obstacle to employment after release.

Next in the causal chain, the third column in Figure 10.1 lists multiple factors that can harm or promote health, sometimes via health-related behaviors. A large body of research sheds light on the relatively direct ways in which aspects of people's physical environments—for instance, access to and quality of housing, transportation, stores, playgrounds, and parks—can either promote or present obstacles to healthy behaviors (Diez Roux and Mair 2010; Pickett and Pearl 2001; Schule and Bolte 2015; Arcaya et al. 2016). Aspects of the social environment, such as peer influences, norms, and social ties, also can shape behaviors, although often in less direct ways.

Access—or lack of access—to resources and opportunities shapes exposure to health-promoting or health-harming conditions-Economic resources (income, occupation, and wealth), for example, affect the extent to which people can afford to live in safe neighborhoods with clean air free of environmental toxins, low crime rates, and safe pleasant places to exercise. Higher-income neighborhoods have healthier food environments, with a low concentration of fast-food outlets. Fresh food typically costs more than processed food and tends to be less available in low-income neighborhoods. A good income makes it possible to live in a neighborhood with adequately funded schools that provide a solid education overall and have sports programs, which presumably could increase the likelihood that young people will exercise. Higher income neighborhoods often have healthier prevailing norms and peer influences (with respect to alcohol, smoking, drug use, physical activity, and doing well in school) (Diez Roux and Mair 2010; Sugiyama et al. 2015; Arcaya et al. 2016). Insufficient income or wealth (largely determined by education and occupation), for example, is an important source of chronic stress for many people as they try to meet daily challenges such as paying for housing, food, child care, getting to and from work on time, and medical expenses, with inadequate resources.

Resources and opportunities such as education, occupation, income, and wealth also play a major role in determining who has access to quality medical care, which can promote health. Most people

> Access—or lack of access—to resources and opportunities such as education, occupation, income, wealth, and racial residential segregation shape access to health-promoting conditions and protection from health-harming conditions, which in turn influence health-related behaviors.

younger than age 65 years in the United States obtain health insurance through their employers if they are employed (Centers for Disease Control and Prevention 2017). Others have coverage only if they can afford to purchase it, and even those who have insurance may be unable to afford the often large deductibles and copayments charged by many private insurance plans (Kaiser Family Foundation 2020).

Stressful conditions and experiences contribute to unhealthy behaviors. Although a growing body of research suggests that chronic stress can have direct physiologic effects on health, stress also can shape health indirectly via its effects on health-related behaviors. For example, children who experience stressful circumstances, particularly on a daily basis, are more likely later in life to adopt—and less likely to discontinue—risky health behaviors such as smoking, drug use, and excess alcohol (Hughes et al. 2017; Rehkopf et al. 2016; Loudermilk et al. 2018; Lee and Chen 2017), which may be coping mechanisms.

Racial discrimination and racial residential segregation (Figure 10.1, column 1), which are examples of systemic racism (Figure 10.1, column 1), systematically constrain the options that people of color—including many with middle incomes (Adelman 2004; Sharkey 2014)—have for where they will reside. Segregation constrains the income, wealth, and often the educational level that a person of color may attain (Figure 10.1, column 2). This exposes them to the health-harming and lack of health-promoting conditions (Figure 10.1, column 3) that, because of racism, prevail in many segregated communities (Cushing, Faust, et al. 2015; Cushing, Morello-Frosch, et al. 2015; Morello-Frosch and Lopez 2006). All of these conditions are stressful. In addition, racism and the unfair treatment that it produces and condones—intentional or not—also directly subject people of color of all economic levels to chronic stress. Chronic stress can harm health directly—for example, through neuroendocrine and immune mechanisms. It also can harm health indirectly through its effects on health-related behaviors. The stress may come not only from experiencing overt incidents of discrimination but also from maintaining a perpetual state of vigilance to be prepared in case incidents occur (Lewis, Cogburn, and Williams 2015; Braveman et al. 2017).

All of the factors listed in the third column of Figure 10.1 can influence health-related behaviors. In the figure, health-related behaviors are categorized in column 3 because they are health-harming or health-promoting factors.

10.3. EXAMPLES OF THE SOCIAL PATTERNING OF HEALTH-RELATED BEHAVIORS

Although economic factors are not the only determinants of behaviors, they have repeatedly been shown to be particularly strong determinants. Economic disadvantage, furthermore, is a major (although not the only) way that systemic racism exerts its ill effects; this makes it important to be aware of and understand the economic patterning of health behaviors in order to interpret data on behavioral differences by race or ethnic group. Furthermore, unlike the highly consistent patterning of behaviors by income or education (including within racial/ethnic groups), patterns are often inconsistent when considering behaviors by race/ethnic group. Blacks, Latinos, and Whites have a higher prevalence of some adverse behaviors but a lower prevalence of others.

American Indians/Alaska Natives appear to consistently rank relatively poorly on use of all of the harmful substances examined in *Health, United States* (National Center for Health Statistics 2019) (cigarette smoking, binge or heavy alcohol use, illicit drugs, and misuse of prescription psychotherapeutics and drugs), although not on physical activity measures. Asians—but not Native Hawaiians and other Pacific Islanders—tend to rank favorably across substance use categories. The socioeconomic gradient pattern of behaviors largely persists when considering each racial/ethnic group separately, and the racial/ethnic differences in behaviors generally appear smaller when comparing people of different racial/ethnic groups who have similar income or education levels (National Center for Health Statistics 2019). Lillie-Blanton, Anthony, and Schuster (1993) observed that higher prevalence rates of crack cocaine use by Blacks and Latinos compared to Whites became nonsignificant after adjusting for residence in socially disadvantaged neighborhoods suggesting that, socioeconomic advantage, rather than race, seemed to explain elevated crack use. The examples shown in this chapter therefore focus on socioeconomic disparities in behaviors.

Many important behavioral risk factors for illness and early death in the United States vary dramatically depending on where people are situated on the ladder of economic success; this is reflected by multiple examples cited in this chapter. The links between health-related behaviors and both education and income—the most common measures of social and economic advantage in the United States—have been well documented. As the examples below illustrate, increases in income and educational attainment generally correspond to decreases in the prevalence of health-harming behaviors and increases in the prevalence of health-promoting behaviors. In many cases, these differences reflect more than just a contrast between those who are poorest or least educated and everyone else; instead, incremental improvements in behaviors with each step up the income or education ladder are often seen. These stepwise gradient patterns have been observed for an array of behaviors, beginning in childhood and continuing throughout life (Braveman et al. 2010; Watts et al. 2016; Siddiqi, Hertzman, and Smith 2018).

The following examples illustrate the links between several health-related behaviors and factors including income, education, and neighborhood economic conditions, beginning in childhood. These basic patterns of behaviors improving as economic resources increase—have been seen in findings from a range of studies, including those that have simultaneously accounted for many other potentially relevant factors (Pampel, Krueger, and Denney 2010; Lantz et al. 1998). Variations in the patterns also have been observed. In some cases, the stepwise gradient does not apply completely and one may see a dichotomy—for example, between the most or least well-off group and all others. Some health-damaging behaviors, moreover, are more prevalent among socioeconomically better-off individuals. These, however, are exceptions.

Physical Activity

Both income and education are associated with physical activity among adults. Lower rates of physical activity (Figure 10.2) and higher rates of sedentary behavior (not shown) generally are seen at lower levels of income and educational attainment. Similar patterns have been observed among adolescents, based on the income or education of their heads of household (Watts et al. 2016).

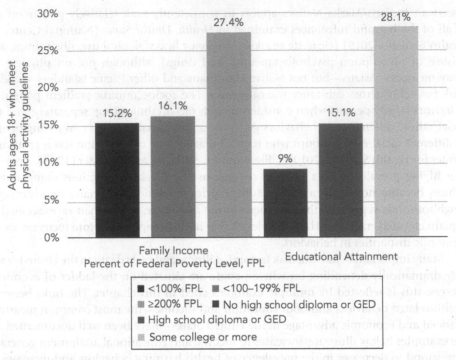

FIGURE 10.2 Adults with higher incomes and more schooling are more physically active. *Source*: National Center for Health Statistics (2019).

Nutrition/Healthy Eating

As illustrated in Figure 10.3, people with higher incomes and more schooling (educational attainment) are generally more likely to eat healthy foods (Darmon and Drewnowski 2008; D. Wang et al. 2014). Exceptions are seen, as illustrated below, where the most socioeconomically disadvantaged group does somewhat better than the next-to-most-disadvantaged group; the overall pattern, however, is consistent. On average, people in lower income households eat fruits and vegetables less frequently (Lorson, Melgar-Quinonez, and Taylor 2009; Hanson and Connor 2014; Drewnowski and Rehm 2015). The lower cost and longer shelf life of processed foods have been identified as important factors influencing the food decisions of low-income individuals and families (Moran et al. 2019).

The built environment—exterior and interior characteristics of buildings—and features of, sidewalks, roads, and other humanly constructed elements of a neighborhood—appears to influence what people eat. Despite widespread beliefs about the role of "food deserts," evidence is in fact mixed on whether or not proximity to or availability of supermarkets influence diet (Caspi et al. 2012; Boone-Heinonen et al. 2011; Mackenbach et al. 2017; Peng and Kaza 2019). Evidence is more consistent about "food swamps"—neighborhoods with a high density of fast-food outlets; the quality of residents' diets worsens significantly with greater neighborhood-level concentration of fast-food outlets (Boone-Heinonen et al. 2011), which are more prevalent in low-income neighborhoods

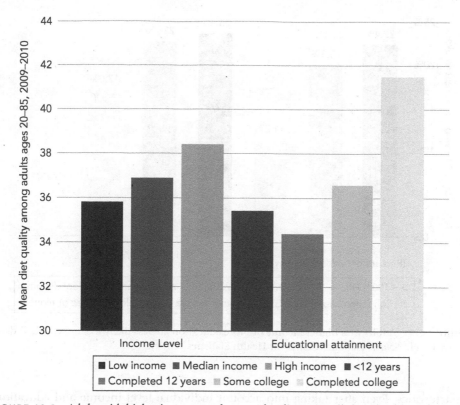

FIGURE 10.3   Adults with higher incomes and more schooling generally have healthier diets. Diet quality was measured by the Alternative Healthy Eating Index (AHEI), which measures intake of 11 key diet components, each ranging from 0 to 10, with higher scores indicating healthier eating. The maximum AHEI score is 110. D. Wang et al. (2014) excluded the trans-fat component of the AHEI from their analysis. *Source*: National Health and Nutrition Examination Survey (NHANES). Chart constructed using NHANES data presented in Table 2 of D. Wang et al. (2014).

(Fleischhacker et al. 2011). Fast-food restaurants in higher-income communities, furthermore, are more likely to offer healthier food options than fast-food restaurants in low- and middle-income communities (Heinert, Isgor, and Powell 2018).

Smoking

As seen in Figure 10.4, both income and education have been associated with cigarette smoking among U.S. adults overall (Hiscock et al. 2012; Jamal et al. 2016), with the lowest rates typically seen in the highest income and most-educated groups. This also has been seen among pregnant women (Drake, Driscoll, and Mathews 2018; Goodwin et al. 2017). Smokers of lower socioeconomic status, furthermore, are more likely to be heavy smokers (20 or more cigarettes per day) (Chen et al. 2019), and their attempts to quit are generally less successful (Hiscock et al. 2012; Pizacani et al. 2018). Although smoking rates have decreased over time, the declines have been most dramatic among the most socially and economically advantaged groups (Drope et al. 2018; Kanjilal et al. 2006). Smoking rates have been associated with neighborhood social and economic

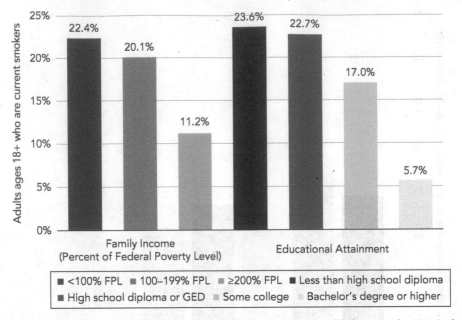

FIGURE 10.4   Adults with higher income or more education are less likely to smoke. FPL, Federal Poverty Level. *Source*: National Center for Health Statistics (2019).

characteristics. Even after taking into account individual-level income and education, rates of smoking are higher in economically disadvantaged neighborhoods (as reflected by more convenience stores, higher crime, and limited access to transportation and exercise facilities) (Chuang et al. 2005; Gary et al. 2008; Jitnarin et al. 2015; X. Wang et al. 2017). Socioeconomic disadvantage during childhood has been associated with smoking later in life (Friedman et al. 2015; Fergusson et al. 2007; Jefferis et al. 2004).

At the same time that rates of traditional cigarette smoking have decreased, use of electronic cigarettes (e-cigarettes) or "vaping" has increased dramatically among adolescents and adults of all income and education levels in recent years (Schaeffer 2019; T. Wang et al. 2018; King et al. 2015). There is inconsistent evidence that e-cigarette use varies by income or education level among adolescents or adults (Hartwell et al. 2017; Simon et al. 2018; Riggs and Pentz 2016; Friedman and Horn 2019; Stallings-Smith and Ballantyne 2019; Wilson and Wang 2017). The long-term health effects of e-cigarette use remain unknown.

Alcohol and Drugs

Alcohol is used by people of all economic levels; however, income, educational level, and neighborhood socioeconomic disadvantage strongly predict alcohol dependence and quantity and frequency of use among U.S. adults (Collins 2016). Socioeconomic disparities in adult alcohol use disorder have been increasing over time (Grant et al. 2017). Socioeconomic patterns of binge drinking and illicit drug use, however, do not paint a clear picture. As shown in Figure 10.5, the Substance Abuse and Mental Health

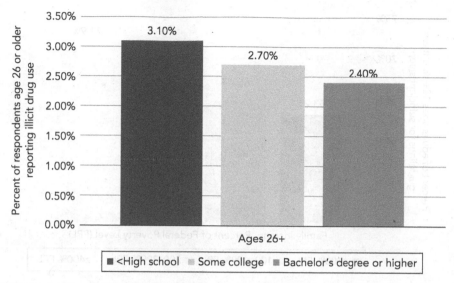

FIGURE 10.5 Use of illicit drugs appears to decrease somewhat with higher levels of education. *Source*: Substance Abuse and Mental Health Services Administration (2018).

Services Administration's (2018) National Survey on Drug Use and Health found that illicit drug use followed a socioeconomic gradient in the expected direction—higher drug use among adults aged 26 years or older of lower education levels. Adults who are unemployed or who did not attend college have disproportionately high rates of illicit drug use disorders (not displayed in Figure 10.5). It is reasonable to question, however, whether some of the association between drug use and unemployment may reflect reverse causation—that is, people becoming unemployed because of problematic drug use. In a departure from the usual pattern in which adverse health-related behaviors are more prevalent among people of lower socioeconomic resources, however, another study found that adolescents from more socioeconomically advantaged households appear more likely to engage in binge drinking and use illicit drugs such as cocaine (Humensky 2010). There is inconsistent evidence that socioeconomic status in childhood predicts use or abuse of illicit drugs later in life (Daniel et al. 2009). There also is limited evidence that neighborhood-level economic disadvantage is associated with alcohol or drug outcomes (Karriker-Jaffe 2011).

Sleep

Sleep may not be the first issue to come to mind when one thinks about health-related behaviors. It appears to have very strong effects on health and well-being, however. Luyster et al. (2012) concluded that "sleep deprivation contributes to a number of molecular, immune, and neural changes that play a role in disease development" (p. 727). As illustrated in Figure 10.6, sleep, like many of the behaviors discussed above, follows a strong socioeconomic gradient, with higher income associated with better sleep (Moore et al. 2002; Patel et al. 2010). Sleep may be an important mediator of the relationship between socioeconomic status and many health outcomes (Papadopoulos et al. 2022)—for

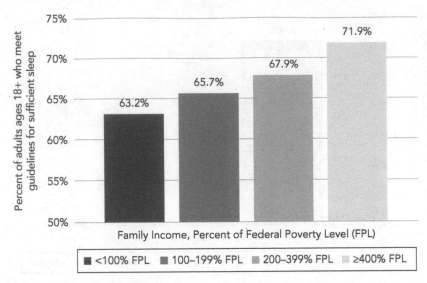

FIGURE 10.6 Adults with higher incomes are more likely to get sufficient sleep. *Source*: National Center for Health Statistics (2019).

example, by mediating the relationship between "stress-related thoughts" and immune function (Moore et al. 2002).

It is important to note that behaviors alone, although important, do not fully account for the observed links between factors such as income and education and many health outcomes. For example, Figure 10.7 shows differences in adult health status by both a person's educational attainment and whether or not they have healthy behaviors (smoking and leisure-time exercise). This figure indicates that a person's chances of being in very good or excellent health are greater at each higher level of educational attainment—whether or not they practice healthy behaviors. This suggests that, socioeconomic resources and opportunities—such as education—can have powerful effects on health, over and above how they shape health-related behaviors.

10.4. STRATEGIES TO IMPROVE HEALTH-RELATED BEHAVIORS: REMOVING OBSTACLES

Much remains to be learned about the most successful strategies for helping people adopt and maintain health-promoting behaviors. Current knowledge does, however, provide a sufficient basis for concluding that improving the health-related behaviors of the population overall and narrowing disparities by income, education, and race will require broadening our focus beyond the individual. Effective interventions must move beyond the necessary but not sufficient step of educating and encouraging individuals to make healthier choices. Many people face daunting obstacles to healthy behaviors that can only be removed by societal action; they, do not have healthy options. Approaches must be found to improve the conditions in people's homes, schools, workplaces, and communities that powerfully shape people's opportunities to make healthy choices

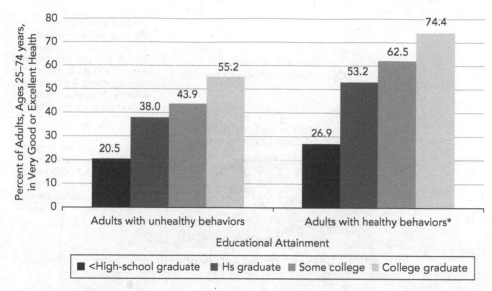

Prepared for the RWJF Commission to Build a Healthier America by the Center on Social Disparities in Health, University of California, San Francisco
Source: 2005–2007 Behavioral Risk Factor Surveillance System Survey Data *Smoking and leisure-time exercise

FIGURE 10.7 Socioeconomic resources and opportunities, such as education, can have powerful effects on health, over and above how they shape health-related behaviors. *Source*: Braveman, Egerter, and Barclay (2011).

(World Health Organization 2008; Frieden 2010; Golden et al. 2015; Marmot 2015; Schroeder 2007). Individuals' efforts will always be important in maintaining healthy behaviors. Many people, however, face obstacles to healthy behaviors that cannot be overcome solely through their own individual efforts; society must act to reduce the obstacles, particularly for those who face the greatest obstacles.

Figure 10.8 is a highly simplified depiction of major influences on health. It is intended to illustrate limitations of the traditional focus, which has been largely to rely on medical care and convincing individuals to engage in healthy behaviors. That narrow focus does not address the major obstacles that many individuals face to adopting and maintaining healthy behaviors.

The traditional focus on motivating individuals to change their behaviors has often appeared least successful in reaching those at high risk (Golden et al. 2015; Laverack 2017). The success of anti-smoking campaigns in reducing overall smoking rates has been largely based on the markedly declining rates of smoking among people in more socially advantaged groups (as indicated by a group's highest level of education) (Drope et al. 2018; Kanjilal et al. 2006; Jamal et al. 2016; de Walque 2010). Figure 10.9, based on data from the Centers for Disease Control and Prevention through 2017, paints a more complicated picture, however: Although it shows widening smoking disparities between the highest and lowest education groups, it also shows substantial improvement in the two lowest as well as the highest education groups. Persistent socioeconomic differences

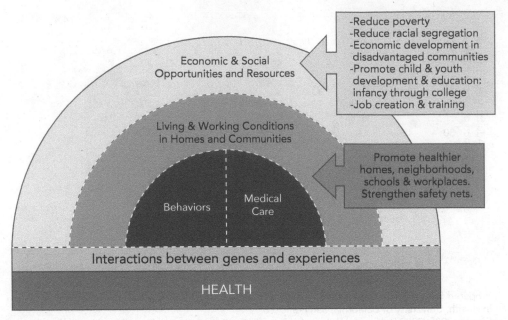

FIGURE 10.8 What influences health? Broadening the focus. *Source*: Adapted from Braveman and Egerter (2008).

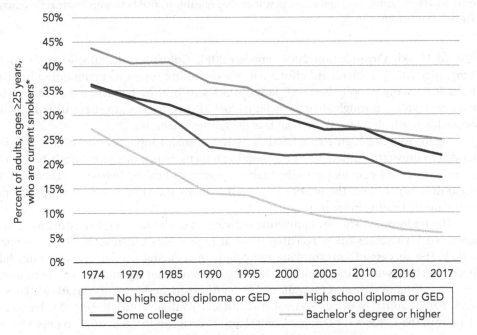

FIGURE 10.9 Persistent gaps in smoking by education. *Age-adjusted. *Source*: National Center for Health Statistics (2019).

in smoking rates—and in receipt of timely, quality medical care (Figure 10.7)—raise concerns about health equity (Graham et al. 2006).

The United States has for some time ranked at or near the bottom among affluent nations on almost all health indicators (Organisation for Economic Co-operation and Development 2019). According to Figure 10.8, perhaps the reason that the United States has been less successful than other affluent nations in achieving good health for its population is that the focus—on medical care and individuals' responsibility for their behaviors—has been too narrow. We have failed to consider that both access to medical care and healthy behaviors are often beyond the reach of individuals alone. They are both determined to a large extent by living and working conditions—health-damaging or health-promoting conditions—which, as illustrated in Figure 10.1, are themselves determined by access to resources and opportunities, such as good jobs with a living wage, good public schools, and a robust social safety net; these resources and opportunities in turn are shaped by public policies, laws, practices, and beliefs, including systemic racism.

Given the important role of behaviors in shaping health (The U.S. Burden of Disease Collaborators 2018; Mokdad et al. 2004), any strategy for improving health must include ensuring that more people have the options and ability to adopt and maintain healthy behaviors, beginning in childhood and throughout their lives. As Thomas R. Frieden, the former head of the Centers for Disease Control and Prevention, has recommended, highest priority should be given to "interventions that change the context to make individuals' default decisions healthy" (Frieden 2010, p. 590). Although no government or private program can take the place of people making healthy choices for themselves and their families, current knowledge indicates the need for societal responsibility as well: to pursue programs and policies that not only encourage but also enable all persons—and particularly those who face the greatest obstacles—to engage in healthy behaviors.

Other chapters in this book explore how income and wealth, education, working conditions, housing, neighborhoods, stress, and early childhood conditions influence health (sometimes, but not always, by influencing health-related behaviors); they provide examples of interventions that appear to have worked in creating healthier environments. In addition to policies focused on expanding social and economic resources and opportunities—including the Earned Income Tax Credit, minimum wage laws, and high-quality Early Head Start programs—the following are several U.S.-based examples of programmatic approaches that appear to show promise for improving health-related behaviors, in part because of their emphasis on providing access to resources and opportunities, including capacity-building:

- Evaluations of programs providing *universal* free breakfast, as opposed to targeted free/reduced price meals only for low-income children, have found higher school meal participation and increased school attendance when serving children across all family income levels rather than only low-income children. The universal model is thought to

> The highest priority should be given to "interventions that change the context to make individuals' default decisions healthy"—Thomas Frieden (2010, p. 590), former head of the Centers for Disease Control and Prevention.

reduce stigma associated with eating free meals at school, a factor contributing to less than optimal participation in non-universal programs (U.S. Department of Agriculture 2004; Leos-Urbel et al. 2013). The stigma often attached to using targeted programs for low-income individuals/households (versus universal programs) should be considered in developing many programs and policies.

- The federal Healthy Food Financing Initiative (HFFI) was first launched in 2010. A partnership between the U.S. Department of Agriculture, Treasury Department, and Department of Health and Human Services, the initiative aims to improve access to healthy food and create jobs through supermarket development in so-called "food deserts." As of 2018, HFFI has awarded $220 million in grants and loans to more than 35 states, and grantees have leveraged an additional $1 billion from private partners (Reinvestment Fund 2018). The program is modeled after Pennsylvania's highly successful Fresh Food Financing Initiative (Evans 2010).

- Since 2005, the U.S. Department of Transportation has allocated more than $1 billion to the Safe Routes to School Program (SRTS), which provides funding for infrastructure improvements and educational programs that promote walking and biking to school. Schools throughout the country have used the funds to create sidewalks, crosswalks, and bicycle parking facilities. They have also used the funds to purchase bicycle helmets and safety vests for students. From 2007 to 2012, one study found that SRTS programs in Eugene, Oregon (10 programs in total) were associated with a 5–20% increase in walking and biking to school (McDonald et al. 2013).

- Recognizing that sugar-sweetened beverages are the largest source of added sugar in Americans' diets, the City of Philadelphia implemented a three-cents-per-ounce tax on sugar-sweetened beverages in 2017 (Bettigole and Farley 2016). Several other cities, such as Chicago, Illinois, and Boulder, Colorado, have since passed their own sugar-sweetened beverages tax. Such a tax is considered by experts as the most cost-effective method for childhood obesity prevention at the population level (Gortmaker et al. 2015). Philadelphia's tax is projected to eliminate 36,000 cases of obesity and save $200 million in health care expenditures over 10 years (CHOICES Project 2016). This approach can be criticized as regressive taxation because the increased prices disproportionately affect those who are socioeconomically worse off. The regressive taxation, however, is on a harmful substance; thus there is substantial consensus in the field of public health that soda taxes are an important tool for reducing health damage among vulnerable groups.

- The Shape Up Somerville program collaborates with community organizations and municipal departments to increase options for physical activity and availability of healthful foods in children's school, home, and community environments in Somerville, Massachusetts. After the first 2 years of the program, participating first-, second-, and third-grade children had significantly decreased body mass index compared with nonparticipating children in two sociodemographically similar Massachusetts communities (Economos et al. 2013).

- In 2007, nearly 50,000 residents of Oklahoma City, Oklahoma—which has one of the highest adult obesity rates in the nation—joined their mayor's campaign to collectively lose 1 million pounds. After launching the campaign, the mayor used funding from the Affordable Care Act, business loans, and a temporary sales tax to develop and improve parks, bike lanes, sidewalks, walking paths, and recreational facilities throughout the city, with a special focus on areas with the highest rates of heart disease. After 5 years of logging their weight-loss journeys online, the residents reached their goal of collectively losing 1 million pounds (Reeve et al. 2015; Cornett and White 2019). Although it is not possible to rigorously evaluate whether the city's infrastructure improvements were causally related to residents' weight loss, the improvements undoubtedly created more opportunities for residents to engage in physical activity, and it is difficult to explain the improvement in another way.

- In 2002, New York City embarked on an ambitious effort to address behavioral causes of chronic disease. After large increases in cigarette taxes, legislation promoting smoke-free workplaces and restaurants, provision of free nicotine replacement therapy to smokers, and an aggressive anti-tobacco advertising campaign, the city saw its first drop in smoking prevalence in a decade. The declines were evident across all age and racial–ethnic groups, at every level of educational attainment, among both U.S.-born and foreign-born persons and in all five boroughs of the city. Declines were especially pronounced among low-income and Hispanic women (Frieden et al. 2005).

10.5. KEY POINTS

- Traditional approaches to improving health-related behaviors have focused on informing people about the importance of healthy behaviors and urging them to engage in those behaviors.
- A large body of knowledge, however, indicates that a person's living and working conditions—and factors such as income, wealth, education, occupation, and racism that shape those conditions—play a fundamental role in shaping health-related behaviors.
- Strategies to improve health-related behaviors must address the obstacles that people, particularly those with limited economic resources, face to adopting and maintaining healthy behaviors. Many of those obstacles can only be addressed by society, not by individuals.

10.6. QUESTIONS FOR DISCUSSION

1. Which of the other social determinants of health has important effects on behaviors? How does this happen? What are the sequential steps in causal pathways leading from these other important social determinants to behaviors?
2. What are two effective "upstream" strategies for addressing behaviors (a) as a social determinant of health and (b) as a social determinant of health disparities?

Why do you think these are of the most effective strategies? How do the strategies to improve health overall differ from those to reduce health disparities?

ACKNOWLEDGMENTS

This chapter builds on

Braveman, P., S. Egerter, and C. Barclay. 2011. "What shapes health-related behaviors? The role of social factors." Robert Wood Johnson Foundation. http://www.nmpha.org/Resources/Docume nts/RWJF%20Issue%20Brief%20-%20The%20Role%20of%20Social%20Factors.pdf.

Julia Acker, Nicole Holm, and Tram Nguyen contributed to the research.

REFERENCES

Adelman, R. M. 2004. "Neighborhood opportunities, race, and class: The Black middle class and residential segregation." *City Community* 3(1): 43–63. doi:10.1111/j.1535-6841.2004.00066.x.

Arcaya, M. C., R. D. Tucker-Seeley, R. Kim, A. Schnake-Mahl, M. So, and S. V. Subramanian. 2016. "Research on neighborhood effects on health in the United States: A systematic review of study characteristics." *Soc Sci Med* 168: 16–29. https://doi.org/10.1016/j.socsci med.2016.08.047.

Artiga, S., and E. Hinton. 2018. *Beyond Health Care: The Role of Social Determinants in Promoting Health and Health Equity.* San Francisco, CA: Kaiser Family Foundation.

Bech, A. B., T. Clausen, H. Waal, J. Š. Benth, and I. Skeie. 2019. "Mortality and causes of death among patients with opioid use disorder receiving opioid agonist treatment: A national register study." *BMC Health Serv Res* 19(1): 440. doi:10.1186/s12913-019-4282-z.

Berkman, N. D., S. L. Sheridan, K. E. Donahue, D. J. Halpern, and K. Crotty. 2011. "Low health literacy and health outcomes: An updated systematic review." *Ann Intern Med* 155(2): 97–107. doi:10.7326/0003-4819-155-2-201107190-00005.

Bettigole, C., and T. A. Farley. 2016. "The Philadelphia story: Attacking behavioral and social determinants of health." *Ann Intern Med* 165(8): 593–594. doi:10.7326/m16-1570.

Biddle, S. 2016. "Physical activity and mental health: Evidence is growing." *World Psychiatry* 15(2): 176–177. doi:10.1002/wps.20331.

Boone-Heinonen, J., P. Gordon-Larsen, C. I. Kiefe, J. M. Shikany, C. E. Lewis, and B. M. Popkin. 2011. "Fast food restaurants and food stores: Longitudinal associations with diet in young to middle-aged adults: The CARDIA Study." *Arch Intern Med* 171(13): 1162–1170. doi:10.1001/archinternmed.2011.283.

Braveman, P., C. Cubbin, S. Egerter, D. R. Williams, and E. Pamuk. 2010. "Socioeconomic disparities in health in the United States: What the patterns tell us." *Am J Public Health* 100(Suppl 1): S186–S196. doi:10.2105/AJPH.2009.166082.

Braveman, P., and S. Egerter. 2008. *Overcoming Obstacles to Health: Report from the Robert Wood Johnson Foundation to the Commission to Build a Healthier America.* Princeton, NJ: Robert Wood Johnson Foundation.

Braveman, P., and S. Egerter. 2013. *Overcoming Obstacles to Health in 2013 and Beyond.* Princeton, NJ: Robert Wood Johnson Foundation.

Braveman, P., S. Egerter, and C. Barclay. 2011. "What shapes health-related factors? The role of social factors." Robert Wood Johnson Foundation. http://www.nmpha.org/Resour ces/Documents/RWJF%20Issue%20Br ief%20-%20The%20Role%20of%20Soc ial%20Factors.pdf.

Braveman, P., K. Heck, S. Egerter, T. P. Dominguez, C. Rinki, K. S. Marchi, and M. Curtis. 2017. "Worry about racial discrimination: A missing piece of the puzzle of Black–White disparities in preterm birth?" *PLoS One* 12(10): e0186151.

Caspi, C. E., I. Kawachi, S. V. Subramanian, G. Adamkiewicz, and G. Sorensen. 2012. "The relationship between diet and perceived and objective access to supermarkets among low-income housing residents." *Soc Sci Med* 75(7): 1254–1262. https://doi.org/10.1016/j.socscimed.2012.05.014.

Centers for Disease Control and Prevention. 2008. "Behavioral risk factor surveillance system." https://www.cdc.gov/brfss/index.html.

Centers for Disease Control and Prevention. 2017. "Workplace health in America 2017." https://www.cdc.gov/workplacehealthpromotion/data-surveillance/docs/2017-Workplace-Health-in-America-Summary-Report-FINAL-updated-508.pdf.

Chan, D.-C., C.-B. Chang, D.-S. Han, C.-H. Hong, J.-S. Hwang, K.-S. Tsai, and R.-S. Yang. 2018. "Effects of exercise improves muscle strength and fat mass in patients with high fracture risk: A randomized control trial." *J Formosan Med Assoc* 117(7): 572–582. https://doi.org/10.1016/j.jfma.2017.05.004.

Chen, A., M. Machiorlatti, N. M. Krebs, and J. E. Muscat. 2019. "Socioeconomic differences in nicotine exposure and dependence in adult daily smokers." *BMC Public Health* 19(1): 375. doi:10.1186/s12889-019-6694-4.

CHOICES Project. 2016. "Brief: Cost-effectiveness of a sugar-sweetened beverage excise tax in Philadelphia, PA." https://choicesproject.org/publications/brief-cost-effectiveness-sugar-sweetened-and-diet-beverage-excise-tax-philadelphia-pa.

Chuang, Y. C., C. Cubbin, D. Ahn, and M. A. Winkleby. 2005. "Effects of neighbourhood socioeconomic status and convenience store concentration on individual level smoking." *J Epidemiol Community Health* 59(7): 568–73. doi:10.1136/jech.2004.029041.

Collins, S. E. 2016. "Associations between socioeconomic factors and alcohol outcomes." *Alcohol Res* 38(1): 83–94.

Cornett, M., and J. White. 2019. "Honest conversations. Better science. Real health outcomes." *Am J Public Health* 109(4): 543–543. doi:10.2105/ajph.2019.304984.

Cushing, L., J. Faust, L. M. August, R. Cendak, W. Wieland, and G. Alexeeff. 2015. "Racial/ethnic disparities in cumulative environmental health impacts in California: Evidence from a statewide environmental justice screening tool (CalEnviroScreen 1.1)." *Am J Public Health* 105(11): 2341–2348. doi:10.2105/AJPH.2015.302643.

Cushing, L., R. Morello-Frosch, M. Wander, and M. Pastor. 2015. "The haves, the have-nots, and the health of everyone: The relationship between social inequality and environmental quality." *Annu Rev Public Health* 36(1): 193–209. doi:10.1146/annurev-publhealth-031914-122646.

Daniel, J. Z., M. Hickman, J. Macleod, N. Wiles, A. Lingford-Hughes, M. Farrell, R. Araya, P. Skapinakis, J. Haynes, and G. Lewis. 2009. "Is socioeconomic status in early life associated with drug use? A systematic review of the evidence." *Drug Alcohol Rev* 28(2): 142–153. doi:10.1111/j.1465-3362.2008.00042.x.

Darmon, N., and A. Drewnowski. 2008. "Does social class predict diet quality?" *Am J Clin Nutr* 87(5): 1107–1117. doi:10.1093/ajcn/87.5.1107.

de Walque, D. 2010. "Education, information, and smoking decisions: Evidence from smoking histories in the United States, 1940–2000." *J Hum Resour* 45(3): 682–717.

Diez Roux, A. V., and C. Mair. 2010. "Neighborhoods and health." *Ann N Y Acad Sci* 1186: 125–145. doi:10.1111/j.1749-6632.2009.05333.x.

Drake, P., A. K. Driscoll, and T. J. Mathews. 2018. "Cigarette smoking during pregnancy: United States, 2016." National Center for Health Statistics. https://www.cdc.gov/nchs/data/databriefs/db305.pdf.

Drewnowski, A., and C. D. Rehm. 2015. "Socioeconomic gradient in consumption of whole fruit and 100% fruit juice among US children and adults." *Nutr J* 14(1): 3. doi:10.1186/1475-2891-14-3.

Drope, J., A. C. Liber, Z. Cahn, M. Stoklosa, R. Kennedy, C. E. Douglas, R. Henson, and J. Drope. 2018. "Who's still smoking? Disparities in adult cigarette smoking prevalence in the United States." *CA Cancer J Clin* 68(2): 106–115. doi:10.3322/caac.21444.

Economos, C. D., R. R. Hyatt, A. Must, J. P. Goldberg, J. Kuder, E. N. Naumova, J. J. Collins, and M. E. Nelson. 2013. "Shape Up Somerville two-year results: A community-based environmental change intervention sustains weight reduction in children." *Prev Med* 57(4): 322–327. https://doi.org/10.1016/j.ypmed.2013.06.001.

Evans, D. 2010, March 4. "Pennsylvania Fresh Food Financing Initiative." Budget Briefing. https://www.ncsl.org/documents/labor/workingfamilies/pa_fffi.pdf.

Fergusson, D. M., L. J. Horwood, J. M. Boden, and G. Jenkin. 2007. "Childhood social disadvantage and smoking in adulthood: Results of a 25-year longitudinal study." *Addiction* 102(3): 475–482. doi:10.1111/j.1360-0443.2006.01729.x.

Fernandez-Mendoza, J., and A. N. Vgontzas. 2013. "Insomnia and its impact on physical and mental health." *Curr Psychiatry Rep* 15(12): 418–418. doi:10.1007/s11920-013-0418-8.

Fleischhacker, S. E, K. R Evenson, D. A Rodriguez, and A. S Ammerman. 2011. "A systematic review of fast food access studies." *Obes Rev* 12(5): e460–e471.

Florence, C., F. Luo, and K. Rice. 2021. "The economic burden of opioid use disorder and fatal opioid overdose in the United States, 2017." *Drug Alcohol Depend* 218: 108350. https://doi.org/10.1016/j.drugalcdep.2020.108350.

Frieden, T. R. 2010. "A framework for public health action: The health impact pyramid." *Am J Public Health* 100(4): 590–595. doi:10.2105/AJPH.2009.185652.

Frieden, T. R., F. Mostashari, B. D. Kerker, N. Miller, A. Hajat, and M. Frankel. 2005. "Adult tobacco use levels after intensive tobacco control measures: New York City, 2002–2003." *Am J Public Health* 95(6): 1016–1023. doi:10.2105/ajph.2004.058164.

Friedman, A. S., and S. J. L. Horn. 2019. "Socioeconomic disparities in electronic cigarette use and transitions from smoking." *Nicotine Tob Res* 21(10): 1363–1370. doi:10.1093/ntr/nty120.

Friedman, E. M., A. S. Karlamangla, T. L. Gruenewald, B. Koretz, and T. E. Seeman. 2015. "Early life adversity and adult biological risk profiles." *Psychosom Med* 77(2): 176–185. doi:10.1097/PSY.0000000000000147.

Friis, K., M. Lasgaard, G. Rowlands, R. H. Osborne, and H. T. Maindal. 2016. "Health literacy mediates the relationship between

educational attainment and health behavior: A Danish population-based study." *J Health Commun* 21(Suppl 2): 54–60. doi:10.1080/10810730.2016.1201175.

Gary, T. L., M. M. Safford, R. B. Gerzoff, S. L. Ettner, A. J. Karter, G. L. Beckles, and A. F. Brown. 2008. "Perception of neighborhood problems, health behaviors, and diabetes outcomes among adults with diabetes in managed care: The Translating Research Into Action for Diabetes (TRIAD) study." *Diabetes Care* 31(2): 273–278. doi:10.2337/dc07-1111.

Glass, T. A., and M. J. McAtee. 2006. "Behavioral science at the crossroads in public health: extending horizons, envisioning the future." *Soc Sci Med* 62(7): 1650–1671. doi:10.1016/j.socscimed.2005.08.044.

Golden, S. D., K. R. McLeroy, L. W. Green, J. A. L. Earp, and L. D. Lieberman. 2015. "Upending the social ecological model to guide health promotion efforts toward policy and environmental change." *Health Educ Behav* 42(1 Suppl): 8S–14S. doi:10.1177/1090198115575098.

Goodwin, R. D., K. Cheslack-Postava, D. B. Nelson, P. H. Smith, M. M. Wall, D. S. Hasin, Y. Nomura, and S. Galea. 2017. "Smoking during pregnancy in the United States, 2005–2014: The role of depression." *Drug Alcohol Depend* 179: 159–166. https://doi.org/10.1016/j.drugalcdep.2017.06.021.

Gortmaker, S. L., M. W. Long, S. C. Resch, Z. J. Ward, A. L. Cradock, J. L. Barrett, D. R. Wright, et al. 2015. "Cost effectiveness of childhood obesity interventions: Evidence and methods for CHOICES." *Am J Prev Med* 49(1): 102–111. doi:10.1016/j.amepre.2015.03.032.

Graham, H., H. M. Inskip, B. Francis, and J. Harman. 2006. "Pathways of disadvantage and smoking careers: Evidence and policy implications." *J Epidemiol Community Health* 60(Suppl 2): 7–12. doi:10.1136/jech.2005.045583.

Grant, B. F., S. P. Chou, T. D. Saha, R. P. Pickering, B. T. Kerridge, W. J. Ruan, B. Huang, et al. 2017. "Prevalence of 12-month alcohol use, high-risk drinking, and DSM-IV alcohol use disorder in the United States, 2001–2002 to 2012–2013: Results from the National Epidemiologic Survey on Alcohol and Related Conditions." *JAMA Psychiatry* 74(9): 911–923. doi:10.1001/jamapsychiatry.2017.2161.

Hahn, R. A., and B. I. Truman. 2015. "Education improves public health and promotes health equity." *Int J Health Serv* 45(4): 657–678. doi:10.1177/0020731415585986.

Hanson, K. L, and L. M. Connor. 2014. "Food insecurity and dietary quality in US adults and children: A systematic review." *Am J Clin Nutr* 100(2): 684–692. doi:10.3945/ajcn.114.084525.

Hartwell, G., S. Thomas, M. Egan, A. Gilmore, and M. Petticrew. 2017. "E-cigarettes and equity: A systematic review of differences in awareness and use between sociodemographic groups." *Tob Control* 26(2): e85–e91. doi:10.1136/tobaccocontrol-2016-053222.

Heinert, S. W., Z. Isgor, and L. M. Powell. 2018. "Availability of healthier food options in fast-food restaurants by community racial/ethnic and socioeconomic composition in a national sample." Illinois Prevention Research Center. https://p3rc.uic.edu/wp-content/uploads/sites/561/2019/11/FoodOptions508v2.pdf.

Hills, A. P., L. B. Andersen, and N. M. Byrne. 2011. "Physical activity and obesity in children." *Br J Sports Med* 45(11): 866–870. doi:10.1136/bjsports-2011-090199.

Hiscock, R., L. Bauld, A. Amos, J. A. Fidler, and M. Munafo. 2012. "Socioeconomic status and smoking: A review." *Ann N Y Acad Sci* 1248: 107–123. doi:10.1111/j.1749-6632.2011.06202.x.

Hong, I., P. Coker-Bolt, K. R. Anderson, D. Lee, and C. A. Velozo. 2016. "Relationship between physical activity and overweight and obesity in children: Findings from the 2012 National Health and Nutrition Examination Survey National Youth Fitness Survey." *Am J Occup Ther* 70(5): 7005180060p1–5. doi:10.5014/ajot.2016.021212.

Hughes, K., M. A. Bellis, K. A. Hardcastle, D. Sethi, A. Butchart, C. Mikton, L. Jones, and M. P. Dunne. 2017. "The effect of multiple adverse childhood experiences on health: A systematic review and meta-analysis." *Lancet Public Health* 2(8): e356–e366. doi:10.1016/s2468-2667(17)30118-4.

Humensky, J. L. 2010. "Are adolescents with high socioeconomic status more likely to engage in alcohol and illicit drug use in early adulthood?" *Subst Abuse Treat Prev Policy* 5: 19–19. doi:10.1186/1747-597X-5-19.

Jamal, A., B. A. King, L. J. Neff, J. Whitmill, S. D. Babb, and C. M. Graffunder. 2016. "Current cigarette smoking among adults—United States, 2005–2015." *MMWR Morb Mortal Wkly Rep* 65(44): 1205–1211. doi:10.15585/mmwr.mm6544a2.

Jefferis, B. J. M. H., C. Power, H. Graham, and O. Manor. 2004. "Effects of childhood socioeconomic circumstances on persistent smoking." *Am J Public Health* 94(2): 279–285. doi:10.2105/ajph.94.2.279.

Jitnarin, N., K. M. Heinrich, C. K. Haddock, J. Hughey, L. Berkel, and W. S. Poston. 2015. "Neighborhood environment perceptions and the likelihood of smoking and alcohol use." *Int J Environ Res Public Health* 12(1): 784–799. doi:10.3390/ijerph120100784.

Kaiser Family Foundation. 2020. "2020 Employer Health Benefits Survey." https://www.kff.org/health-costs/report/2020-employer-health-benefits-survey.

Kanjilal, S., E. W. Gregg, Y. J. Cheng, P. Zhang, D. E. Nelson, G. Mensah, and G. L. Beckles. 2006. "Socioeconomic status and trends in disparities in 4 major risk factors for cardiovascular disease among US adults, 1971–2002." *Arch Intern Med* 166(21): 2348–2355. doi:10.1001/archinte.166.21.2348.

Karriker-Jaffe, K. J. 2011. "Areas of disadvantage: A systematic review of effects of area-level socioeconomic status on substance use outcomes." *Drug Alcohol Rev* 30(1): 84–95. doi:10.1111/j.1465-3362.2010.00191.x.

King, B. A., R. Patel, K. H. Nguyen, and S. R. Dube. 2015. "Trends in awareness and use of electronic cigarettes among US adults, 2010–2013." *Nicotine Tob Res* 17(2): 219–227. doi:10.1093/ntr/ntu191.

Laniado-Laborín, R. 2009. "Smoking and chronic obstructive pulmonary disease (COPD): Parallel epidemics of the 21 century." *Int J Environ Res Public Health* 6(1): 209–224. doi:10.3390/ijerph6010209.

Lantz, P. M., J. S. House, J. M. Lepkowski, D. R. Williams, R. P. Mero, and J. Chen. 1998. "Socioeconomic factors, health behaviors, and mortality results from a nationally representative prospective study of US adults."

JAMA 279(21): 1703–1708. doi:10.1001/jama.279.21.1703.

Laverack, G. 2017. "The challenge of behaviour change and health promotion." *Challenges* 8(2): 25.

Lee, R. D., and J. Chen. 2017. "Adverse childhood experiences, mental health, and excessive alcohol use: Examination of race/ethnicity and sex differences." *Child Abuse Negl* 69: 40–48. doi:10.1016/j.chiabu.2017.04.004.

Leos-Urbel, J., A. E. Schwartz, M. Weinstein, and S. Corcoran. 2013. "Not just for poor kids: The impact of universal free school breakfast on meal participation and student outcomes." *Econ Educ Rev* 36: 88–107. doi:10.1016/j.econedurev.2013.06.007.

Lewis, T. T., C. D. Cogburn, and D. R. Williams. 2015. "Self-reported experiences of discrimination and health: Scientific advances, ongoing controversies, and emerging issues." *Annu Rev Clin Psychol* 11(11): 407–440.

Lillie-Blanton, M., J. C. Anthony, and C. R. Schuster. 1993. "Probing the meaning of racial/ethnic group comparisons in crack cocaine hnic group comparisons in crack cocaine smoking." *JAMA Smoking* 269(8): 993–997. doi:10.1001/JAMA 1993. 03500080041029.

Lorson, B. A., H. R. Melgar-Quinonez, and C. A. Taylor. 2009. "Correlates of fruit and vegetable intakes in US children." *J Am Diet Assoc* 109(3): 474–478. doi:10.1016/j.jada.2008.11.022.

Lortet-Tieulent, J., A. Goding Sauer, R. L. Siegel, K. D. Miller, F. Islami, S. A. Fedewa, E. J. Jacobs, and A. Jemal. 2016. "State-level cancer mortality attributable to cigarette smoking in the United States." *JAMA Intern Med* 176(12): 1792–1798. doi:10.1001/jamainternmed.2016.6530.

Lortet-Tieulent, J., I. Kulhanova, E. J. Jacobs, J. W. Coebergh, I. Soerjomataram, and A. Jemal. 2017. "Cigarette smoking-attributable burden of cancer by race and ethnicity in the United States." *Cancer Causes Control* 28(9): 981–984. doi:10.1007/s10552-017-0932-9.

Loudermilk, E., K. Loudermilk, J. Obenauer, and M. A. Quinn. 2018. "Impact of adverse childhood experiences (ACEs) on adult alcohol consumption behaviors." *Child Abuse Negl* 86: 368–374. doi:10.1016/j.chiabu.2018.08.006.

Luyster, F. S., P. J. Strollo, Jr., P. C. Zee, and J. K. Walsh. 2012. "Sleep: A health imperative." *Sleep* 35(6): 727–734. doi:10.5665/sleep.1846.

Lynch, J. W., G. A. Kaplan, and J. T. Salonen. 1997. "Why do poor people behave poorly? Variation in adult health behaviours and psychosocial characteristics by stages of the socioeconomic lifecourse." *Soc Sci Med* 44(6): 809–819. doi:10.1016/s0277-9536(96)00191-8.

Ma, J., R. L. Siegel, E. J. Jacobs, and A. Jemal. 2018. "Smoking-attributable mortality by state in 2014, U.S." *Am J Prev Med* 54(5): 661–670. doi:10.1016/j.amepre.2018.01.038.

Mackenbach, J. D., T. Burgoine, J. Lakerveld, N. G. Forouhi, S. J. Griffin, N. J. Wareham, and P. Monsivais. 2017. "Accessibility and affordability of supermarkets: Associations with the DASH diet." *Am J Prev Med* 53(1): 55–62. https://doi.org/10.1016/j.amepre.2017.01.044.

Marmot, M. 2015. "The health gap: The challenge of an unequal world." *Lancet* 386(10011): 2442–2444.

McDonald, N. C., Y. Yang, S. M. Abbott, and A. N. Bullock. 2013. "Impact of the Safe Routes to School program on walking and biking: Eugene, Oregon study." *Transport Policy* 29: 243–248. https://doi.org/10.1016/j.tranpol.2013.06.007.

Mokdad, A. H., J. S. Marks, D. F. Stroup, and J. L. Gerberding. 2004. "Actual causes of death in the United States, 2000." *JAMA* 291(10): 1238–1245. doi:10.1001/jama.291.10.1238.

Moore, P., N. Adler, D. Williams, and J. Jackson. 2002. "Socioeconomic status and health: The role of sleep." *Psychosom Med* 64: 337–344. doi:10.1097/00006842-200203000-00018.

Moran, A. J., N. Khandpur, M. Polacsek, and E. B. Rimm. 2019. "What factors influence ultra-processed food purchases and consumption in households with children? A comparison between participants and non-participants in the Supplemental Nutrition Assistance Program (SNAP)." *Appetite* 134: 1–8. https://doi.org/10.1016/j.appet.2018.12.009.

Morello-Frosch, R., and R. Lopez. 2006. "The riskscape and the color line: Examining the role of segregation in environmental health disparities." *Environs Res* 102(2): 181–196. https://doi.org/10.1016/j.envres.2006.05.007.

Nathan, A., K. Villanueva, J. Rozek, M. Davern, L. Gunn, G. Trapp, C. Boulangé, and H. Christian. 2018. "The role of the built environment on health across the life course: A call for collaborACTION." *Am J Health Promot* 32(6): 1460–1468. doi:10.1177/0890117118779463a.

National Center for Health Statistics. 2019. *Health, United States, 2018.* Hyattsville, MD: National Center for Health Statistics.

O'Keeffe, L. M., G. Taylor, R. R. Huxley, P. Mitchell, M. Woodward, and S. A. E. Peters. 2018. "Smoking as a risk factor for lung cancer in women and men: A systematic review and meta-analysis." *BMJ Open* 8(10): e021611. doi:10.1136/bmjopen-2018-021611.

Organisation for Economic Co-operation and Development. 2019. *Health at a Glance 2019.* Paris, France: OECD Publishing.

Osna, N. A., T. M. Donohue, Jr., and K. K. Kharbanda. 2017. "Alcoholic liver disease: Pathogenesis and current management." *Alcohol Res* 38(2): 147–161.

Ozlü, T., and Y. Bülbül. 2005. "Smoking and lung cancer." *Tuberk Toraks* 53(2): 200–209.

Pampel, F. C., P. M. Krueger, and J. T. Denney. 2010. "Socioeconomic disparities in health behaviors." *Annu Rev Sociol* 36(1): 349–370. doi:10.1146/annurev.soc.012809.102529.

Papadopoulos, D., F. A. Sosso, T. Khoury, and S. Surani. 2022. "Sleep disturbances are mediators between socioeconomic status and health: A scoping review." *Int J Mental Health Addict* 20: 480–504. doi:10.1007/s11469-020-00378-x.

Patel, N. P., M. A. Grandner, D. Xie, C. C. Branas, and N. Gooneratne. 2010. "'Sleep disparity' in the population: Poor sleep quality is strongly associated with poverty and ethnicity." *BMC Public Health* 10(1): 475. doi:10.1186/1471-2458-10-475.

Peng, K., and N. Kaza. 2019. "Availability of neighbourhood supermarkets and convenience stores, broader built environment context, and the purchase of fruits and vegetables in US households." *Public Health Nutr* 22(13): 2436–2447. doi:10.1017/s1368980019000910.

Petrovic, D., C. de Mestral, M. Bochud, M. Bartley, M. Kivimäki, P. Vineis, J. Mackenbach, and S. Stringhini. 2018. "The contribution of health behaviors to socioeconomic inequalities in health: A systematic review." *Prev Med* 113: 15–31. https://doi.org/10.1016/j.ypmed.2018.05.003.

Pickett, K. E., and M. Pearl. 2001. "Multilevel analyses of neighbourhood socioeconomic context and health outcomes: A critical review." *J Epidemiol Community Health* 55(2): 111–122. doi:10.1136/jech.55.2.111.

Pizacani, B., K. Pickle, J. Maher, K. Rohde, and A. Fenaughty. 2018. "Smoking cessation patterns by socioeconomic status in Alaska." *Prev Med Rep* 10: 24–28. https://doi.org/10.1016/j.pmedr.2018.01.007.

Reeve, B., M. Ashe, R. Farias, and L. Gostin. 2015. "State and municipal innovations in obesity policy: Why localities remain a necessary laboratory for innovation." *Am J Public Health* 105(3): 442–450. doi:10.2105/ajph.2014.302337.

Rehkopf, D. H., I. Headen, A. Hubbard, J. Deardorff, Y. Kesavan, A. K. Cohen, D. Patil, L. D. Ritchie, and B. Abrams. 2016. "Adverse childhood experiences and later life adult obesity and smoking in the United States." *Ann Epidemiol* 26(7): 488–492.e5. doi:10.1016/j.annepidem.2016.06.003.

Reinvestment Fund. 2018. "HFFI bill would expand healthy food access, revitalize communities." https://www.healthyfoodacc ess.org/perspectives-hffi-bill-healthy-food-acc ess-revitalize-communities.

Riggs, N. R., and M. A. Pentz. 2016. "Inhibitory control and the onset of combustible cigarette, e-cigarette, and hookah use in early adolescence: The moderating role of socioeconomic status." *Child Neuropsychol* 22(6): 679–691. doi:10.1080/09297049.2015.1053389.

Rycroft, C. E., A. Heyes, L. Lanza, and K. Becker. 2012. "Epidemiology of chronic obstructive pulmonary disease: A literature review." *Int J Chron Obstruct Pulmon Dis* 7: 457–494. doi:10.2147/COPD.S32330.

Schaeffer, K. 2019. "Before recent outbreak, vaping was on the rise in U.S., especially among young people." Pew Research Center. https://www.pewresearch.org/fact-tank/2019/09/26/vaping-survey-data-roundup.

Schroeder, S. A. 2007. "We can do better—Improving the health of the American people." *N Engl J Med* 357(12): 1221–1228.

Schule, S. A., and G. Bolte. 2015. "Interactive and independent associations between the socioeconomic and objective built environment on the neighbourhood level and individual health: A systematic review of multilevel studies." *PLoS One* 10(4): e0123456. doi:10.1371/journal.pone.0123456.

Sharkey, P. 2014. "Spatial segmentation and the Black middle class." *Am J Sociol* 119(4): 903–954.

Siddiqi, A., C. Hertzman, and B. T. Smith. 2018. "The fundamental role of socioeconomic resources for health and health behaviors." In *Principles and Concepts of Behavioral Medicine: A Global Handbook*, edited by E. B. Fisher, L. D. Cameron, A. J. Christensen, U. Ehlert, Y. Guo, B. Oldenburg and F. J. Snoek, 389–413. New York, NY: Springer.

Simon, P., D. R. Camenga, M. E. Morean, G. Kong, K. W. Bold, D. A. Cavallo, and S. Krishnan-Sarin. 2018. "Socioeconomic status and adolescent e-cigarette use: The mediating role of e-cigarette advertisement exposure." *Prev Med* 112: 193–198. https://doi.org/10.1016/j.ypmed.2018.04.019.

Singh, R. K., H.-W. Chang, D. Yan, K. M. Lee, D. Ucmak, K. Wong, M. Abrouk, et al. 2017. "Influence of diet on the gut microbiome and implications for human health." *J Transl Med* 15(1): 73–73. doi:10.1186/s12967-017-1175-y.

Stallings-Smith, S., and T. Ballantyne. 2019. "Ever use of e-cigarettes among adults in the United States: A cross-sectional study of sociodemographic factors." *Inquiry* 56: 46958019864479. doi:10.1177/0046958019864479.

Substance Abuse and Mental Health Services Administration. 2018. "National Survey on Drug Use and Health." https://www.datafiles.samhsa.gov/dataset/national-survey-drug-use-and-health-2018-nsduh-2018-ds0001.

Sugiyama, T., N. J. Howard, C. Paquet, N. T. Coffee, A. W. Taylor, and M. Daniel. 2015. "Do relationships between environmental attributes and recreational walking vary according to area-level socioeconomic status?"

J Urban Health 92(2): 253–264. doi:10.1007/s11524-014-9932-1.

The U.S. Burden of Disease Collaborators. 2018. "The state of US health, 1990–2016: Burden of diseases, injuries, and risk factors among US states." *JAMA* 319(14): 1444–1472. doi:10.1001/jama.2018.0158.

Toro, P. A., C. J. Tompsett, S. Lombardo, P. Philippot, H. Nachtergael, B. Galand, N. Schlienz, et al. 2007. "Homelessness in Europe and the United States: A comparison of prevalence and public opinion." *J Soc Issues* 63(3): 505–524. https://doi.org/10.1111/j.1540-4560.2007.00521.x.

Turecki, G., and M. J. Meaney. 2016. "Effects of the social environment and stress on glucocorticoid receptor gene methylation: A systematic review." *Biol Psychiatry* 79(2): 87–96. https://doi.org/10.1016/j.biopsych.2014.11.022.

Umberson, D., R. Crosnoe, and C. Reczek. 2010. "Social relationships and health behavior across the life course." *Annu Rev Sociol* 36: 139–157.

U.S. Department of Agriculture. 2004. "Evaluation of the School Breakfast Program Pilot Project: Final report." https://fns-prod.azureedge.us/sites/default/files/sbp/SBPPFinal.pdf.

Wang, D. D., C. W. Leung, Y. Li, E. L. Ding, S. E. Chiuve, F. B. Hu, and W. C. Willett. 2014. "Trends in dietary quality among adults in the United States, 1999 through 2010." *JAMA Intern Med* 174(10): 1587–1595. doi:10.1001/jamainternmed.2014.3422.

Wang, T. W., A. Gentzke, S. Sharapova, K. A. Cullen, B. K. Ambrose, and A. Jamal. 2018. "Tobacco product use among middle and high school students—United States, 2011–2017." *MMWR Morb Mortal Wkly Rep* 67(22): 629–633. doi:10.15585/mmwr.mm6722a3.

Wang, X., A. H. Auchincloss, S. Barber, S. L. Mayne, M. E. Griswold, M. Sims, and A. V. Diez Roux. 2017. "Neighborhood social environment as risk factors to health behavior among African Americans: The Jackson Heart Study." *Health Place* 45: 199–207. doi:10.1016/j.healthplace.2017.04.002.

Watts, A. W., S. M. Mason, K. Loth, N. Larson, and D. Neumark-Sztainer. 2016.

"Socioeconomic differences in overweight and weight-related behaviors across adolescence and young adulthood: 10-year longitudinal findings from Project EAT." *Prev Med* 87: 194–199. https://doi.org/10.1016/j.ypmed.2016.03.007.

Wilson, F. A., and Y. Wang. 2017. "Recent findings on the prevalence of e-cigarette use among adults in the U.S." *Am J Prev Med* 52(3): 385–390. doi:10.1016/j.amepre.2016.10.029.

Woolf, S. H., and L. Aron. 2013. "The National Academies Collection: Reports funded by National Institutes of Health." In *U.S. Health in International Perspective: Shorter Lives, Poorer Health*, edited by S. H. Woolf and L. Aron. Washington, DC: National Research Council and Institute of Medicine.

Woolf, S. H., M. M. Dekker, F. R. Byrne, and W. D. Miller. 2011. "Citizen-centered health promotion: Building collaborations to facilitate healthy living." *Am J Prev Med* 40(1 Suppl 1): S38–S47. doi:10.1016/j.amepre.2010.09.025.

World Health Organization. 2008. *Closing the Gap in a Generation: Health Equity Through Action on the Social Determinants of Health: Final Report of the Commission on Social Determinants of Health*. Geneva, Switzerland: World Health Organization.

Yen, I. H., and S. L. Syme. 1999. "The social environment and health: A discussion of the epidemiologic literature." *Annu Rev Public Health* 20(1): 287–308. doi:10.1146/annurev.publhealth.20.1.287.

Young, D. R., M.-F. Hivert, S. Alhassan, S. M. Camhi, J. F. Ferguson, P. T. Katzmarzyk, C. E. Lewis, N. Owen, C. K. Perry, and J. Siddique. 2016. "Sedentary behavior and cardiovascular morbidity and mortality: A science advisory from the American Heart Association." *Circulation* 134(13): e262–e279.

Zimmerman, E., and S. H. Woolf. 2014. *Understanding the Relationship Between Education and Health*. Washington, DC: Institute of Medicine.

INDEX

For the benefit of digital users, indexed terms that span two pages (e.g., 52–53) may, on occasion, appear on only one of those pages.

Figures and boxes are indicated by *f* and *b* following the page number